Recent Advances in

Surgery
29

Recent Advances in Surgery 28
Edited by I. Taylor & C. D. Johnson

ISBN 1-85315-610–8
ISSN 0143 8395

Recent Advances in

Surgery
29

Edited by

C. D. Johnson MChir FRCS
Reader and Consultant Surgeon, University Surgical Unit, Southampton
General Hospital, Southampton, UK

I. Taylor MD ChM FRCS FMedSci FRCPS(Glas)Hon
Vice-Dean and Director of Clinical Studies
David Patey Professor of Surgery, Royal Free and University College London
Medical School, University College London, London, UK

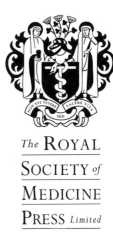

The ROYAL
SOCIETY *of*
MEDICINE
PRESS *Limited*

Published by the Royal Society of Medicine Press Ltd
1 Wimpole Street, London W1G 0AE, UK
Tel: +44 (0)20 7290 2921
Fax: +44 (0)20 7290 2929
Email: publishing@rsm.ac.uk
Website: www.rsmpress.co.uk

British Library Cataloguing in Publication Data
A catalogue record for this book is available from the British Library
ISBN 1-85315-692-2

Distribution in Europe and Rest of World:

Marston Book Services Ltd
PO Box 269, Abingdon
Oxon OX14 4YN, UK
Tel: +44 (0)1235 465500
Fax: +44 (0)1235 465555
Email: direct.order@marston.co.uk

Distribution in the USA and Canada:

Royal Society of Medicine Press Ltd
c/o BookMasters Inc
30 Amberwood Parkway
Ashland, OH 44805, USA
Tel: +1 800 247 6553/+1 800 266 5564
Fax: +1 419 281 6883
Email: order@bookmasters.com

Distribution in Australia and New Zealand:

Elsevier Australia
30-52 Smidmore Street
Marrikville NSW 2204, Australia
Tel: +61 2 9517 8999
Fax: +61 2 9517 2249
Email: service@elsevier.com.au

Editorial services and typesetting by GM & BA Haddock, Ford, Midlothian, UK

Printed in Great Britain by Bell & Bain, Glasgow, UK

Contents

Contributors

Mohammad Abu Hilal MD
Specialist Registrar in General Surgery, Department of Surgery, University Surgical Unit,
Southampton University Hospitals, Southampton, UK

Jens Anderson MD
Consultant Surgeon and Head of Colorectal Surgery, Department of Surgical Gastroenterology,
Hvidovre University Hospital, Hvidovre, Denmark

Nicholas C. Armitage DM FRCS
Consultant Surgeon, Queen's Medical Centre, University Hospital NHS Trust, Nottingham, UK

Gary Atkin MD MRCS
Specialist Registrar in General Surgery, North West Thames Region, London, UK

Stephen J. Beningfield FF Rad(D) (SA)
Professor and Head, Division of Radiology, Groote Schuur Hospital and University of Cape Town
Health Sciences Faculty, Cape Town, South Africa

Philip C. Bornman MMed(Surg) FCRS(Edin) FRCS(Glasg) FCS(SA)
Professor and Head, Surgical Gastroenterology Unit, Department of Surgery, Groote Schuur
Hospital and University of Cape Town Health Sciences Faculty, Cape Town, South Africa

John R. Bottomley MBChB FRANZCR
Consultant Vascular Radiologist, Sheffield Vascular Institute, Northern General Hospital, Sheffield,
UK

David J. Breen MRCP FRCR
Consultant Abdominal Radiologist, Department of Radiology, Southampton University Hospitals,
Southampton, UK

Ross Carter MBChB FRCS MD FRCS(Gen)
Consultant Surgeon and Honorary Senior Lecturer, West of Scotland Pancreatic Unit, Lister
Department of Surgery, Glasgow Royal Infirmary, Glasgow, UK

Richard A. Cassell BSc
Medical Student, University Surgical Unit, Southampton General Hospital, Southampton, UK

Sohail A. Choksy BSc MBBS FRCS
Senior Registrar in Vascular Surgery, Sheffield Vascular Institute, Northern General Hospital,
Sheffield, UK

Abhay Chopada MS FRCS FRCSI
Consultant Colorectal Surgeon, Department of Surgery, Ealing Hospital NHS Trust, London, UK

Louise Cousens MB ChB MRCP
Specialist Registrar in Anaesthetics, Yorkshire Deanery, Leeds, UK

Chris P. Driver
Consultant Paediatric Surgeon and Urologist, Royal Aberdeen Children's Hospital, Aberdeen, UK

Jonathan Fawcett DPhil FRCS FRACS
Professor of Surgery University of Queensland, Consultant General and HPB surgeon, Deputy

Director, Queensland Liver Transplant Service, Princess Alexandra Hospital, Brisbane, Queensland, Australia

Michael J. Gough ChM FRCS
Consultant Vascular Surgeon, The General Infirmary at Leeds, Leeds, UK

Henry Hook BSc MBBS FRACS
Lister Surgical Fellow, West of Scotland Pancreatic Unit, Lister Department of Surgery, Glasgow Royal Infirmary, Glasgow, UK

Colin D. Johnson MChir FRCS
Reader and Consultant Surgeon, University Surgical Unit, Southampton General Hospital, Southampton, UK

James Keir DOHNS MRCS
Specialist Registrar, Queen's Medical Centre, Nottingham University Hospital NHS Trust, Nottingham, UK

Mohammed Keshtgar BSc MBBS FRCSI FRCS(Gen) PhD
Senior Lecturer in Surgery and Consultant Surgical Oncologist, Department of Surgery, University College London, London, UK

Jake E.J. Krige FACS FRCS(Edin) FCS(SA)
Associate Professor and Head, HPB Surgical Unit, Department of Surgery, Groote Schuur Hospital and University of Cape Town Health Sciences Faculty, Cape Town, South Africa

Adarsh Kumar FRCS MS DM FRCS(Gen Surg)
Senior Fellow in Laparoscopic Colorectal Surgery, University Department of Colorectal Surgery, The Queen Elizabeth Hospital, Adelaide, Australia

Emma-Kate Lacey BM
Senior House Officer, University Surgical Unit, Southampton General Hospital, Southampton, UK

Reza Mansouri MD
Senior House Officer, Department of Surgery, University College London, London, UK

Abdul-Wahed N. Meshikhes MBChB FRCSI
Consultant Surgeon and Chairman, Department of Surgical Specialties, King Fahad Specialist Hospital, Dammam, Eastern Province, Saudi Arabia

Rowan W. Parks MD FRCSI FRCS(Ed)
Senior Lecturer in Surgery and Honorary Consultant Surgeon, Edinburgh Royal Infirmary, Edinburgh, UK

Adel H. Rateme MB BCh FRCS(Glasg)
Senior Specialist Registrar in Breast and General Surgery, Department of Surgery, University College London, London, UK

John H. Scholefield MB ChB ChM FRCS
Professor of Surgery, Queen's Medical Centre, University Hospital NHS Trust, Nottingham, UK

Kellee Slater FRACS
Fellow in HPB Surgery, Queensland Liver Transplant Service, Princess Alexandra Hospital, Brisbane, Queensland, Australia

Irving Taylor MD ChM FRCS FMedSci FRCPS(Glas)Hon
David Patey Professor of Surgery, Vice-Dean and Director of Clinical Studies, Royal Free and University College Medical School, London, UK

Brendan C. Visser MD
Clinical Fellow, Edinburgh Royal Infirmary, Edinburgh, UK

Jonathan Wilson BSc MB ChB FRCA
Consultant Anaesthetist, York Hospital, Wiggington Road, York , UK

George G. Youngson
Honorary Professor of Paediatric Surgery, Royal Aberdeen Children's Hospital, Aberdeen, UK

Bashar Zeidan MD
Senior House Officer, University Surgical Unit, Southampton General Hospital, Southampton, UK

George G. Youngson   Chris P. Driver

1

Paediatric surgery in the district general hospital

Paediatric surgery, uniquely amongst the surgical specialties, is a specialty defined by age rather than a body system or topographical area. The diversity of pathology, the extent of the operative repertoire, and the specific needs of communicating with children from babies to adolescents, together with the delicacies of dealing with their families, comprise the challenges of delivering this form of surgical care.

Whilst much is made of the vulnerable nature of the young who undergo surgery, as a consequence of size, prematurity and immaturity of body systems, children comprise 20% of the UK population and also feature as part of service provision in most surgical specialties. Whilst, there is a clear need for specialist paediatrics to be appropriately located in specialist children's hospitals, there is also good reason for the care of acute and common general surgical conditions of childhood to be delivered in their own locality.

Whilst wholesale provision of surgical care of all children by specialist paediatric surgeons remains a controversial proposal, current practice would dictate a need for general surgeons being appropriately trained in disease recognition and the management of common conditions.

This chapter will not attempt to detail the basic signs and symptoms of paediatric surgical disease processes but instead will favour a practice-based approach. It is acknowledged that there will be many conditions outwith the scope of this chapter but it should also be recognised that a surgeon whose practice is based in adult general surgery, given the appropriate additional preparatory training, has the attributes and potential to deal with children

George G. Youngson PhD FRCS (for correspondence)
Honorary Professor of Paediatric Surgery, Royal Aberdeen Children's Hospital, Westburn Road, Aberdeen AB25 2ZG, UK
E-mail: ggyrach@abdn.ac.uk

Chris P. Driver FRCS paed surg
Consultant Paediatric Surgeon and Urologist, Royal Aberdeen Children's Hospital, Westburn Rd, Aberdeen AB25 2ZG, UK

Table 1 Clinical areas relevant to service provision for children

- The child in the out-patient department
- The child in the medical ward
- The child in the emergency department
- The child in theatre
- The child in the in-patient ward
- The child during transfer

across the age spectrum. Moreover, a surgeon with an interest in children is ideally placed to provide good transitional care for teenagers and young adults.

This chapter, therefore, approaches the topic of children's surgery from the perspective of the clinical sites where children present and the appropriate treatment therein (Table 1).

SERVICE REQUIREMENTS

Given the need to distinguish between specialist and general surgery of childhood, it is important that a surgeon working in a non-specialist unit identifies the constraints and limitations placed on the ability of that unit to deal with children suffering from surgical conditions. In that regard, the operative ability and familiarity with surgical procedures in children is but one limitation. It is equally important that the skills of the anaesthetic and nursing teams are taken into consideration when contemplating surgical care of the child, particularly the very young.

Whilst there are no absolute exclusions for care outwith the neonatal period,[1] a children's surgeon should be aware of the standards of care to which his team can contribute. A child with complex needs or co-morbidity can make challenging demands on management, which exceed the ability of the unit to deliver appropriate care though the surgical procedure itself poses no particular technical challenges. The care of a neurologically compromised child with gastro-oesophageal reflux in need of a fundoplication is one example.

Much has been made, therefore, of the limitations placed on adult general surgeons to deliver children's care, but if elective surgery is to be provided then it is important that there are dedicated sessions for children in the out-patient department and in the operating theatre.[2] There needs to be a full awareness of the rights of the child, the issues of consent in relation to children, the specific needs of the teenage population and the contributions that can be made to patient care by play therapists and other allied health professionals. Similarly, parental involvement in care, including attendance in the anaesthetic room and recovery room, are but a few examples of the standards that should be expected of children's surgery irrespective of whether delivered in a specialist children's hospital or a district general hospital.[3]

EMERGENCY SURGERY PROVISION

Whilst discretion can be exercised over undertaking elective surgery or not, emergency presentations provide the biggest challenge to district general hospitals. Occasionally, the urgency of the situation obligates management by a surgeon who would not otherwise have chosen to be involved in children's care. It is important, therefore, that all surgeons who take part in emergency rotas in district general hospitals have an awareness of the principles of surgical practice in children.

In addition, the district general hospital surgeon should be comfortable managing the initial stages of surgical trauma and be aware of the principles of resuscitation and stabilisation of a child who may subsequently need transfer to a specialist centre. ATLS and APLS training are valuable in this regard.

Whilst it is recognised that paediatricians are useful partners in these situations, there is no substitute for the surgical skills needed in assessment and stabilisation, if not in surgical intervention itself. The ability to recognise the child with an intussusception, the atypical presentation of appendicitis, or the baby with an incarcerated inguinal hernia all require a competent children's surgeon working in partnership with a paediatrician.

Key point 1

- In the planning of district hospital services for children. it is essential to recognise the competence of the whole team and the need for skills training in resuscitation, stabilisation and transfer to a specialist centre (if required).

THE CHILD IN THE OUT-PATIENT DEPARTMENT

The prime domains of clinical practice exercised in outpatients are clinical assessment, diagnosis and management planning, all of which need to be done in a brief time interval. Good practice would suggest that referral letters should be screened in advance so maximal preparation can be achieved. The venue is also an excellent opportunity for teaching medical students on the core clinical material in children's surgery. The wide array of problems which present include functional problems such as constipation and urinary sepsis, hernias, preputial pathology, labial fusion, rectal bleeding, and recurrent non-specific abdominal pain. A good understanding and familiarity with the natural history of these conditions is mandatory for confident and effective management.

HERNIAS IN CHILDREN

Body wall hernias are common in childhood and are frequently found in the inguinal canal, umbilicus and epigastrium. Femoral hernia, by comparison, is unusual and seldom an elective presentation. Other variants (Richter's hernia and Littre's hernia) rarely present electively.

Inguinal hernia
The incidence of complications in inguinal hernia is age-related and should be considered an urgent referral in infants, requiring expeditious management.

Indeed, the referral process should recognise this urgency and, once the diagnosis is confirmed, operative treatment on a day-care basis should likewise be prioritised.

While controversy exists over whether bilateral exploration is required in those children presenting with a unilateral hernia, majority opinion favours an approach restricted to the site of presentation in boys although in girls bilateral groin exploration is to be recommended.[4] A particular awareness of the potential for bilateral inguinal hernia in infant girls to be the first presentation of androgen insensitivity syndrome is required. Current practice recommends confirmation of female gender by karyotype or by identification of mullerian structures such as a fallopian tube or ovary by inspection through the internal ring at the time of groin exploration. Sensitive handling of this issue is required for the purposes of pre-operative consent. The incidence of this gender anomaly in such a clinical scenario is estimated at about 1%.[5]

Special care must also be taken in the event of infant herniotomy for a previous premature infant with a significant risk of apnoea up to age 56 weeks after conception.[6] Appropriate monitoring (oximetry and apnoea monitoring) and, in particular, the potential for ventilatory support in the postoperative period would suggest that this group of patients are best treated in specialist centres.

In the absence of any co-morbidity, geographical considerations or family concerns, the operative care of the child requiring inguinal herniotomy should be performed on a day-care basis. Intra-operative and postoperative analgesia is best supplemented through regional blockade performed after induction or at the time of operative repair with 2 mg/kg (0.8 ml/kg of 0.25% bupivacaine) the recommended dose to block the ileo-inguinal and ileo-hypogastric nerves.

Umbilical hernia

In the vast majority of children, even umbilical hernia of substantial dimensions will regress with growth, and the indications for repair are simply cosmetic. There is a high incidence of this condition in Afro-Caribbean races and a conservative approach is warranted in all. The expectation that resolution will take place has its confidence in the fact that the umbilical hernial sac is protruding directly through the defect at the umbilicus to the umbilical skin cicatrix and, as such, there is no potential for visceral entrapment. This is not true of the supra-umbilical hernia, which by contradistinction has an oblique defect and displaces the umbilicus inferiorly. Incarceration is associated with the supra-umbilical variant and elective repair of these hernias is recommended at the time of diagnosis.

Epigastric hernia

The defect in this condition is typically extremely small (1–2 mm) and only allows pre-peritoneal fat to protrude. There is, therefore, often difficulty in even visualising the lump. Nonetheless, in some cases, symptoms appear to be related to this hernia; whilst controversy exists over the merits of repair, suture closure of the defect is common practice. It should be noted that the lump may disappear after palpation under anaesthesia and it is essential that pre-operative localisation by skin marking is performed to enable precise intra-operative identification of the defect.

HYDROCELE

The aetiology of hydrocele in childhood is persistent patency of the processus vaginalis. As a consequence, the hydrocele volume fluctuates, with the scrotum being full by evening after a day's activity but relatively empty in the morning after the fluid has drained back into the peritoneal cavity through the patent processus. It is common after birth and through infancy.

The refraction of light passing through the hydrocele fluid can often give it a bluish discolouration that may cause the parents some alarm, but it is a non-tender and otherwise asymptomatic condition. Spontaneous resolution will usually occur and this lesion requires no operative intervention until consistent patency is obvious after age 2 years. Thereafter, ligation of the patent processus vaginalis is recommended as a day-case.

SURGERY TO THE FORESKIN

Definitive recommendations on the management of requests for religious circumcision have generally been avoided in the surgical literature. The General Medical Council has set out guidelines on the factors that constitute good surgical practice in relation to religious circumcision: adherence to sound surgical technique in the presence of full aseptic precautions with adequate analgesia is mandatory. The recommendation of dual signatures (mother and father) on consent forms is highlighted.[7]

In the district general hospital setting, there is just one absolute indication for circumcision – balanitis xerotica obliterans. (Other relative indications, reserved for children with complex urinary tract abnormalities are those with massively dilated upper urinary tracts or those on clean intermittent catheterisation in whom the prepuce is producing technical difficulties).

The ballooning foreskin and the non-retractile foreskin are not of themselves an indication for circumcision. The assessment of the dimensions of the preputial opening is best made by forward traction of the margin of the prepuce rather than retraction. Inspection of the median raphe on the ventral aspect reveals a spiral course and forward traction on this helix of tissue allows the surgeon to demonstrate the potential calibre of the preputial meatus to parent and child alike so re-inforcing the lack of any obstruction to forward flow. Hence circumcision is unnecessary since spontaneous change to the adult tubular prepucial shape will occur spontaneously with growth.

In troublesome recurrent balanitis and in boys with preputial adhesions, maturation of the separation between the fused epithelial surface of the glans and preputial epithelium can be expedited with the use of steroid cream. Betamethasone cream (0.1%) applied over a 4-month period is successful in about 50% of such cases.[8]

Key point 2
- Greater than 95% of boys with a non-retractile foreskin are normal and do not require a circumcision. Balanitis xerotica obliterans is the only absolute indication for circumcision.

TESTICULAR MALDESCENT

It is mandatory that the examining clinician be able to distinguish between a retractile testis, which is a variant of normal, and an undescended testis in need of operative intervention. The former category should be excluded by gentle but firm bi-manual examination of the groin with gentle traction on the testis overcoming the reflex spasm of the cremaster muscle. The middle of the testis should come 4 cm below the pubic tubercle located by palpation rather than inspection.

There are three variants to the maldescended testis – undescended testis, ectopic testis and testicular ascent

Undescended testis

Undescended testis will be present at birth in about 3% of boys and this will persist in 1% beyond the 3-month mark.[9] No further descent will occur beyond this time and a diagnosis can be confidently made at any time thereafter. The optimal time for orchidopexy is 1 year of age and postponement beyond age 3 years results in germ cell atrophy.[10] An undescended testis is always found in conjunction with an inguinal hernia sac. Orchidopexy in the second year of life is a technically challenging procedure and significant experience in paediatric groin surgery is to be recommended before attempting this operation.

If the testis is impalpable then the child should be prepared for two possible options. An initial step is to perform an examination under anaesthesia and, if the testis is palpable, the surgeon can proceed to orchidopexy. If, however, there is still no palpable testis, the next appropriate step is laparoscopy, which will determine if the testis is intra-abdominal or if testicular regression has occurred. The finding of a closed internal ring with a vas entering the internal ring along with spermatic vessels would suggest a prior testicular torsion at some antecedent time with subsequent regression. There is no merit in further surgery in this circumstance. The finding of an intra-abdominal testis on laparoscopy should prompt either a two-stage Fowler-Stevens procedure or, preferably, a pre-peritoneal orchidopexy which retains the integrity of the vascular pedicle to the testis.[11]

Bilateral impalpable testes require referral to an endocrinologist and a specialist paediatric surgical unit.

Ectopic testis

The anomaly in this condition is the location of the otherwise normal testis which, instead of being scrotal in position, is in the superficial inguinal pouch. This is an operative finding and is indistinguishable pre-operatively from an undescended testis. There is no associated hernia and the testis is not at risk of the associations with undescended testis, *i.e.* malignancy and infertility. The potential for torsion, however, still exists.

Testicular ascent

This increasingly recognised condition is a consequence of attenuation of growth of the spermatic cord by a fibrosed processus vaginalis; hence as the child grows, the distance from the internal ring to the testis remains constant and there is ascent of the testis out of the scrotum. It is, therefore, generally only recognised after age 5 years and requires a cord dissection and orchidopexy for correction.

LABIAL FUSION

This condition is not present at birth and is thought to develop as a consequence of oestrogen deficiency through the loss of maternal oestrogenic influence.[12] A frequent concern of parents, often replicated by primary care physicians, is that this represents an absence of the vagina. The labial fusion can be demonstrated to parents by flexing the baby's hips, separating the labia majora and demonstrating the presence of the dark line of fusion. The sequential appearance of multiple small apertures, which eventually coalesce, allowing separation of the labia minora, can be confidently predicted. In those girls where deflection of the urinary stream and vaginal voiding are resulting in urinary irritation, the process of separation can be expedited by the application of 0.1% dienoestrol cream for a 1-week period. Failure of this intervention is an indication for separation of the labia. In early infancy this can be done after the application of topical local anaesthetic cream but in older girls the procedure will require a brief general anaesthetic.

TONGUE TIE

Speech impediment in children with tongue-tie is not prevented or relieved by division of the frenulum and these children are best referred for speech and language therapy assessment. The indications for intervention include poor feeding, ulceration from the incisor teeth and separation of the lower incisor dentition.

However, the majority of children will obtain no benefit and a fully informed consultation should emphasise this. It is the practice in some specialist units, when the child has difficulties in bottle- or breast-feeding attributed to the tongue-tie, to proceed with division of the frenulum without anaesthesia under temporary restraint with adjuvant oral analgesia and using a grooved dissector to displace the tongue, thus allowing an expeditious scissor division. This is only appropriate in infants under 6 months of age.

RECTAL BLEEDING

The implications of this symptom are entirely different from those of rectal bleeding seen in adult life. Whilst there are numerous causes, those that run the most benign course and hence are seen in out-patient referrals include anal fissure, peri-anal cellulitis, juvenile polyp, food allergy and threadworm infestation. Whilst there are numerous other causes including Meckel's diverticulum, intussusception, duplication of the gastrointestinal tract *etc.*, these will all have a more acute presentation.

Anal fissure

This is associated with pain on defaecation. The diagnosis is made by inspection on parting the buttocks and no attempt should be made to perform digital rectal examination. The presence of an anal skin tag is pathognomonic of the fissure, which is commonly seen in the 12- or 6-o'clock position. Virtually all fissures will respond to stool softening by increasing the fluid intake and the use of a purgative such as Senokot syrup or Movicol Paediatric®. Osmotic laxatives such as lactulose are unhelpful because of their bulking effect, which causes distress and pain consequent to the anal spasm. In exceptional circumstances, examination under anaesthesia and anal dilatation will relieve the symptoms.

Peri-anal cellulitis

This condition characterised by maceration of the peri-anal skin, numerous superficial ulcers, rectal bleeding, mucous discharge and a ring of erythema around the anal margin, is caused by Group A *Streptococcus* spp. It is under-diagnosed and responds well to penicillin-based antibiotics such as Co-Amoxyclav. It is a slowly responding condition that may require up to 6 weeks of antibiotic therapy.[13]

Juvenile polyp

Whilst normally singular, 10% are associated with multiple lesions which are hamartomatous in origin. The history is typically one of intermittent painless passage of bright red blood of approximately egg-cup volume. The natural history is one of auto-amputation but, in the interim, a significant amount of bleeding can occur and colonoscopic removal under general anaesthetic is recommended. This approach also allows identification of more proximal co-existing polyps.

Enterobiasis

Threadworm infection can produce an allergic proctitis and the friability of the mucosa can result in rectal bleeding in a proportion of children. The diagnosis can be made in some instances by a Sellotape test but may only ultimately be diagnosed on flexible endoscopy.

IN-GROWING TOENAIL

The management of this condition is indistinguishable from that in teenage and adult life, the difference being the reduced tolerance of children to isolated ring blocks and performance of the procedure in an operating theatre environment. Brief general anaesthesia with concomitant ring block to permit phenol wedge resection is recommended to reduce the risk of recurrence. A Zadek's procedure is only used for recurrences.

Key point 3

- The following conditions can be expected to resolve without surgical intervention: non-retractile/ballooning foreskin; tongue tie; labial fusion; anal fissure; and umbilical hernia.

Key point 4

- Interventions in some conditions are best performed at certain ages: hernia – on presentation (but elective repair of an inguinal hernia in children < 1 year of age must be considered urgent); undescended testis – aged 1 year; hydrocele – aged 2 years; and umbilical hernia – aged 5 years.

MISCELLANEOUS

Many other conditions such as recurrent non-specific abdominal pain, constipation and lumps in the head and neck will present in the out-patient clinic and readers are referred to standard paediatric texts for conventional management.

THE CHILD IN THE PAEDIATRIC WARD

MEDICAL PRESENTATION OF SURGICAL CONDITIONS

The request for a surgical opinion in the medical paediatric ward generally indicates either a surgical complication of a medical condition but, equally as likely, a medical presentation of a surgical condition. In this regard there are two important diagnoses of which the surgeon must be aware, which may present as gastroenteritis. Of cases of intussusception, 50% will have an antecedent history of diarrhoea prompting admission to a medical unit.[14] Similarly, diarrhoea as a consequence of rectal irritation from late appendicitis with a pelvic abscess is a clinical scenario which the surgeon must suspect. This particular instance is one of the few situations in clinical surgery where a rectal examination in a child may be indicated. It is useful, however, to confer this examination the status of an investigation rather than routine clinical practice, and to perform it only with parental assent.[15]

SURGICAL COMPLICATIONS OF MEDICAL CONDITIONS

Whilst a number of children with medical conditions have a surgical presentation and may find themselves being admitted directly to a surgical ward (*e.g.* lower lobe pneumonia, measles, diabetic keto-acidosis), surgical complications of medical conditions require special consideration. Testicular pain complicating Henoch Schönlein purpura, typhlitis in an immuno-suppressed child undergoing chemotherapy and abdominal complications of cystic fibrosis, such as meconium ileus equivalent, are all challenging conditions to manage and are not for the occasional practitioner in surgical paediatrics.

Wide-spread familiarity with the ultrasound findings of hypertrophic infantile pyloric stenosis has now removed the dependency upon clinical judgement of the vomiting infant when distinguishing this condition from gastro-oesophageal reflux. Nonetheless, many surgeons will still wish to palpate the pyloric olive personally before committing a child to pyloromyotomy. This operation, now performed through a supra-umbilical incision, is perhaps the one which best defines the ability of the surgical team and should only be performed if there is universal competence within the operating team to manage fluid balance, pain control and the operative and anaesthetic implications of abdominal surgery in young infants.

Surgical assessment of an infant with symptoms suggestive of an intussusception also requires confident management by the surgical team. Again, the contribution of ultrasound examination is paramount, but false-negative examinations do occur and primacy should be given to clinical assessment. Successful pneumostatic reduction is the expected outcome in 70%

of infants[16] and the unavailability of a radiologist familiar with this technique should prompt referral to a specialist team. Indeed, the surgical team must be prepared to contend with the consequences of failure of pneumostatic reduction and any potential complications ensuing from this procedure. A high level of confidence with abdominal surgery in children is required; therefore, before progressing to in-house management of intussusception and in the absence of any of these abilities, referral to a specialist unit is recommended. It should be remembered that intussusception has a real risk of mortality, usually from atypical presentation.[17]

Key point 5

- Rectal examination should be performed selectively during clinical examination of a child with abdominal pain and should not be considered routine, but instead be conferred the status of an investigation.

THE CHILD IN THE EMERGENCY DEPARTMENT

HEAD INJURY

This is the commonest cause for admission of a child to hospital. The Glasgow Coma Scale is difficult to apply to children under 5 years and needs to be interpreted with care although there are age-appropriate modifications. (Adelaide Coma Scale).

Skull fractures in children are not as predictive as in adults and significant intracranial injury occurs more frequently in the absence of a skull fracture. There are other features in infancy, *e.g.* tense fontanelle, that are equally important in determining the need for a CT scan. If clinical experience is unavailable in an urgent situation, a CT scan would be required.[18]

Key point 6

- The indications for admission to hospital for observation after head injury include any of: (i) a history of loss of consciousness; (ii) neurological abnormality; (iii) persistent headache and/or vomiting; (iv) difficulty in making a full assessment; (v) suspicion of non-accidental injury; (vi) significant co-morbidity; (vii) adverse social circumstances; and (viii) no responsible carer available.

The child can be discharged if none of the above factors apply but with written instructions for parents. In children less than 12 months, the possibility of non-accidental injury must be considered, particularly if the family is on the At-Risk Register.[19]

Haematoma may overlie a skull fracture and may become substantial in size. These should always be left to resolve with no attempt at aspiration or drainage.

ABDOMINAL TRAUMA

The prime considerations are of resuscitation and stabilisation with virtually all abdominal injuries being managed conservatively, even in the presence of significant solid organ injury. Ultrasound examination can reliably detect free fluid in the peritoneal cavity but is unreliable in identifying its source.[20] The mechanism of injury is important, however, and seatbelt injuries, particularly with visible abdominal bruising, have a high association with intra-abdominal injury. The case for a laparotomy in childhood on the basis of abdominal trauma is exceptionally rare – the exception being those cases where hollow organ perforation has occurred. All cases of significant abdominal trauma should be stabilised according to APLS guidelines and transferred to a specialist unit.

TESTICULAR PAIN

Whilst most texts refer to the importance of excluding testicular torsion, this condition comprises only 20% of all cases of testicular pain presenting in childhood and torsion of the hydatid of Morgagni is a much more common condition.[21] The differentiating features between the two are the duration of symptoms and the lack of constitutional upset associated with hydatid torsion. Epididymo-orchitis is extremely rare in children and is usually limited to infants (where it is found in association with a urinary tract infection and requires urological evaluation) and in boys with a co-existing viral infection, e.g. mumps. Extension of the inflammation into the peri-anal area and up the groin is pathognomonic of idiopathic scrotal oedema, a condition which should be managed by observation alone. If testicular torsion cannot be excluded clinically, then urgent surgical exploration is mandatory.

ABSCESSES

These occur in a variety of sites and are common in the first year of life. Peri-anal abscess is virtually always a condition of infant males, the majority of whom have a congenital abnormality of the crypt of Morgagni and will develop a fistula, subsequently requiring fistulotomy.[22] Abscesses in the limbs and in the cervical region, if fluctuant, will respond well to aspiration performed either under general anaesthesia or under topical local anaesthetic cream. Particular care should be taken with the 'cold' abscess of chronic duration on the face. These should be aspirated with a suspicion of a mycobacterium or atypical mycobacterium being the causative organism. In the event of atypical mycobacterium being diagnosed, excision of the lymph node is the prime treatment with particular attention to the portion of the node deep to the deep cervical fascia; chemotherapy should be held in reserve if lymph node excision fails to deal with the problem.[23]

INCARCERATED INGUINAL HERNIA

The majority of incarcerated inguinal hernias in infants can be initially managed by non-operative reduction. Achieving a successful reduction requires technical skill rather than strenuous force with pressure applied over the deep ring and a squeezing manoeuvre – directed initially towards the scrotum – rather than a pushing action. Once reduced, repair should follow within 24 h. The significant (5%) risk of testicular ischaemia in this situation indicates that the receiving surgeon should attempt reduction, irrespective of whether or not they will proceed to herniotomy. Sedation is usually withheld in these circumstances because of the persistence of its action once the hernia is reduced. Surgical correction of an irreducible hernia is a very difficult procedure and should probably be done in a specialist centre.

Key point 7

- Non-operative reduction of an incarcerated hernia is the preferred initial manoeuvre. If successful, definitive repair should be achieved before discharge.

THE CHILD IN THE WARD

The majority of children in a children's surgical ward in a district general hospital will be for observation of abdominal pain. Readers are referred to the diagnostic and treatment algorithms involved in this, but generally for each case of appendicectomy there are 3 cases of non-specific abdominal pain.[24] There are no routine investigations for abdominal pain of childhood and active observation, rather than radiological and laboratory investigations, is the single most useful discriminant in correctly identifying those caused by appendicitis.[25]

Key point 8

- Diagnostic accuracy of appendicitis in childhood can be best achieved by repeated clinical examination rather than laboratory or imaging investigations.

Pain control should not be withheld during the period of active observation and similarly postoperative pain control is an important element of paediatric surgical care. Multimodality treatment using a 'pain ladder' approach (utilising visual analogue pain scoring methods) with intra-operative regional blocks should be the basis for a paediatric pain management protocol.

Key point 9

- Children are susceptible to postoperative dilutional hyponatraemia and should be prescribed isotonic crystalloid (0.45% saline/5% dextrose).

Particular care should be given to postoperative fluids. Children are more sensitive than adults to the adverse effects of dilutional hyponatraemia and intracellular swelling. As a consequence, the routine use of hypotonic intravenous fluids as found in paediatric conditions (4% dextrose, 0.18% NaCl) is to be discouraged in the postoperative period and 0.45% NaCl/5% dextrose with 10 mmol/l potassium should be the fluid of choice.[26] All fluid losses should be measured and replaced with 0.9% saline and potassium solution.

THE CHILD IN THEATRE

In contradistinction to adult practice, parental attendance in theatre is to be encouraged with a parent present at induction and in the recovery room.

In keeping with good surgical technique in adult practice, open operative surgery in children requires careful consideration to haemostasis, gentle tissue dissection, careful temperature control, and generally benefits from optimal illumination through the use of a co-axial headlight and magnification through optical loupes.

The surgeon should give intra-operative consideration to postoperative pain control with the use of regional blockade.

The principles of laparoscopic surgery in children are similar to those in adults but there are some specific differences. The open Hassan technique is recommended for initial port insertion as the smaller abdominal size makes intra-abdominal injury more likely. Similarly, intra-abdominal pressures are age-related but should be kept as low as possible to achieve a satisfactory visual field. In addition, differing age – and hence different sized – children require careful consideration before port placement to aid dissection.

The laparoscopic approach should be considered for assessment of the impalpable testis, appendicectomy and in a diagnostic role for suspected ovarian pathology. More complex procedures are not for the occasional paediatric practitioner and should probably be reserved for specialist centres.

OPERATION UNDER LOCAL ANAESTHESIA

This is generally not well tolerated in children under 10 years of age, and diagnostic procedures such as endoscopy, that are often carried out under sedation in adults, are preferably carried out under general anaesthesia in childhood.

THE CHILD DURING TRANSFER

Resuscitation and stabilisation of children is a multidisciplinary event. The particular role of the surgeon is in assessment and, if required, placement of catheters and drains, *e.g.* intercostal tube drains.[27]

Increasingly, critical care retrieval is in itself a sub-specialty. The surgeon's responsibility in addition to the above is to ensure that there is good communication with the surgical team at the receiving hospital. This, apart from professional etiquette, ensures continuity of care. Written protocols, preferably with a 'checklist' approach for the transfer of children should be locally available. Repatriation arrangements should occur during step-down care back into the district general hospital setting.

Key points for clinical practice

- In the planning of district hospital services for children. it is essential to recognise the competence of the whole team and the need for skills training in resuscitation, stabilisation and transfer to a specialist centre (if required).

- Greater than 95% of boys with a non-retractile foreskin are normal and do not require a circumcision. Balanitis xerotica obliterans is the only absolute indication for circumcision.

- The following conditions can be expected to resolve without surgical intervention: non-retractile/ballooning foreskin; tongue tie; labial fusion; anal fissure; and umbilical hernia.

- Interventions in some conditions are best performed at certain ages: hernia – on presentation (but elective repair of an inguinal hernia in children < 1 year of age must be considered urgent); undescended testis – aged 1 year; hydrocele – aged 2 years; and umbilical hernia – aged 5 years.

- Rectal examination should be performed selectively during clinical examination of a child with abdominal pain and should not be considered routine, but instead be conferred the status of an investigation.

- The indications for admission to hospital for observation after head injury include any of: (i) a history of loss of consciousness; (ii) neurological abnormality; (iii) persistent headache and/or vomiting; (iv) difficulty in making a full assessment; (v) suspicion of non-accidental injury; (vi) significant co-morbidity; (vii) adverse social circumstances; and (viii) no responsible carer available.

- Non-operative reduction of an incarcerated hernia is the preferred initial manoeuvre. If successful, definitive repair should be achieved before discharge.

- Diagnostic accuracy of appendicitis in childhood can be best achieved by repeated clinical examination rather than laboratory or imaging investigations.

- Children are susceptible to postoperative dilutional hyponatraemia and should be prescribed isotonic crystalloid (0.45% saline/5% dextrose).

References

1. Lloyd DA. (ed) *Paediatric Surgery: Standards of Care*. London: British Association of Paediatric Surgeons, 2002.
2. The Royal College of Surgeons of England. *Children's Surgery. A First Class Service: Report of Paediatric Forum of The Royal College of Surgeons of England*. London: RCSE, 2000.
3. The Royal College of Anaesthetists. *Guidance on the Provision of Paediatric Anaesthetic Services*, Bulletin 8. London: The Royal College of Anaesthetists, 2001.
4. Manoharan S, Samarakkody U, Kulkarni M *et al*. Evidence-based change of practice in the management of unilateral inguinal hernia. *J Pediatr Surg* 2005; **40**: 1163–1166.
5. Deeb A, Hughes, I. Inguinal hernia in female infants: a cue to check the sex chromosomes. *BJU Int* 2005; **96**: 401–403.

6. Steward DJ. Pre-term infants are more prone to complications following minor surgery than are term infants. *Anaesthesiology* 1982: **56**: 304–306.
7. General Medical Council. *Guidance for doctors who are asked to circumcise male children.* London: General Medical Council, 1997.
8. Vincent MV, Mackinnon E. The response of clinical balanitis xerotica obliterans to the application of topical steroid-based creams. *J Pediatr Surg* 2005; **40**: 709–712.
9. Heyns CF, Hutson JM. Historical review of the theories on testicular descent. *J Urol* 1995; **153**: 754–767.
10. Mengel W, Heinz H, Sippell WG *et al*. Studies on cryptorchidism: a comparison of histological findings in the germinative epithelium before and after the second year of life. *J Pediatr Surg* 1974; **9**: 445–450.
11. Youngson GG, Jones PF. Management of impalpable testis: long-term results of the pre-peritoneal approach. *J Pediatr Surg* 1991; **26**: 618–620.
12. Leung A, Robson WL, Kao C *et al*. Treatment of labial fusion with topical oestrogen therapy. *Clin Paediatr* 2005; **44**: 245–247.
13. Grant HW, Bisset WH, Mackinlay GA *et al*. Perianal cellulitis in children caused by Group A *Streptococcus*. *Pediatr Surg Int* 1993; **8**: 410–416.
14. Macdonald IA, Beattie TF. Intussusception presenting to a paediatric accident & emergency department. *J Accident Emerg Med* 1995; **12**: 182–186.
15. Jesudason EC, Walker J. Rectal examination in paediatric surgical practice. *Br J Surg* 1999; **86**: 376–378.
16. British Society of Paediatric Radiology. Intussusception reduction, British Society of Paediatric Radiology draft guidelines for suggested safe practice. *Radiology* 1994; **191**: 781–785.
17. Stringer MD, Pledger G, Drake DP. Childhood deaths from intussusception in England and Wales 1984–1989. *BMJ* 1992; **304**: 737–739.
18. Scottish Intercollegiate Guideline Network (SIGN). *Early Management of Patients with a Head Injury*, 2000. <http://www.sign.ac.uk>.
19. Carty H. Non-accidental injury: a review of the radiology. *Eur Radiol* 1997; **7**: 1365–1376.
20. Coley BD, Mutabagani KH, Martin LC *et al*. Focused abdominal sonography for trauma (FAST) in children with blunt abdominal trauma. *J Trauma* 2000; **48**: 902–906.
21. Davenport M. ABC of general surgery in children: acute problems of the scrotum. *BMJ* 1996; **312**: 435–437.
22. Poenaru D, Yazbek S. Anal fistula in children: etiology, features management. *J Pediatr Surg* 1993; **28**: 1194–1195.
23. Davenport M. ABC of general surgery in children: lumps and swelling of the head and neck. *BMJ* 1996; **312**: 368–371.
24. Driver CP, Youngson GG. Abdominal pain in children. *Scot Health Bull* 1995; **53**: 113–118.
25. Jones PF. Active observation and management of acute abdominal pain in children. *BMJ* 1976; **ii**: 551–553.
26. Duke T, Molynieux EM. Intravenous fluids for seriously ill children: time to reconsider. *Lancet* 2003; **362**: 1320–1323.
27. Driver CP, Robinson C, De Caluwe DO *et al*. The quality of inter-hospital transfer of the surgical neonate. *Today's Emerg* 2000; **6**: 102–105.

Jonathan Wilson Louise Cousens

2

Pre-operative cardiac assessment and interventions in high-risk elective surgical patients

A high-risk surgical procedure can be considered as one in which there is a significant risk of life-threatening complications. If we consider 'significant' as a mortality rate of 1% or greater, for elective surgery this would include abdominal aortic aneurysm surgery, colorectal cancer surgery, and upper gastrointestinal cancer surgery. Recent, large-scale UK audits demonstrate mean elective mortality rates of 6.1%, 5.6% and 12%, respectively, for these operations,[1-3] which many larger hospitals will be carrying out on a regular basis. Aside from mortality, there is a significant incidence of complications which may lead to prolonged hospital stay, and use of critical care facilities.

A recent comprehensive meta-analysis has demonstrated that the mortality from high-risk surgery can be reduced by a strategy of monitoring cardiac output and optimising tissue perfusion in the peri-operative period,[4] with a risk reduction of 0.66 (95% CI 0.54–0.81). (These treatment strategies have been covered in the previous book in this series[5]). Moreover, the same meta-analysis showed that once complications leading to sepsis and multi-organ failure were established, initiating the same strategies was an ineffective treatment (RR 0.92; 95% CI 0.75–1.11). Therefore, there is compelling evidence that peri-operative optimisation strategies should be directed at the correctly identified high-risk patient, and initiated before or during surgery, to prevent complications occurring.

There will always be a small number of otherwise fit patients who die from purely surgical complications, but the majority of postoperative deaths occur in elderly patients with known significant co-morbidities. Indeed, *Then and*

Jonathan Wilson BSc MB ChB FRCA (for correspondence)
Consultant Anaesthetist, York Hospital, Wiggington Road, York YO31 8HE, UK
E-mail: rjtwilson@doctors.org.uk

Louise Cousens MB ChB MRCP
Specialist Registrar in Anaesthetics, Yorkshire Deanery, Leeds, UK

Now, the 2000 report of the National Confidential Enquiry into Perioperative Deaths (NCEPOD), demonstrated clearly that this an increasing problem.[6] Comparing non-survivors from 1998–1999 to those from the 1990 report, they stated that the incidence of cardiac co-morbidity had increased from 54% to 66%, respiratory co-morbidity from 33% to 37% and neurological morbidity from 18% to 33%.

Most patients who die after major elective surgery will do so as a result of cardiac events such as myocardial infarction, thrombo-embolic disease and cardiac failure leading to multi-organ dysfunction and failure through inadequate tissue perfusion. The assessment of adequacy of cardiac function, and improvement where necessary, is therefore of paramount importance in the preparation of patients undergoing high-risk surgery

The aim of this chapter is to review recent advances in the pre-operative assessment and identification of the high-risk surgical patient, and the effects of pre-admission interventions in this patient group, particularly those that aim to improve cardiac function or reduce cardiac risk.

Key point 1

- The majority of patients who die after major elective surgery have significant cardiac and respiratory co-morbidity.

IDENTIFICATION OF THE HIGH-RISK PATIENT AT PRE-ASSESSMENT

THE PRE-ASSESSMENT CLINIC

The majority of UK Hospital Trusts now have Pre-Assessment Clinics, although these are largely nurse-led, and, when medical staff are present, they are often junior trainees with little experience. The 2005 NCEPOD report highlighted that only 79% of patients awaiting elective aneurysm repair attended a pre-operative assessment; of these, 30% were seen by a nurse or preregistration house officer, without any senior assessment.[1] It seems self-evident that any initial form of risk assessment should be straightforward enough to be undertaken by relatively inexperienced staff.

PREDICTING POSTOPERATIVE CARDIAC COMPLICATIONS

Cardiac Risk Index

Pre-operative assessment is based upon the traditional findings of history, examination and investigations. From these findings, a risk assessment in the form of a scoring system can be derived, from which a patient can be given an overall percentage risk of particular complications or mortality occurring.

For predicting postoperative cardiac complications in non-cardiac surgery, Lee's Cardiac Risk Index[7] is a simple score based on the presence or absence of six factors (Table 1). Fifty-six major cardiac complications occurred in the derivation cohort of 2893 patients, from which the six independent predictive variables were identified. The rate of cardiac complications in patients with 0,

Table 1 Risk factors for postoperative cardiac complications

- High-risk type of surgery
- Ischaemic heart disease
- History of congestive cardiac failure
- History of cerebrovascular disease
- Insulin therapy for diabetes
- Pre-operative serum creatinine >177 µmol/l

1, 2 or 3 or more of these variables was 0.5%, 1.3%, 4% and 9%, respectively. In the validation population of 1422 patients, the incidence was 0.4%, 0.9%, 7% and 9%, respectively. This is a relatively simple score to consider at the pre-assessment clinic, and for patients with two or more of these risk factors the risk of a major cardiac complication is significant. However, the score and percentage risk are not particularly helpful in identifying any particular factors that can be improved pre-operatively, but the index can be used as a trigger to identify higher-risk patients, and direct them towards more specialised investigations of cardiac function.

The recently updated American Heart Association *Guideline for Perioperative Cardiovascular Evaluation for Noncardiac Surgery*[8] suggests a stepwise strategy that relies on the assessment of clinical markers, prior coronary evaluation and treatment, functional capacity and surgery-specific risk.

Functional status

Emphasis is now increasingly placed on assessing functional capacity, and the response of the cardiorespiratory unit when stressed. These assessments can initially be questionnaire-based, using a tool such as the Duke Activity Status Index (DASI).[9] The DASI questionnaire gives a reasonable estimate of measured peak oxygen consumption, which reflects cardiovascular fitness. When used to assess 100 vascular patients, the DASI score correlated with the ability to complete a simple exercise test, and was inversely correlated with the time taken to complete the test.[10]

Stair-climbing has been used to predict postoperative cardiopulmonary complications after high-risk surgery. In a series of 83 patients undergoing either thoracotomy, sternotomy or upper abdominal laparotomy, 89% of those unable to climb one flight of stairs developed a postoperative complication, compared to none in the group able to climb seven flights.[11] Inability to climb two flights of stairs had a positive predictive value of 82% for development of a postoperative complication.

So far, the tests described above are simple to do in the pre-assessment setting, and will go some way to identifying patients at risk of postoperative cardio-respiratory complications. However, whilst useful screening tools, none of them provide the assessing physician with any specific clues as to what exactly is limiting exercise capacity, and hence what treatment strategies to employ.

Cardiopulmonary exercise testing

Cardiopulmonary exercise testing (CPX testing) is increasingly used as a pre-operative assessment investigation to gain objective physiological data of functional status. CPX testing examines the ability of the cardiorespiratory systems to deliver oxygen to tissues under stress, in this case the exercising limb muscles as the patient pedals at a constant rate on a specialised cycle ergometer. As the work-rate increases, the oxygen demands of the exercising muscle increase, leading to an increase in cardiac output. Eventually, the energy demands outstrip the supply of oxygen and aerobic metabolism is supplemented by anaerobic metabolism, with the consequent generation of lactate. The oxygen consumption at which this occurs is known as the anaerobic threshold (AT), and can be identified easily in most individuals. Older et al.[12] measured AT in 187 elderly patients before major abdominal surgery. The overall non-surgical mortality from the cohort was 5.9%. Patients who had an AT < 11 ml/kg/min ($n = 55$) had a mortality of 18% compared with those who had an AT > 11 ml/kg/min ($n = 132$) whose mortality was 0.8%. In patients who also had ischaemic heart disease, the mortality was 42% for patients whose AT was < 11 ml/kg/min, whilst it was only 4% for those whose AT was > 11 ml/kg/min. From these data, it is seen that poor ventricular function and hence poor oxygen delivery, as measured by AT, predicted a high-risk for major surgery, particularly when coupled with evidence of myocardial ischaemia. In a second study of 548 consecutive patients undergoing major abdominal surgery, Older et al.[13] used AT to stratify risk and to direct peri-operative interventions accordingly. In this study, 153 patients (28%) had an AT < 11 ml/kg/min and were admitted to the intensive care unit (ICU) pre-operatively and had haemodynamic optimisation before surgery; 115 patients (21%) with an AT > 11 ml/kg/min but with evidence of myocardial ischaemia on testing were admitted to HDU postoperatively, and those with an AT > 11 ml/kg/min with no evidence of ischaemia were cared for on a normal ward postoperatively. Of the 21 patients who died, 19 had been triaged to ICU or HDU as a result of CPX testing, and the two deaths in the ward group were due to disease progression. Through pre-admission to ICU and use of invasive monitoring to optimise cardiac function, the mortality in the high-risk group (low AT) had been reduced from 18% to 8.9%.

Measuring anaerobic threshold accurately identifies a population that is less able to mount the appropriate increase in oxygen delivery demanded after major surgery, and in which a strategy of invasive monitoring and optimisation of cardiac function is more likely to improve outcome. It is a non-invasive test, and safe in the elderly surgical population. It is currently being established in some UK pre-assessment clinics, including the authors' own, where some 460 patients have undergone testing. The data from CPX testing can differentiate the causes of poor functional status, and allow pre-operative interventions to be made, such as β-blockade to improve heart failure or ischaemia. In such patients, the test can then be repeated to see whether the patient's status has improved.

Key point 2

- The patient at risk of poor peri-operative cardiac function can best be identified by dynamic tests of functional cardiac performance such as CPX testing or dobutamine stress echocardiography.

Stress echocardiography

When dobutamine is administered to increase heart rate and myocardial oxygen demand, echocardiography can identify developing areas of ventricular wall motion abnormality, indicating the likelihood of underlying coronary artery stenoses causing ischaemia. As an assessment tool prior to major vascular surgery, dobutamine stress echocardiography (DSE) has a strong negative predictive value: 96 patients with no wall motion abnormality had no postoperative cardiac complications.[14] However, 15 of 35 patients with a positive DSE had major cardiac complications.

Compared to thallium scanning, a recent meta-analysis has shown that DSE is a significantly better predictive and negative test.[15] The size of the lesion identified is an important factor in the likelihood of cardiac complications, and both techniques are equally efficacious at identifying the subgroup who have moderate-to-large abnormalities (14–16% of patients tested).

The main disadvantage of DSE is reproducibility, being a user-dependent test, but it is a continually evolving technique and refinements are allowing more objective measures to be made.[16] The availability of DSE in the UK is still limited though, and resource limitations mean it is unlikely to be a routine test for patients undergoing major high-risk surgery.

PRE-OPERATIVE INTERVENTIONS IN THE HIGH-RISK SURGICAL PATIENT

Having assessed a patient as being at significant risk of cardiac problems postoperatively, and identified a correctable lesion, interventions can be made to improve cardiac function and/or minimise risk of postoperative ischaemia. Much recent interest has been directed at pharmacological interventions, and at pre-operative coronary artery revascularisation, either surgical or percutaneous.

PHARMACOLOGICAL INTERVENTION

β_1-Blockade

There has been much interest in the use of β_1-adrenergic blockade to reduce tachycardic cardiovascular responses to surgery, and hence minimise the postoperative incidence of myocardial ischaemia and adverse cardiovascular events. The exact mode of action of these agents is unclear, with several possible mechanisms.

During surgery and in the postoperative period, there is a persistent increase in heart rate and myocardial contractility. This can, particularly in susceptible patients, cause prolonged mismatch of coronary perfusion and demand, resulting in ischaemia and infarction of the myocardium. β-Blockers can attenuate this mismatch in two ways. First, supply is improved when the heart rate falls. This is because left ventricular coronary perfusion occurs mainly during diastole, the length of which increases rapidly below about 75 beats/min. Second, β-blockers reduce contractility, reducing demand.

Demand may also be reduced by suppressing lipolysis, which switches the myocardium to the use of glucose as a substrate. This metabolic pathway requires less oxygen for the same energy output, and so demand falls.

β-Blockers are not thought to have any impact on the formation of atherosclerotic plaques, but may help to prevent plaque rupture by reducing some of the mechanical stresses placed on the vessel. β-Blockers are also thought to raise the threshold for ventricular tachycardias and other arrhythmias in the presence of ischaemia, conferring a protective effect in the peri-operative period.[17,18]

However, the evidence for peri-operative β-blockade remains inconclusive. Several studies have been conducted which appear to show a beneficial effect, while others demonstrate no effect, or even a harmful effect within certain patient sub-groups.

Mangano et al.[19] performed a randomised, controlled, double-blinded study looking at the use of atenolol in non-cardiac surgery patients with, or at risk from, coronary artery disease. The study was unique in assessing not just the peri-operative period, but also the long-term outcomes up to 2 years postoperatively. Existing coronary artery disease was indicated by previous myocardial infarction, angina, or atypical angina with a positive stress test. 'At risk' was defined as having two of the following risk factors: age > 65 years, hypertension, smoking, cholesterol > 6.2 mmol/l and diabetes mellitus. A total of 200 patients were randomised to receive either a placebo or atenolol at induction of anaesthesia, immediately postoperatively, and every day for up to 7 days (determined by the length of hospital stay). Holter monitoring was used for the first 48 h postoperatively, and in the atenolol group, a 50% reduction in ischaemia was demonstrated. Post-discharge mortality was reduced in the atenolol group from 8% to 0% at 6 months, 14% to 3% in the first year and 21% to 10% at 2 years. The greatest reduction in mortality and morbidity was in the first 6 months, and this survival benefit was maintained in the long term. However, atenolol did not appear to reduce the risk of death from cardiac causes during hospital stay, or reduce peri-operative myocardial infarctions, despite the reduction in ischaemia seen on Holter monitoring. It is possible that this is a reflection of the low incidence of these events, with consequent under powering of the study. In patients identified as high risk through dobutamine stress testing, there is an expected cardiac event rate of 28% peri-operatively;[20] however, the study of Mangano et al.[19] included patients who merely had risk factors, with no proven cardiovascular disease. In this lower risk group, the event rate is only around 3%.

In 1999, Poldermans and Boersma[20] reported a randomised, controlled, multicentre study of peri-operative β-blockade in vascular surgery. The patients were selected on the basis of clinical risk factors and a positive dobutamine stress test (see above), and therefore constituted a high-risk group. Clinical risk factors were essentially the same as for the Mangano et al. study. Patients who were already taking β-blockers were excluded from the study. Bisoprolol, a cardioselective β-blocker, was started at least 1 week before surgery and continued for up to 30 days postoperatively. Primary end points were cardiac-cause death and non-fatal myocardial infarction. The combined incidence of these end-points was reduced from 34% in the standard care group to 3.4% in the bisoprolol group. Given the magnitude of this difference, the trial was stopped early. The conclusion drawn by the authors was that the use of bisoprolol peri-operatively, commencing 1–2 weeks before surgery, significantly reduces the risk of non-fatal myocardial infarction and death from cardiac cause in high-risk patients undergoing vascular surgery.

Key point 3

- Techniques which optimise cardiac function, tissue perfusion and oxygen delivery in the peri-operative period reduce mortality and morbidity.

Lindenhauer et al.[21] challenged some of these findings in a later study. The authors conducted a multicentre, retrospective cohort study of patients undergoing major non-cardiac surgery in the US. The information was derived from billing and other administrative data, and patients were classified according to Lee's Revised Cardiac Risk Index (see above). If the patient received β-blockers within the first 2 days of hospital stay, they were considered to have received 'prophylactic' treatment and were entered into the study. For each such patient there were two matched patients from the non-β-blocker group. The 2% of patients with an RCRI score of 3 or above (i.e. highest risk group) had the greatest benefit from β-blockers, with an adjusted odds ratio for death of between 0.71 and 0.58. Patients with an RCRI of 2 showed less benefit (odds ratio 0.88), and the lowest risk patients, RCRI 0 or 1, showed no advantage from use of β-blockers. Indeed, there was evidence that treatment in this group may be harmful; the number needed to harm was calculated at 208. The cause for this is not clear. It seems likely that low-risk patients who received β-blockers did so because of an unexpected cardiac event in the first two hospital days – hence were misclassified as low risk. A further limitation is that owing to the data source, there was no reliable data about incidence of non-fatal infarction and ischaemia, only deaths. The authors concluded that until large randomised trials were completed, β-blockers in high-risk patients were still warranted, but their use in low-risk patients may be harmful.

In 2005, Devereaux et al.[22] performed a meta-analysis of 22 trials, totalling 2437 patients, assessing the use of peri-operative β-blockers in non-cardiac surgery. Trials were included if they met specific criteria, including the use of control groups. The 1999 Poldermans and Boersma study was excluded as it was stopped early. The outcomes used included total deaths, cardiovascular deaths, non-fatal myocardial infarction and cardiac arrest, heart failure, bronchospasm and hypotension needing treatment. In all but one study, the β-blocker was given at the time of anaesthesia and the treatment period lasted up to 30 days postoperatively. The meta-analysis appeared to show that for any individual outcome, there was no significant reduction, but that the reduction in relative risk for the composite of cardiovascular mortality, non-fatal myocardial infarction and non-fatal cardiac arrest was 0.56. However, the relative risk for bradycardia needing treatment was 2.3, and for hypotension needing treatment 1.3.

In conclusion, there is good evidence that among high-risk patients having non-cardiac surgery, the use of peri-operative β-blockers can reduce the incidence of adverse cardiac events, but in the lower risk patients the evidence is not clear for their use and may actually be harmful. In addition, there is an increased risk of bradycardia and hypotension needing treatment. The results of a very large multicentre trial currently underway, assessing peri-operative ischaemia, POISE, may help clarify some of these issues.

Key point 4

- Instituting cardioselective β-blocker treatment may protect against cardiac complications in the highest-risk patients.

Statins

Inhibitors of 3-hydroxy-3-methylglutaryl coenzyme A (HMACo-A) reductase have been shown to have a class effect of significant reduction in cardiovascular disease and complications. More recently, they have been found to have beneficial effects on tumour growth inhibition and prevention of bony fractures. As yet, there appear to be very few adverse effects from these drugs and their use is increasing in medicine and surgery. The main side effect noted is a derangement of liver enzyme function tests.

The substrate for HMACo-A reductase, mevalonate, is the precursor for cholesterol as well as many non-steroidal compounds. Inhibition of this enzyme, therefore, results in a wide range of actions. Cholesterol biosynthesis is inhibited and the low-density lipoprotein (LDL) profile improved; in addition, statins cause increased nitric oxide release (a powerful vasodilator), reduction of inflammation, increased stability of atherosclerotic plaques and improvements in platelet function.[23] These factors combine to reduce the progression and even promote regression, of the atherosclerotic plaques, which are at the root of coronary artery disease.

A large meta-analysis in 1996 by Cheung-Bernard et al.[24] evaluated the effect of statins on cardiovascular outcomes in a wide range of patient groups, with a follow-up period of 3 years. They found that the use of statins reduced the incidence of coronary events by up to 29%, and all-cause mortality by 15%.[24] The reduction in events was independent of gender, presence of hypertension and diabetes. The greatest reduction was seen in smokers.

More recently, in 2003, Poldermans et al.[25] studied the effect of peri-operative statins in vascular patients. This was a retrospective, case-controlled study, with data sourced from the hospital information system. Patients ($n = 160$) were each matched to two controls, with 'case' being defined as in-hospital death, from any cause, up to 30 days postoperatively. The cholesterol and LDL measurements were considered raised if above 5.5 total and 3.5, respectively. This study found that peri-operative mortality was reduced in statin users by 4.5-fold (from 5–6% at 30 days). This reduction was consistent in across subgroups formed by surgery type, cardiac risk factors and use of aspirin and β-blockers.

These findings support previous work from a retrospective study by O'Neil-Callahan et al.[26] in 2001, which also looked at outcomes in vascular patients. These outcomes included death, myocardial infarction, ischaemia, heart failure and ventricular arrhythmias. It was found that the complication rate fell from 16.5% in non-statin users to 9.9% in those treated with statins. This difference was mostly due to a reduction in myocardial infarction and heart failure. This protective effect was consistent across very diverse subgroups of patients, and persisted after adjustment for other known predictors of peri-operative complications (such as diabetes and emergency surgery).

In 2005, Biccard *et al.*[27] demonstrated the cost-effectiveness of statin therapy by analysing prospective studies of statin administration in major elective vascular surgery. Using the 2004 NHS reference costs for statins, he calculated that around 60% of the total cost of atorvastatin was recovered through the reduction in peri-operative adverse events.[18]

In summary, the use of statins is likely to have a significant impact on the event rate for cardiovascular complications in the peri-operative period, which is consistent across diverse patients subgroups.

Key point 5

- Statin therapy is likely to prevent cardiac complications postoperatively.

INTERVENTIONS: CORONARY ARTERY REVASCULARISATION

Studies have been recently published which examine the effect of deliberate coronary artery revascularisation in patients awaiting non-cardiac surgery (usually vascular), who have been classified as high-risk on clinical grounds, then found to have stenotic lesions on coronary angiography.

The CARP study assessed 5859 patients at US Veterans' Affairs medical centres who were scheduled for vascular surgery.[28] Coronary angiography was recommended if a cardiologist considered the patient at increased risk of cardiac problems. Patients were then eligible for the study if angiography showed one or more major vessels with greater than 70% stenoses, which were suitable for revascularisation. A total of 510 patients were subsequently randomised to revascularisation, either surgical or percutaneous, or to best medical therapy. There were considerable numbers of excluded patients, for instance 215 had coronary artery disease not amenable to revascularisation, and 54 patients had > 50% stenosis of the left main coronary artery; 74% of randomised patients had two or more of Lee's Cardiac Risk Index factors (see above).[7] In the revascularisation group, of 258 patients, 59% underwent percutaneous intervention, and 41% had bypass surgery.

After the definitive vascular procedure there were no differences in the mortality rates and infarction rates, which were 3.1% and 11.6% in the revascularisation group, and 3.4% and 14.3% in the control group, respectively. Additionally, long-term follow-up at 2.7 years after randomisation showed no difference at all in mortality with 22% in the revascularisation group and 23% in the control group. On the basis of these results, the authors concluded that a strategy of coronary artery revascularisation before elective vascular surgery among patients with stable cardiac symptoms cannot be recommended.

Key point 6

- Pre-operative coronary artery revascularisation, either by bypass surgery or by angioplasty and stenting, does not significantly reduce postoperative cardiac complications in patients with stable cardiac disease.

In a retrospective, propensity-scored, controlled trial, patients who had had percutaneous coronary intervention prior to abdominal aortic surgery had a similar incidence of postoperative infarction or death compared to the expected incidence.[29] Therefore, percutaneous coronary intervention did not seem to limit cardiac risk or death after aortic surgery.

SUMMARY

Mortality rates from major elective surgery remain significant, and the majority of deaths occur in patients with cardiac disease. High-risk patients can be screened pre-operatively through simple scoring systems or by more sophisticated and accurate methods such as cardiopulmonary exercise testing, or dobutamine stress echocardiography. Emphasis should be placed on assessing the functional capacity of the patient.

Pre-emptive coronary artery revascularisation in otherwise stable patients does not confer a survival advantage, and may unnecessarily delay the required surgery. Pre-operative treatment with cardioselective β-blockers and statins may reduce cardiac risk in higher-risk patients, but more studies are required in lower risk patient groups. The mainstay of peri-operative care of the high-risk patient remains careful monitoring and optimisation of tissue perfusion.

Key points for clinical practice

- The majority of patients who die after major elective surgery have significant cardiac and respiratory co-morbidity.

- The patient at risk of poor peri-operative cardiac function can best be identified by dynamic tests of functional cardiac performance such as CPX testing or dobutamine stress echocardiography.

- Techniques which optimise cardiac function, tissue perfusion and oxygen delivery in the peri-operative period reduce mortality and morbidity.

- Instituting cardioselective β-blocker treatment may protect against cardiac complications in the highest-risk patients.

- Statin therapy is likely to prevent cardiac complications postoperatively.

- Pre-operative coronary artery revascularisation, either by bypass surgery or by angioplasty and stenting, does not significantly reduce postoperative cardiac complications in patients with stable cardiac disease.

References

1. National Confidential Enquiry into Perioperative Deaths. *Abdominal Aortic Aneurysm: a service in need of surgery?* NCEPOD 2005. <http://www.ncepod.org.uk/2005b.htm>.
2. Tekkis P, Poloniecki J, Thompson M, Stamatakis J. Operative mortality in colorectal cancer: prospective national study. *BMJ* 2003; **327**: 1196–1201.

3. McCulloch P, Ward J, Tekkis P. Mortality and morbidity in gastro-oesophageal cancer surgery: initial results of ASCOT multicentre prospective cohort study. *BMJ* 2003; **327**: 1192–1197.

4. Poeze M, Greve JWM, Ramsay G. Meta-analysis of haemodynamic optimization: relationship to methodological quality. *Crit Care* 2005; **9**: 771–779.

5. Boyd O. Optimization of the high-risk surgical patient. Taylor I, Johnson CD. (eds) *Recent Advances in Surgery*, vol 28. London: Royal Society of Medicine Press, 2005; 33–45.

6. National Confidential Enquiry into Perioperative Deaths. *Then And Now: The 2000 Report of the National Confidential Enquiry into Perioperative Deaths.* NCEPOD 2000. <http://www.ncepod.org.uk/20001.htm>.

7. Lee T, Marcantonio E, Mangione C *et al.* Derivation and validation of a simple index for prediction of cardiac risk of major non-cardiac surgery. *Circulation* 1999; **100**: 1043–1049.

8. Eagle KA, Berger PB, Calkins H *et al.* ACC/AHA Guideline Update for Perioperative Cardiovascular Evaluation for Noncardiac Surgery – Executive Summary. *Anesth Analg* 2002; **94**: 1052–1064.

9. Hlatky MA, Boineau RE, Higginbotham ME *et al.* A brief self-administered questionnaire to determine functional capacity (the Duke Activity Status Index). *Am J Cardiol* 1989; **64**: 651–654.

10. McGlade DP, Poon AB, Davies MJ. The use of a questionnaire and simple exercise test in the preoperative assessment of vascular surgery patients. *Anaesth Intensive Care* 2001; **29**: 520–526.

11. Girish M, Trayner E, Dammann O *et al.* Symptom-limited stair climbing as a predictor of postoperative cardiopulmonary complications after high-risk surgery. *Chest* 2001; **120**: 1147–1151.

12. Older P, Smith R, Courtney P *et al.* Preoperative evaluation of cardiac failure and ischaemia in elderly patients by cardiopulmonary exercise testing. *Chest* 1993; **104**: 701–704.

13. Older P, Hall A, Hader R. Cardiopulmonary exercise testing as a screening test for perioperative management of major surgery in the elderly. *Chest* 1999; **116**: 355–362.

14. Poldermans D, Fioretti PM, Forster T *et al.* Dobutamine stress echocardiography for assessment of perioperative cardiac risk in patients undergoing major vascular surgery. *Circulation* 1993; **87**: 1506–1512.

15. Beattie WS, Abdelnaem E, Wijeysundera DN *et al.* A meta-analytic comparison of preoperative stress echocardiography and nuclear scintigraphy imaging. *Anesth Analg* 2006; **102**: 8–16.

16. Poldermans D, Bax JJ. Dobutamine echocardiography: a diagnostic tool comes of age. *Eur Heart J* 2003; **24**: 1541–1542.

17. Poldermans D, Boersma E. Beta-blocker therapy in non-cardiac surgery. *N Engl J Med* 2005; **353**: 4.

18. London M, Zaugg M, Schaub M *et al.* Perioperative beta-adrenergic receptor blockade. *Anaesthesiology* 2004; **100**: 170–175.

19. Mangano D, Layug E, Wallace A *et al.* Effect of atenolol on mortality and cardiovascular morbidity after noncardiac surgery. Multicenter study of Perioperative Ischemia Research Group. *N Engl J Med* 1996; **335**: 1713–1720.

20. Poldermans D, Boersma E. The effect of bisoprolol on perioperative mortality and myocardial infarction in high-risk patients undergoing vascular surgery. *N Engl J Med* 1999; **341**: 1789–1795.

21. Lindenauer P, Pekow P, Wang K *et al.* Perioperative beta-blockade therapy and mortality after major non-cardiac surgery. *N Engl J Med* 2005; **353**: 349–361.

22. Devereaux PJ, Beattie WS, Choi P *et al.* How strong is the evidence for the use of perioperative beta-blockers in non-cardiac surgery? Systematic review and meta-analysis of randomised controlled trials. *BMJ* 2005; **331**: 313–321.

23. Stancu C, Sima A. Statins: mechanism of action. *J Cell Mol Med* 2001; **5**: 378–387.

24. Cheung-Bernard MY, Lau-Chu-Pak, Kumana C. Meta-analysis of large randomised controlled trials to evaluate impact of statins on cardiovascular outcomes. *Br J Clin Pharmacol* 2004; **57**: 640–651.

25. Poldermans D, Bax JJ, Kertai MD *et al.* Statins are associated with a reduced incidence of perioperative mortality in patients undergoing major non-cardiac vascular surgery.

Circulation 2003; **107**: 1848–1851.

26. O'Neil-Callahan K, Katsimaglis G, Tepper M *et al*. The statins for risk reduction in surgery study. *J Am Coll Cardiol* 2005; **45**: 336–342.

27. Biccard B, Sear J, Foex P. The pharmaco-economics of perioperative statin therapy. *Anaesthesia* 2005; **60**: 1059–1063.

28. McFalls EO, Ward HB, Moritz TE *et al*. Coronary artery revascularisation before elective major vascular surgery. *N Engl J Med* 2004; **351**: 2795–2804.

29. Godet G, Riou B, Bertrand M *et al*. Does preoperative coronary angioplasty improve perioperative cardiac outcome? *Anesthesiology* 2005; **102**: 739–746.

Gary Atkin Abhay Chopada

3

Recent advances in angiogenesis and their surgical implications

The process of new blood vessel formation from pre-existing vessels, such as capillaries and venules, is termed angiogenesis.[1] Vasculogenesis refers to the process of embryonic vascular development whereby vessels are formed *de novo* from progenitor cells.[2] Both processes are important in a range of physiological and pathological conditions relevant to surgeons. Tumour growth is intimately related to the process of new blood vessel formation. Clinicians treating cancer patients need to be aware of the steps involved to allow comprehension of the disease process and to interpret the results of anti-angiogenic therapies appropriately. The process of angiogenesis is also intimately related to fundamental processes like wound healing.

Angiogenesis may be a physiological phenomenon associated with wound healing, inflammation and menstruation, or it may be a pathological process (when it is often termed neovascularisation), in conditions such as diabetic retinopathy, rheumatoid arthritis, and cancer.[3] In normal tissues, there is a balance between pro- and anti-angiogenic mediators, such that little new vessel formation occurs. However, in these physiological and pathological conditions, there is a shift in the equilibrium towards stimulation of angiogenesis and hence new vessel generation.[2] In the physiological situation, angiogenesis is tightly controlled; in the pathological setting, it escapes regulation and excessive neovascularisation ensues.[4] In recent years, there has been an intense investigation into the field of angiogenesis. This is because it appears to be fundamental to cancer progression, and is being extensively studied in the hope that it may predict prognosis in a range of malignancies,

Gary Atkin MD MRCS (for correspondence)
Specialist Registrar in General Surgery, North West Thames Region, London, UK
E-mail: gkatkin@blueyonder.co.uk

Abhay Chopada MS FRCS FRCSI
Consultant Colorectal Surgeon, Department of Surgery, Ealing Hospital NHS Trust, Uxbridge Road, Southall, Middlesex UB1 3EW, UK

as well as permitting tumour-targeted therapy. As the mechanisms of cancer growth via the angiogenic pathway are further elucidated, it is hoped multiple windows of therapeutic opportunity will become available through anti-angiogenic therapies.

COMPONENTS OF THE ANGIOGENIC CASCADE

The angiogenic cascade involves the complex interaction between tumour cells and host immune cells and stromal cells, in particular the cells that form the building blocks for new vessel formation, namely endothelia and modified smooth muscle cells called pericytes. Throughout the angiogenic process, the cellular and molecular mediators are regulated by autocrine and paracrine mechanisms, resulting in a coherent interplay between pro- and anti-angiogenic factors (Table 1).

The most extensively studied angiostimulatory molecule is vascular endothelial growth factor (VEGF). This plays an important role in many of the steps of the angiogenic cascade. It is a protein secreted by nearly all cells[2] and is expressed as 4 isoforms.[5] Its release is stimulated by hypoxia and is under the control of cytokines, oncogenes, and tumour suppressor genes.[6] It acts on endothelia to increase the vascular permeability (hence it was originally named vascular permeability factor), which permits the escape of proteins into the extravascular space to provide the lattice needed for subsequent endothelial migration. It is also an endothelial cell-specific mitogen and angiogenic factor.[7]

It is thought the new vessels formed under the influence of VEGF are immature, in that they lack a covering of smooth muscle cells.[8] The formation of mature vessels requires the action of angiopoietin-1, which causes vessel stabilisation by inducing the expression of platelet-derived growth factors (PDGFs) that stimulate the migration of pericytes and other accessory cells. The angiopoietins are a family of mediators that are endothelial cell-specific. Angiopoietin-1 binds to the Tie-2 receptor causing endothelial stabilisation, whereas the binding of angiopoietin-2 to the same receptor leads to endothelial

Table 1 Pro- and anti-angiogenic agents[4,9]

Angiostimulators	Angio-inhibitors
Vascular endothelial growth factor (VEGF)	Thrombospondins-1,2
Basic and acidic fibroblast growth factors (bFGF, aFGF)	Endostatin
Platelet-derived endothelial cell growth factor	Angiostatin
Matrix metalloproteinases (MMPs)	Interferons α and β
Insulin-like growth factor (IGF)	Interleukin-12 (IL-12)
Epidermal growth factor (EGF)	Tamoxifen
Interleukins (IL-1, IL-4, IL-6, IL-8, IL-15)	Thalidomide
Angiogenin	Captopril
Integrins $\alpha v_1\beta_3$ and $\alpha v_1\beta_5$	Dexamethasone
Endotoxin	Indomethacin
Endothelin-1	Diclofenac
Angiopoietin-1 (Ang-1)	Angiopoietin-2 (Ang-2)
Tumour necrosis factor (TNF)-α (*in vivo*)	TNF-α (*in vitro*)

Key points 1–3

- Angiogenesis is a fundamental process important for tissue growth and survival.

- Normally a balance between pro- and anti-angiogenic mediators prevents neo-angiogenesis.

- Angiogenesis is an end result of interaction between several different mediators.

destabilisation and vascular regression.[9] The endothelins are another family of growth factors implicated in the pathophysiology of a number of tumour types. Endothelin-1 is involved in several steps of the angiogenic cascade, as well as playing a role in tumour cell survival and invasion.[10] Other, non-specific angiogenic mediators have been investigated and shown to have numerous actions including endothelial activation and migration, extracellular matrix invasion and capillary tube formation (Table 1). The important thing to consider is that these effects are not the result of a single mediator, but result from the interaction of multiple factors acting together.

ANGIOGENESIS AND CANCER FORMATION

Angiogenesis is fundamental to tumour growth, invasion and metastasis. For a cancer to grow more than 2–3 mm^3, it requires its own blood supply to meet the demands of tumour cell metabolism.[11] The rich vascular network typical of solid tumours allows entry of tumour cells into the circulation, thereby facilitating the metastatic process.[2] Similarly, micrometastases need to acquire a circulation at a site distant to the primary tumour in order to survive. Angiogenesis is, therefore, associated with primary tumour progression, as well as the components throughout the metastatic cascade.[12] It has always been considered the main mechanism of tumour blood vessel formation. Recently, however, it has been shown that 40% of tumour vessels are derived from endothelial progenitor cells and not from pre-existing vessels.[13] This suggests the process of vasculogenesis may contribute significantly to the development of the tumour vasculature.

Tumour angiogenesis involves a gradual loss of cell-cycle regulation, with an imbalance of pro- and anti-angiogenic factors. For most tumours, the switch to an angiogenic phenotype is a discrete step in the malignant process.[14] In fact, for cancer progression, a lack of angiogenesis will keep the neoplastic cell in a state of dormancy until the angiogenic switch has occurred.[15] For a few tumour types, for example cervical carcinoma, the angiogenic phenotype may actually precede the malignant phenotype, such that neovascularisation appears at the premalignant dysplastic stage.[16]

With dormant tumours, the actions of pro- and anti-angiogenic mediators are in equilibrium, and the rate of cellular proliferation is balanced by tumour cell apoptosis. For the switch to an angiogenic phenotype to occur, the angiostimulators must outweigh the angio-inhibitors. Generally, this is brought about by changes in the local tumour environment, such as inflammation,

Table 2 Mechanisms possibly involved in the initiation of angiogenesis[17]

- The need for continued growth of avascular tumours beyond 2–3 mm^3. This is the most common angiogenic switch mechanism, and occurs in 95% of human cancers.[15] It is mediated by an increase in angiostimulators released by tumour cells

- Co-option of existing vessels, whereby tumours at their periphery grow towards, and then infiltrate, existing vessels,[18] thus forming hybrids of tumour and endothelial cells. The central part of the tumour undergoes necrosis as new vessels surround, and induce regression of, pre-existing vessels by secretion of angiopoietin-2. This causes local hypoxic conditions, and hence stimulation of gene expression (for example VEGF) via hypoxia-mediated pathways, resulting in new vessel formation at the tumour periphery

- New vessel formation from circulating haemopoietic progenitor cells (for example, CD4$^+$ endothelial cell precursors)

- Vascular mimicry, the theory which suggests that new vessels are formed from tumour cells rather than endothelia

hypoxia, and acidosis, as well as altered gene expression by tumour and host cells, such as the loss of the tumour suppressor gene p53.[9] Specific mechanisms suggested to explain the onset of the angiogenic switch are shown in Table 2.[17]

Once the angiogenic switch has occurred, tumours grow exponentially. This is due, in part, to a reduced apoptotic rate and the symbiotic relationship that exists between tumour and endothelial cells. Angiogenic factors secreted by tumour cells result in an increase in the number of local blood vessels, the endothelia of which, in turn, secrete paracrines that increase tumour growth.[19]

STAGES OF THE ANGIOGENIC CASCADE

Angiogenic factors produced by tumour and host cells diffuse to nearby existing vessels (venules and capillaries), and bind to endothelial receptors. This stimulates signal transduction pathways, resulting in endothelial activation and anti-apoptotic molecule expression (*e.g.* BCl-2 and survivin), an effect mediated primarily by VEGF and bFGF.[20,21]

It has been suggested that the proliferation of activated endothelial cells leads to the formation of 'mother' vessels which are 3–4 times larger in cross-sectional area than the progenitor vessel.[22] The mother vessels have a thinner lining of endothelium and pericytes, and exhibit basement membrane degradation. They are also more permeable, as they form vesicle–vacuolar organelles under the influence of VEGF, which are an interconnected network of cytoplasmic vesicles and vacuoles.[23] The mother vessels only last a few days and then change morphology (Table 3).

The sprouting of angiogenic microvessels is the characteristic feature of tumour angiogenesis, and initially involves basement membrane degradation around the mother vessel by the action of proteases such as MMPs and plasminogen activator.[24] These are released mainly by pericytes. VEGF and angiopoietin-2 then destabilise the endothelial lining of the mother vessel and allow sprouting and migration of activated endothelia away from the mother vessel through the degraded basement membrane.[25] The endothelial cells move along a fibrin skeleton of extracellular matrix towards the source of the

Table 3 New characteristics which develop in 'mother' vessels after a few days

- Become muscular arteries or veins, whereby they retain a large size and acquire smooth muscle cells and an internal elastica
- Form vascular bridges composed of cytoplasmic projections into the lumen. These divide the main lumen and form daughter vessels or occasionally a disorganised vascular body
- Demonstrate intussusceptive microvascular growth, in which longitudinal invagination of connective tissue pillars divides the lumen into two (termed 'non-sprouting' angiogenesis)
- Exhibit sprouting of angiogenic microvessels

stimulus, facilitated by the autocrine release of adhesion molecules (for example, $\alpha v_1\beta_3$ and $\alpha v_1\beta_5$ integrins). The tips of the growing vessels secrete MMPs that enable further invasion of the extracellular matrix. Aligned cords of cells are thus formed due to interactions between endothelial cell surface proteins (*e.g.* PECAM-1, galectin-2) and the extracellular matrix.[26,27] These cords become lined by a second population of endothelia that cause remodelling and hence lumen formation. These vascular tubes differentiate into vascular loops, and represent the arterial and venous ends of the neovasculature. The new vessels formed are leaky as they have an incomplete basement membrane, and so are stabilised by recruitment of smooth muscle cells and pericytes via cytokines such as PDGF.[28] Endothelial cell and pericyte contact has been shown to release the angio-inhibitor transforming growth factor–β (TGF–β),[29] suggesting an autoregulatory feedback loop whereby vascular stabilisation inhibits further angiogenesis. The stages of new vessel formation are depicted in Figure 1.

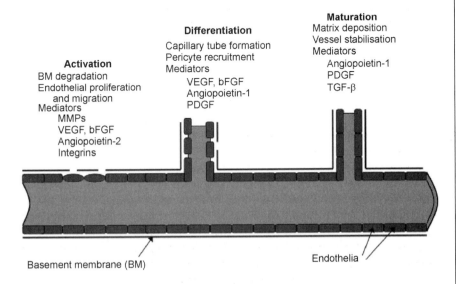

Maturation
Matrix deposition
Vessel stabilisation
Mediators
  Angiopoietin-1
  PDGF
  TGF-β

Differentiation
Capillary tube formation
Pericyte recruitment
Mediators
  VEGF, bFGF
  Angiopoietin-1
  PDGF

Activation
BM degradation
Endothelial proliferation
  and migration
Mediators
  MMPs
  VEGF, bFGF
  Angiopoietin-2
  Integrins

Basement membrane (BM)

Endothelia

Fig. 1 The stages of neovascularisation.

ASSESSMENT OF ANGIOGENESIS

There has been considerable interest in methods to measure the angiogenic potential of a tumour, in order to predict prognosis, monitor the tumour burden, and assess the response to anti-angiogenic therapy.

Tumour angiogenesis can be assessed by direct and indirect methods.[64] Direct methods assess angiogenic mediators in actual tumour samples. This is limited by the need for repeated invasive procedures to obtain tumour biopsies, and would be impractical for the large number of patients needed for clinical trials of anti-angiogenic therapy.

Indirect methods have been suggested, therefore, that do not require tumour tissue, and measure surrogate markers of tumour angiogenesis. These include circulating angiogenic mediator levels, and radiological imaging techniques to obtain estimates of the tumour vasculature.

The direct methods have traditionally been considered the gold standard for angiogenesis assessment. Immunohistochemical staining of tumour sections for endothelial markers has been extensively used to derive microvessel density (MVD) scores. This reflects the number of vessels present within the tumour, but does not provide data on the functional status of the vasculature.[65] In other words, it provides no indication on vessel perfusion, or the angiogenic activity of the vasculature.

The measurement of surrogate angiogenic markers present within body fluids has not been validated in the assessment of angiogenesis, hence this approach is not established in clinical practice.[3] There has been considerable interest in a number of imaging modalities as indirect methods of angiogenic assessment. These have the advantage of being non-invasive and can be repeated on multiple occasions in order to monitor disease progression and the response to anti-angiogenic therapy. The drive to modify standard imaging techniques for the assessment of angiogenesis stems from the need to use widely-available methods and the requirement to continue standard oncological imaging, for example, measurement of tumour size.

Conventional angiography is too insensitive for accurate visualisation of tumour microvessels,[3] and so other imaging techniques have been investigated. Ultrasonography is non-ionising, and has been used to measure tumour blood flow and volume, as well as deriving a vascularity index.[66] Vessel diameter resolutions of 200 μm have been reported,[67] and this can be increased by the ultrasonic destruction of microbubbles.[3] The technique is limited by the inability to image tumours in inaccessible sites, such as the lungs and brain, as well as the operator dependency.

The principle of computed tomography (CT) and magnetic resonance imaging (MRI) in angiogenesis assessment involves observation of changes in tissue enhancement following intravascular contrast administration, with quantification of tumour vascular estimates derived by mathematical modelling of the enhancement patterns. CT has good spatial resolution, and has been used to provide estimates of tumour blood flow and volume, mean contrast transit time across the vascular bed, and capillary permeability.[68] Observation of changes in tissue enhancement is limited to only a few representative tumour slices,[69] but has the advantage over MRI in that the spatial resolution is maintained even at high data acquisition rates, making it valuable for imaging of liver lesions.[70]

MRI also has excellent spatial resolution, and is non-ionising, thereby allowing repeated imaging without biological effects. It has been used to derive similar vascular estimates as for CT, but it is possible to image simultaneously a greater tumour volume. In an attempt to validate the technique, MRI has been correlated against MVD scores and other histological angiogenic measurements in several tumour types.[71] It has also been investigated as a tool to monitor the efficacy of anti-angiogenic therapy, and has been shown to detect decreases in vascular permeability in a mouse model of breast cancer following treatment with anti-VEGF monoclonal antibody.[72]

Nuclear medicine techniques have also been investigated as angiogenic imaging modalities.[73] Positron emission tomography (PET) and single photon emission computed tomography (SPECT) using radiolabelled tracers have both been used to evaluate tumour metabolism, as well as providing estimates of blood flow and volume. In particular, PET imaging appears promising for the measurement of tumour tissue perfusion and hypoxia.[74,75]

Future directions for angiogenic imaging may involve targeting the contrast agent against components of the angiogenic cascade, or visualisation techniques that are based on the infrared signatures of tumour vessels.[3] There is a continued need for validation of the imaging modalities against the current gold standards of angiogenic assessment, and a requirement for a consensus agreement regarding the most appropriate imaging method, so that it can be validated and subsequently used to dictate therapeutic strategy.

Key points 4 & 5

- Direct assessment of angiogenesis uses tissue samples to measure microvessel density by immunohistochemistry.

- Indirect assessment of angiogenesis can be achieved using magnetic resonance imaging, contrast computed tomography, positron emission tomography scanning or single photon emission computed tomography.

ANTI-ANGIOGENIC THERAPY

There has been considerable interest and research in the field of anti-angiogenic therapy recently, and a wide range of agents have been devised that target one or more steps of the angiogenic process.[3] Most therapies inhibit tumour growth rather than induce regression,[2] and the aims of treatment are to hold tumours as dormant cell clusters, as well as to make tumours more susceptible to attack by immunological and chemotherapeutic processes.

Standard chemotherapy agents have been shown to have anti-angiogenic properties when given at a dose lower than that used for tumour cell killing.[30] This has been seen with cyclophosphamide and doxorubicin,[30,31] and frequent or continuous low-dose scheduling appeared to enhance the anti-angiogenic effect.[30] Other standard agents, such as the cyclooxygenase inhibitors, have also been shown to have anti-angiogenic properties,[30] probably through the inhibition of prostaglandin synthesis.

Key point 6

- Anti-angiogenic therapy may be utilised for supplementing standard oncological treatment with chemotherapy and radiotherapy.

There are several classifications of anti-angiogenic therapies. They can be considered **direct** agents if they specifically inhibit endothelial cell proliferation, or **indirect** agents if they affect the availability of the angiogenic mediators by altering the tumour micro-environment.[4] Another system of classification defines the agents as: (i) **true angiogenic inhibitors**, which halt vessel sprouting but have no effect on established vessels; (ii) **vascular targeting agents**, that target pre-existing vessels and result in tumour necrosis; and (iii) **non-selective anti-angiogenic agents**, which exert a range of effects on a number of cell types, not just tumour vessel endothelia.[3] In addition, specific therapies can be considered on the basis on their target cells or molecules. These include growth factor antagonists (*e.g.* anti-VEGF monoclonal antibodies), endothelial cell signal transduction and proliferation inhibitors, and inhibitors of extracellular matrix invasion (*e.g.* MMP antagonists). Table 4 lists some of the recently reported clinical trials of angiogenesis inhibitors. For a review of the current status of anti-angiogenic therapies, see Zhang *et al.*[32]

Key point 7

- Anti-angiogenic therapy may be direct (agents which inhibit endothelial cell proliferation) or indirect (agents which alter the tumour micro-environment and affect availability of angiogenic mediators).

Optimal agent selection as well as the best dosing schedule and timing of administration of these agents have yet to be determined. Combinations of anti-angiogenic agents, each with a different mechanism of action, may be synergistic;[33] similarly, combining anti-angiogenic agents with standard chemotherapy[34] and radiotherapy[35] regimens may be beneficial. Further clinical studies are needed to optimise patient selection for anti-angiogenic therapies, and determine their contribution alongside standard treatment modalities.

Limitations of anti-angiogenic therapy stem from the knowledge that inhibition of a single agent is unlikely to affect the complex interaction of multiple factors that characterises the angiogenic process. It may be that the anti-angiogenic therapy can be tailored to the individual patient by measuring the predominant angiogenic mediators in tumour and blood samples taken at various stages of the disease, and then targeting these mediators with the appropriate therapy. This technique has been termed angiogenic profiling and may provide a customised treatment approach for individual patients.

Table 4 Recently reported clinical trials of angiogenesis inhibitors

Agent	Mechanism	Trial	Developer
Direct inhibitors of endothelial cells/receptors			
Thalidomide	Decrease, TNF-α, bFGF, VEGF	Phase II ovarian cancer, hepatocellular carcinoma, advanced melanoma, breast and colorectal cancers; phase III NSCLC, non-metastatic prostate, renal cancer	Celgene, NJ, USA
SU6668	Blocks VEGF-R2, FGF-R, PDGF-R	Phase I advanced solid tumours	Sugen, CA, USA
Squalamine	Inhibits sodium–hydrogen exchanger (NHE3)	Phase I advanced cancers; phase II NSCLC, ovarian, brain	Genaera Corp., PA, USA
ZD1839	Inhibits EGF-R	Phase II advanced breast, renal, brain; phase III NSCLC	AstraZeneca, London, UK
Erbitux (C225)	EGF-R monoclonal antibody	Phase II advanced renal, pancreatic, colorectal; phase II/III advanced solid tumours	ImClone, NY, USA
IMC-1C11	Inhibits VEGF-R2	Phase I metastatic colorectal	ImClone, NY, USA
Angiozyme	Inhibits VEGF-R2 and VEGF-R1	Phase II breast and colorectal cancer	Ribozyme Pharma-ceuticals, CO, USA
Endostatin	Glypicans, tropomyosin, $\alpha v_1 \beta_3$ integrin, MMP	Phase II neuroendocrine tumours and metastatic melanoma	EntreMed, MD, USA
Angiostatin	ATP synthase, angiomotin, $\alpha v_1 \beta_3$	Phase I advanced tumours	EntreMed, MD, USA
Indirect agents			
Bevacizumab	VEGF monoclonal antibody	Phase II prostate, renal, acute myeloid leukaemia; phase II/III NSCLC; phase III breast, advanced colorectal	Genentech, CA, USA
BMS-275291	Synthetic MMP inhibitor	Phase II breast; phase II/III advanced NSCLC	Bristol-Myers Squibb, NY, USA
COL-3	Inhibits MMP-2 and MMP-9	Phase I advanced solid tumours; phase I/II brain, Kaposi's sarcoma	CollaGenex, PA, USA
Vitaxin	Integrin $\alpha v_1 \beta_3$ monoclonal antibody	Phase I/II in irinotecan-refractory advanced colorectal cancer	MedImmune MD, USA
EMD121974	Small molecule blocker of integrin $\alpha v_1 \beta_3$	Phase I HIV-related Kaposi's sarcoma, phase III recurrent anaplastic glioma	Merck KGaA, Darmstadt, Germany
Non-specific agents			
Interferon α-2a	Decrease bFGF, VEGF	Phase II penile, advanced renal, breast, cervical cancers; phase III advanced ovarian, and with chemotherapy for advanced colorectal cancer	Commercially available
Celecoxib	COX-2 inhibitor	Phase I prostate; phase I/II cervical; phase II metastatic breast	Pharmacia, NJ, USA
IL-12	Up-regulation of interferon γ and IL-10	Phase I TCC bladder, melanoma; phase II advanced renal and cervical cancers	Genetics Institute, MA, USA
CAI	Inhibitor of calcium influx	Phase I refractory solid tumours; phase II advanced ovarian and renal cancers	National Cancer Institute, USA

Adapted from Scappaticci.[17] NSCLC, non small cell lung cancer.

A further limitation of anti-angiogenic therapy is that, for any specific agent, theoretical *in vitro* anti-angiogenic activity may not translate into overt clinical benefit.[17] In addition, a balance of pro- and anti-angiogenic properties is needed to limit the toxic effects of physiological angiogenesis inhibition in situations such as wound healing and ovulation.[36] An exacerbation of myocardial and cerebral ischaemia has been reported during anti-angiogenic therapy,[37] and haemorrhage secondary to endothelial cell disruption is a concern.[38] It has also been suggested the end-points for assessment of treatment success need to be redefined,[17] in that a diminution in tumour volume is unlikely with most anti-angiogenic therapies, and so would be deemed a failure with current treatment scoring systems.

PRO-ANGIOGENIC THERAPY IN BENIGN DISEASE

Promotion of angiogenesis may actually be therapeutically desirable in ischaemic conditions such as coronary and peripheral artery disease. Recently, there has been considerable interest in gene therapy techniques aimed at increasing the concentration of angiogenic mediators such as VEGF and FGF in ischaemic tissues, in order to augment new vessel formation in response to ischaemia.[39] In contrast, the inhibition of deleterious genes has been investigated in vasoproliferative disorders, such as those occurring after vascular bypass procedures leading to restenosis and graft failure.[40]

A viral or plasmid vector containing the target gene is administered to the region of interest, either by intravascular infusion or intramuscular injection, and the vector DNA encoding the gene becomes incorporated into the host tissue DNA. An alternative approach is to deliver recombinant protein directly to the ischaemic tissue. However, prolonged administration of high concentration protein is needed to ensure adequate tissue uptake, thereby increasing the likelihood of adverse effects.[39]

It has been suggested that promotion of angiogenesis may also be beneficial in some plastic surgical procedures.[41] Flap viability has been shown to improve following VEGF[42,43] and angiopoietin-1[44] gene therapy in animal models, and tissue expansion techniques may be facilitated by pro-angiogenic therapy, as VEGF is up-regulated in expanded skin when compared with native skin.[45]

Safety concerns regarding pro-angiogenic therapy have been raised.[46] From the preceding sections, it is clear that angiostimulators are important mediators of neoplastic progression and metastasis. Non-specific vascular stimulation may result in conditions such as angiomas and diabetic retinopathy.[47] Infection resulting from administration of an adenoviral vector has been related to the death of a patient.[48] In addition, local effects of VEGF administration have been documented, such as increased vascular permeability leading to oedema following intramuscular injection.[46] Controlled clinical trials are being conducted into the efficacy of gene therapy techniques for ischaemic heart and brain diseases as well as peripheral vascular disease (for recent reviews, see Diaz-Sandoval *et al.*[49] and Saitoh *et al.*[50]). The area appears promising although more work is needed before such an approach becomes incorporated into the routine clinical armamentarium.

SURGERY AND THE ANGIOGENIC CASCADE

Healing surgical wounds are perfect environments for tumour growth and metastases.[51] A colonic anastomosis or laparotomy wound is a thousand times more likely to develop a metastatic deposit from circulating tumour cells than normal tissue.[4] This is because the physiological angiogenesis evident in surgical wounds creates suitable conditions for implantation and subsequent proliferation of circulating cancer cells, thereby increasing the likelihood of local tumour recurrence.[52]

In addition, primary tumours may inhibit the growth of metastases through the actions of the anti-angiogenic mediators angiostatin and endostatin,[53] which act to keep a metastatic cell cluster in a state of dormancy. Subsequent resection of the primary tumour may, therefore, favour metastatic growth by creating a pro-angiogenic environment. This has been demonstrated in renal cell carcinomas, as well as melanoma and breast cancers.[54] Similarly, accelerated growth of metastatic deposits in the residual liver has been reported following resection of colorectal metastases.[55] The regeneration following liver resection is associated with an increase in local growth factor production as part of the healing response to tissue injury.[56] This includes a range of pro-angiogenic mediators, such as VEGF which is thought to have a role in the reconstruction of the sinusoids.[57] A similar increase in VEGF levels has been seen following major gastrointestinal and lung surgery.[58,59] It may be, therefore, that as well as a reduction in angio-inhibitor levels, the pro-angiogenic effects of surgery also have a role in the metastatic progression seen following primary tumour resection.[54]

For patients undergoing major surgery, there appears to be a theoretical balance between the beneficial aspects of angiogenesis in terms of wound healing, and the concurrent detrimental facilitation of tumour progression secondary to angiogenic promotion. This latter concern might suggest the need for adjuvant anti-angiogenic therapy during cancer surgery, administered intra- or peri-operatively. However, this raises the possibility of impaired

---

Key points 8–12

- Anti-angiogenic treatment is synergistic to chemotherapy and radiotherapy.

- Angiogenic profiling may provide a customised treatment approach for individual patients.

- Anti-angiogenic treatment does not affect skin wound healing in animal models but may affect anastamotic healing in the colon .Further studies are awaited.

- Anti-angiogenic treatments have a potential to exacerbate myocardial and cerebral ischaemia.

- Pro-angiogenic therapy has a role in treatment of ischaemic diseases but potentially carries a risk of stimulating neoplasia, angioma formation and diabetic retinopathy.

wound healing as a result of suppression of physiological angiogenesis. Animal studies suggest that treatment with anti-angiogenic agents does not have a significant impact on the efficacy of cutaneous wound healing, although it is difficult to draw firm conclusions as human data are lacking.[54] The impact on intestinal anastamotic healing, however, is less clear. Angiogenesis plays a vital role in the healing of colonic anastomosis,[60] and treatment with anti-angiogenic agents has been shown to have a significant impact on anastamotic healing in animal studies.[61] This was not seen after treatment with the angio-inhibitor tamoxifen,[62] however, and inhibitors of MMPs were found to be associated with enhanced colonic anastomotic breaking strength.[63] These findings suggest the need for clinical studies involving human subjects to investigate the matter further.

CONCLUSIONS

Angiogenesis is an important aspect of tumour biology. There is an ever-increasing depth of knowledge and understanding of the angiogenic process, and how it relates to the many physiological and pathological conditions presenting to clinicians. Anti-angiogenic therapy in particular is being widely investigated, with the hope of incorporating it into the standard oncological repertoire. Surgeons need to be aware of these angiogenic mechanisms, in order to permit comprehension of many of the disease processes encountered in surgical practice, as well as understanding the effects of anti-angiogenic therapies on patients undergoing surgery.

Key points for clinical practice

- Angiogenesis is a fundamental process important for tissue growth and survival.

- Normally a balance between pro- and anti-angiogenic mediators prevents neo-angiogenesis.

- Angiogenesis is an end result of interaction between several different mediators.

- Direct assessment of angiogenesis uses tissue samples to measure microvessel density by immunohistochemistry.

- Indirect assessment of angiogenesis can be achieved using magnetic resonance imaging, contrast computed tomography, positron emission tomography scanning or single photon emission computed tomography.

- Anti-angiogenic therapy may be utilised for supplementing standard oncological treatment with chemotherapy and radiotherapy.

- Anti-angiogenic therapy may be direct (agents which inhibit endo-thelial cell proliferation) or indirect (agents which alter the tumour micro-environment and affect availability of angiogenic mediators).

Key points for clinical practice (continued)

- Anti-angiogenic treatment is synergistic to chemotherapy and radiotherapy.

- Angiogenic profiling may provide a customised treatment approach for individual patients.

- Anti-angiogenic treatment does not affect skin wound healing in animal models but may affect anastamotic healing in the colon .Further studies are awaited.

- Anti-angiogenic treatments have a potential to exacerbate myocardial and cerebral ischaemia.

- Pro-angiogenic therapy has a role in treatment of ischaemic diseases but potentially carries a risk of stimulating neoplasia, angioma formation and diabetic retinopathy.

References

1. Noden DM, Embryonic origins and assembly of blood vessels. *Am Rev Respir Dis* 1989; **140**: 1097–1103.
2. Ellis LM, Liu W, Ahmad SA *et al*. Overview of angiogenesis: biologic implications for antiangiogenic therapy. *Semin Oncol* 2001; **28 (Suppl 16)**: 94–104.
3. Li WW. Tumor angiogenesis: molecular pathology, therapeutic targeting, and imaging. *Acad Radiol* 2000; **7**: 800–811.
4. McNamara DA, Harmey JH, Walsh TN, Redmond HP, Bouchier-Hayes DJ *et al*. Significance of angiogenesis in cancer therapy. *Br J Surg* 1998; **85**: 1044–1055.
5. Tischer E, Mitchell R, Hartman T *et al*. The human gene for vascular endothelial growth factor. Multiple protein forms are encoded through alternative exon splicing. *J Biol Chem* 1991; **266**: 11947–11954.
6. Boedefeld 2nd WM, Bland KI, Heslin MJ. Recent insights into angiogenesis, apoptosis, invasion, and metastasis in colorectal carcinoma. *Ann Surg Oncol* 2003; **10**: 839–851.
7. Ferrara N. The role of vascular endothelial growth factor in pathological angiogenesis. *Breast Cancer Res Treat* 1995; **36**: 127–137.
8. Bikfalvi A, Bicknell R. Recent advances in angiogenesis, anti-angiogenesis and vascular targeting. *Trends Pharmacol Sci* 2002; **23**: 576–582.
9. Poon RT, Fan ST, Wong J. Clinical significance of angiogenesis in gastrointestinal cancers: a target for novel prognostic and therapeutic approaches. *Ann Surg* 2003; **238**: 9–28.
10. Bagnato A, Natali PG. Endothelin receptors as novel targets in tumor therapy. *J Translat Med* 2004; **2**: 16.
11. Folkman J. Tumor angiogenesis: therapeutic implications. *N Engl J Med* 1971; **285**: 1182–1186.
12. Folkman J. What is the evidence that tumors are angiogenesis dependent? *J Natl Cancer Inst* 1990; **82**: 4–6.
13. Lyden D, Hattori K, Dias S *et al*. Impaired recruitment of bone-marrow-derived endothelial and hematopoietic precursor cells blocks tumor angiogenesis and growth. *Nat Med* 2001; **7**: 1194–1201.
14. Hanahan D, Folkman J. Patterns and emerging mechanisms of the angiogenic switch during tumorigenesis. *Cell* 1996; **86**: 353–364.
15. Hanahan D, Christofori G, Naik P, Arbeit J *et al*. Transgenic mouse models of tumour angiogenesis: the angiogenic switch, its molecular controls, and prospects for preclinical therapeutic models. *Eur J Cancer* 1996; **32A**: 2386–2393.
16. Smith-McCune KK, Weidner N. Demonstration and characterization of the angiogenic properties of cervical dysplasia. *Cancer Res* 1994; **54**: 800–804.

17. Scappaticci FA. Mechanisms and future directions for angiogenesis-based cancer therapies. *J Clin Oncol* 2002; **20**: 3906–3927.

18. Holash J, Maisonpierre PC, Compton D *et al.* Vessel cooption, regression, and growth in tumors mediated by angiopoietins and VEGF. *Science* 1999; **284**: 1994–1998.

19. Rak J, Filmus J, Kerbel RS. Reciprocal paracrine interactions between tumour cells and endothelial cells: the 'angiogenesis progression' hypothesis. *Eur J Cancer* 1996; **32A**: 2438–2450.

20. Nor JE, Christensen J, Mooney DJ, Polverini PJ. Vascular endothelial growth factor (VEGF)-mediated angiogenesis is associated with enhanced endothelial cell survival and induction of Bcl-2 expression. *Am J Pathol* 1999; **154**: 375–384.

21. O'Connor DS, Schechner JS, Adida C *et al.* Control of apoptosis during angiogenesis by survivin expression in endothelial cells. *Am J Pathol* 2000; **156**: 393–398.

22. Paku S, Paweletz N. First steps of tumor-related angiogenesis. *Lab Invest* 1991; **65**: 334–346.

23. Pettersson A, Nagy JA, Brown LF *et al.* Heterogeneity of the angiogenic response induced in different normal adult tissues by vascular permeability factor/vascular endothelial growth factor. *Lab Invest* 2000; **80**: 99–115.

24. Pepper MS, Ferrara N, Orci L, Montesano R. Vascular endothelial growth factor (VEGF) induces plasminogen activators and plasminogen activator inhibitor-1 in microvascular endothelial cells. *Biochem Biophys Res Commun* 1991; **181**: 902–906.

25. Zetter BR. Migration of capillary endothelial cells is stimulated by tumour-derived factors. *Nature* 1980; **285**: 41–43.

26. Yang S, Graham J, Kahn JW, Schwartz EA, Gerritsen ME. Functional roles for PECAM-1 (CD31) and VE-cadherin (CD144) in tube assembly and lumen formation in three-dimensional collagen gels. *Am J Pathol* 1999; **155**: 887–895.

27. Nangia-Makker P, Honjo Y, Sarvis R *et al.* Galectin-3 induces endothelial cell morphogenesis and angiogenesis. *Am J Pathol* 2000; **156**: 899–909.

28. Darland DC, D'Amore PA. Blood vessel maturation: vascular development comes of age. *J Clin Invest* 1999; **103**: 157–158.

29. Antonelli-Orlidge A, Saunders KB, Smith SR, D'Amore PA. An activated form of transforming growth factor beta is produced by cocultures of endothelial cells and pericytes. *Proc Natl Acad Sci USA* 1989; **86**: 4544–4548.

30. Miller KD, Sweeney CJ, Sledge Jr GW. Redefining the target: chemotherapeutics as antiangiogenics. *J Clin Oncol* 2001; **19**: 1195–1206.

31. Benbow U, Maitra R, Hamilton JW, Brinckerhoff CE. Selective modulation of collagenase 1 gene expression by the chemotherapeutic agent doxorubicin. *Clin Cancer Res* 1999; **5**: 203–208.

32. Zhang HT, Bicknell R. Therapeutic inhibition of angiogenesis. *Mol Biotechnol* 2003; **25**: 185–200.

33. Scappaticci FA, Smith R, Pathak A *et al.* Combination angiostatin and endostatin gene transfer induces synergistic antiangiogenic activity *in vitro* and antitumor efficacy in leukemia and solid tumors in mice. *Mol Ther* 2001; **3**: 186–196.

34. Sweeney CJ, Miller KD, Sissons SE *et al.* The antiangiogenic property of docetaxel is synergistic with a recombinant humanized monoclonal antibody against vascular endothelial growth factor or 2-methoxyestradiol but antagonized by endothelial growth factors. *Cancer Res* 2001; **61**: 3369–3372.

35. Mauceri HJ, Hanna NN, Beckett MA *et al.* Combined effects of angiostatin and ionizing radiation in antitumour therapy. *Nature* 1998; **394**: 287–291.

36. Bloch W, Huggel K, Sasaki T *et al.* The angiogenesis inhibitor endostatin impairs blood vessel maturation during wound healing. *FASEB J* 2000; **14**: 2373–2376.

37. Kuenen BC, Rosen L, Smit EF *et al.* Dose-finding and pharmacokinetic study of cisplatin, gemcitabine, and SU5416 in patients with solid tumors. *J Clin Oncol* 2002; **20**: 1657–1667.

38. Margolin K, Gordon MS, Holmgren E *et al.* Phase Ib trial of intravenous recombinant humanized monoclonal antibody to vascular endothelial growth factor in combination with chemotherapy in patients with advanced cancer: pharmacologic and long-term safety data. *J Clin Oncol* 2001; **19**: 851–856.

39. Freedman SB, Isner JM Therapeutic angiogenesis for coronary artery disease. *Ann Intern Med* 2002; **136**: 54–71.

40. Mann MJ, Whittemore AD, Donaldson MC *et al. Ex-vivo* gene therapy of human vascular

bypass grafts with E2F decoy: the PREVENT single-centre, randomised, controlled trial. *Lancet* 1999; **354**: 1493–1498.

41. Taub PJ, Silver L, Weinberg H. Plastic surgical perspectives on vascular endothelial growth factor as gene therapy for angiogenesis. *Plast Reconstr Surg* 2000; **105**: 1034–1042.

42. Padubidri A, Browne Jr E. Effect of vascular endothelial growth factor (VEGF) on survival of random extension of axial pattern skin flaps in the rat. *Ann Plast Surg* 1996; **37**: 604–611.

43. Taub PJ, Marmur JD, Zhang WX *et al.* Locally administered vascular endothelial growth factor cDNA increases survival of ischemic experimental skin flaps. *Plast Reconstr Surg* 1998; **102**: 2033–2039.

44. Jung H, Gurunluoglu R, Scharpf J, Siemionow M. Adenovirus-mediated angiopoietin-1 gene therapy enhances skin flap survival. *Microsurgery* 2003; **23**: 374–380.

45. Lantieri LA, Martin-Garcia N, Wechsler J, Mitrofanoff M, Raulo Y, Baruch JP. Vascular endothelial growth factor expression in expanded tissue: a possible mechanism of angiogenesis in tissue expansion. *Plast Reconstr Surg* 1998; **101**: 392–398.

46. Epstein SE, Kornowski R, Fuchs S, Dvorak HF. Angiogenesis therapy: amidst the hype, the neglected potential for serious side effects. *Circulation* 2001; **104**: 115–119.

47. Freedman SB. Clinical trials of gene therapy for atherosclerotic cardiovascular disease. *Curr Opin Lipidol* 2002; **13**: 653–661.

48. Ferber D. Gene therapy. Safer and virus-free? *Science* 2001; **294**: 1638–1642.

49. Diaz-Sandoval LJ, Losordo DW. Gene therapy for cardiovascular angiogenesis. *Expert Opin Biol Ther* 2003; **3**: 599–616.

50. Saitoh Y, Kato A, Hagihara Y, Kaneda Y, Yoshimine T. Gene therapy for ischemic brain diseases. *Curr Gene Ther* 2003; **3**: 49–58.

51. Murthy MS, Scanlon EF, Silverman RH, Goodheart CR, Goldschmidt RA, Jelachich ML. The role of fibronectin in tumor implantation at surgical sites. *Clin Exp Metastasis* 1993; **11**: 159–173.

52. Hofer SO, Molema G, Hermens RA, Wanebo HJ, Reichner JS, Hoekstra HJ. The effect of surgical wounding on tumour development. *Eur J Surg Oncol* 1999; **25**: 231–243.

53. O'Reilly MS, Holmgren L, Chen C, Folkman J. Angiostatin induces and sustains dormancy of human primary tumors in mice. *Nat Med* 1996; **2**: 689–692.

54. van der Bilt JD, Borel Rinkes IH. Surgery and angiogenesis. *Biochim Biophys Acta* 2004; **1654**: 95–104.

55. Picardo A, Karpoff HM, Ng B, Lee J, Brennan MF, Fong Y. Partial hepatectomy accelerates local tumor growth: potential roles of local cytokine activation. *Surgery* 1998; **124**: 57–64.

56. Court FG, Wemyss-Holden SA, Dennison AR, Maddern GJ. The mystery of liver regeneration. *Br J Surg* 2002; **89**: 1089–1095.

57. Mochida S, Ishikawa K, Toshima K *et al.* The mechanisms of hepatic sinusoidal endothelial cell regeneration: a possible communication system associated with vascular endothelial growth factor in liver cells. *J Gastroenterol Hepatol* 1998; **13 (Suppl)**: S1–S5.

58. Ikeda M, Furukawa H, Imamura H *et al.* Surgery for gastric cancer increases plasma levels of vascular endothelial growth factor and von Willebrand factor. *Gastric Cancer* 2002; **5**: 137–141.

59. Maniwa Y, Okada M, Ishii N, Kiyooka K. Vascular endothelial growth factor increased by pulmonary surgery accelerates the growth of micrometastases in metastatic lung cancer. *Chest* 1998; **114**: 1668–1675.

60. Thornton FJ, Barbul A. Healing in the gastrointestinal tract. *Surg Clin North Am* 1997; **77**: 549–573.

61. Hendriks JM, Hubens G, Wuyts FL, Vermeulen P, Hubens A, Eyskens E. Experimental study of intraperitoneal suramin on the healing of colonic anastomoses. *Br J Surg* 1999; **86**: 1171–1175.

62. McNamara DA, Walsh TN, Kay E, Bouchier-Hayes DJ. Neoadjuvant antiangiogenic therapy with tamoxifen does not impair gastrointestinal anastomotic repair in the rat. *Colorect Dis* 2003; **5**: 335–341.

63. Syk I, Agren MS, Adawi D, Jeppsson B. Inhibition of matrix metalloproteinases enhances breaking strength of colonic anastomoses in an experimental model. *Br J Surg* 2001; **88**: 228–234.

64. George ML, Dzik-Jurasz AS, Padhani AR *et al*. Non-invasive methods of assessing angiogenesis and their value in predicting response to treatment in colorectal cancer. *Br J Surg* 2001; **88**: 1628–1636.

65. Eberhard A, Kahlert S, Goede V, Hemmerlein B, Plate KH, Augustin HG. Heterogeneity of angiogenesis and blood vessel maturation in human tumors: implications for antiangiogenic tumor therapies. *Cancer Res* 2000; **60**: 1388–1393.

66. Cheng WF, Lee CN, Chu JS *et al*. Vascularity index as a novel parameter for the *in vivo* assessment of angiogenesis in patients with cervical carcinoma. *Cancer* 1999; **85**: 651–657.

67. Ferrara KW, Merritt CR, Burns PN, Foster FS, Mattrey RF, Wickline SA. Evaluation of tumor angiogenesis with US: imaging, Doppler, and contrast agents. *Acad Radiol* 2000; **7**: 824–839.

68. Miles KA, Charnsangavej C, Lee FT, Fishman EK, Horton K, Lee TY. Application of CT in the investigation of angiogenesis in oncology. *Acad Radiol* 2000; **7**: 840–850.

69. Padhani AR, Husband JE. Dynamic contrast-enhanced MRI studies in oncology with an emphasis on quantification, validation and human studies. *Clin Radiol* 2001; **56**: 607–620.

70. Miles KA, Leggett DA, Kelley BB, Hayball MP, Sinnatamby R, Bunce I. *In vivo* assessment of neovascularization of liver metastases using perfusion CT. *Br J Radiol* 1998; **71**: 276–281.

71. Mayr NA, Hawighorst H, Yuh WT, Essig M, Magnotta VA, Knopp MV *et al*. MR microcirculation assessment in cervical cancer: correlations with histomorphological tumor markers and clinical outcome. *J Magn Reson Imaging* 1999; **10**: 267–276.

72. Pham CD, Roberts TP, van Bruggen N *et al*. Magnetic resonance imaging detects suppression of tumor vascular permeability after administration of antibody to vascular endothelial growth factor. *Cancer Invest* 1998; **16**: 225–230.

73. Blankenberg FG, Eckelman WC, Strauss HW *et al*. Role of radionuclide imaging in trials of antiangiogenic therapy. *Acad Radiol* 2000; **7**: 851–867.

74. Lehtio K, Eskola O, Viljanen T *et al*. Imaging perfusion and hypoxia with PET to predict radiotherapy response in head-and-neck cancer. *Int J Radiat Oncol Biol Phys* 2004; **59**: 971–982.

75. Barthel H, Wilson H, Collingridge DR *et al*. *In vivo* evaluation of [^{18}F]-fluoroetanidazole as a new marker for imaging tumour hypoxia with positron emission tomography. *Br J Cancer* 2004; **90**: 2232–2242.

Abdul-Wahed N. Meshikhes

4

General surgical aspects of sickle cell disease

Sickle cell disease (SCD) is the most common inherited haematological disorder affecting man. The first reported case in the literature was in 1910 by Herrick in a medical student from the West Indies.[1] Mason, however, was the first to use the term 'sickle cell anaemia' in 1922.[2] In 1949, the genetic basis for SCD was demonstrated, in which homogeneity of the sickle cell gene leads to sickle cell anaemia while heterogeneity results in sickle cell trait.[3]

In SCD, the red cells undergo sickling when deoxygenated due to decreased solubility and polymerisation of sickle haemoglobin (haemoglobin-S), thereby increasing the intracellular viscosity and deforming the shape of the red cells. This abnormal haemoglobin molecule results from substitution of the amino acid valine for glutamine at the sixth position from the amino terminus of the β-globin chain. As the susceptibility of red cells to sickle correlates well with the concentration of haemoglobin-S within the red blood cells, the clinical problems of SCD are related to the high level of haemoglobin-S. Factors such as dehydration, infection, acidosis and hypothermia also precipitate vaso-occlusive and sequestration crises that are commonly encountered in SCD.

In highly malarial equatorial Africa, SCD is prevalent and sickle cell mutations were named after the areas where they were first described: the Senegal, Benin, Bantu and Cameroon haplotypes. The sickle cell gene seen in North and South America, the UK, the Caribbean, some Mediterranean countries and the western region of the Arabian Peninsula is also of African origin, mostly of the Benin haplotype. However, in eastern Saudi Arabia, other Gulf States and central India, there is a different sickle cell gene – the Asian haplotype – which is generally associated with α-thalassaemia and high levels of fetal haemoglobin (haemoglobin-F), both are believed to ameliorate the severity of the disease.

Abdul-Wahed N. Meshikhes MBChB FRCSI
Consultant Surgeon and Chairman, Department of Surgical Specialties, King Fahad Specialist Hospital, Dammam, Eastern Province, Saudi Arabia
E-mail: meshikhes@doctor.com

Key points 1 & 2

- Greater population mobility in recent years makes recognition of the disease and its various surgical manifestations of paramount importance in clinical practice.

- The clinical problems of sickle cell disease are related to the high level of sickle haemoglobin (haemoglobin-S).

Although SCD is endemic in certain parts of the world and in ethnic minorities of the inner city areas of the western world, greater population mobility in recent years makes recognition of this disease and its surgical manifestations of paramount importance in clinical surgical practice.[4] Furthermore, as surgery in homozygous individuals is associated with high morbidity and mortality, special multi-disciplinary care is needed in management of patients presenting to various surgical specialties. This chapter highlights some important general surgical aspects of sickle cell disease.

CLINICAL MANIFESTATIONS

The clinical manifestation of SCD is quite variable and includes repeated painful vaso-occlusive, haemolytic, aplastic episodes and sequestration crises. Complications affect various systems mainly skeletal, gastrointestinal, spleen, hepatobiliary, cardiopulmonary and central nervous system (CNS). Moreover, chronic hypoxia may eventually damage the heart and kidneys, producing high output cardiac failure and chronic renal failure. Susceptibility to infections with certain organisms is also common and is attributed to a defect in complement activation, asplenia or autosplenectomy and impaired neutrophil function. Sepsis secondary to infection is the most common precipitating factor for sickle cell crisis and the leading cause of death. Hence, measures to prevent or treat infections constitute an important step in the comprehensive care of SCD.[5] Immunisation against infections to which patients are susceptible complements the benefits of prophylactic antibiotics and are directed against *Pneumococcus* spp., *Meningococcus* spp., *Haemophilus influenzae*, and the hepatitis B and influenza viruses.[5] Affected female patients are susceptible to complications during pregnancy, such as increase in painful crises, gestational hypertension, and preterm birth, which increase the maternal and fetal morbidity and mortality.

Key point 3

- Sepsis secondary to infection is the most common precipitating factor for sickle cell crisis and the leading cause of death.

DIAGNOSIS OF SICKLE CELL DISEASE

Sickle erythrocytes are easily detected in a peripheral blood smear and the diagnosis is confirmed by haemoglobin electrophoresis. A sickle solubility test, which is dependent on the insolubility of deoxygenated haemoglobin-S in a high molarity phosphate buffer can be used to screen for the presence of haemoglobin-S in patients undergoing emergency surgery. However, false positive and negative results may occur. Recently, a new technique adopting a modification of the gel technology used for blood grouping has become available.[6]

SURGERY AND ANAESTHESIA IN SCD

General anaesthesia and surgical trauma add additional risk of complications because of changes in temperature, pH, oxygen tension, and fluid volume. Furthermore, circulatory stasis or suboptimal ventilation during surgery allows haemoglobin-S to polymerise in the capillaries with subsequent ischaemic infarcts in many tissues. Thus, understanding the pathophysiology of SCD can minimise complications from anaesthesia and surgery; the reported morbidity for SCD patients having major operations approaches 40%[7] and, despite standard peri-operative care, children with SCD frequently have serious complications, which can be decreased by prophylactic blood transfusions that are frequently given as part of pre-operative management.[7]

Key point 4

- General anaesthesia and surgical trauma add additional risk of complications.

Patients with SCD are usually admitted 2–3 days before elective surgery. A decision on a pre-operative transfusion regimen is made based on the frequency and severity of sickle cell crises. It has been demonstrated that lowering haemoglobin-S levels to < 35% diminishes the blood viscosity and improves the circulation and thus decreases the morbidity and mortality associated with surgery.[8] Attempts, however, must be made to avoid overtransfusion and appropriate prophylactic antibiotics may be prescribed and administered at the time of premedication. Adequate intravenous hydration must be maintained the night before surgery, and pharmacological thromboprophylaxis is prescribed except for patients receiving pre-operative transfusion in whom there may be troublesome intra-operative bleeding.[9]

Knowledge of the patient's history and the actual haemoglobin-S level helps to estimate the individual peri-operative risks and facilitate safe anaesthesia, and surgery.[5,7,10] Sickle-associated damage to liver, spleen, bones, lung and CNS increases the peri-operative risk and, in such patients, general anaesthesia seems to be better than regional anaesthesia.[5,7] Careful peri-operative monitoring should help avoid factors that trigger vaso-occlusive crises such as hypoxaemia, hypovolaemia, hypothermia, acidosis and overtransfusion, decreasing the incidence of vaso-occlusive and haemolytic crises.[10]

In the postoperative period, nursing in an intensive care unit is rarely needed and all patients should receive oxygen supplementation and intravenous hydration, together with thromboprophylaxis.[7] It cannot be overemphasised that proper peri-operative care helps to minimise postoperative complications in patients undergoing surgery. The two most feared complications are acute chest syndrome (ACS) and vaso-occlusive crisis (VOC). ACS, a phenomenon of pulmonary sequestration, is frequently missed in the postoperative period. The symptoms range from fever and respiratory distress to abdominal discomfort. In the fulminant state, it carries a 25–50% mortality rate in the postoperative patient. The incidence of ACS in paediatric patients undergoing minimally invasive surgery remains high at 10% despite avoidance of known risk factors for development of postoperative complications.[11] Painful VOCs, which require long hospital stays, are often precipitated by the stress of surgery. Poorly controlled postoperative pain also can worsen an impending painful crisis and effective postoperative pain control is, therefore, essential. Non-steroidal anti-inflammatory drugs can be an excellent adjunct to opioids and epidural analgesia can minimise respiratory depression. The use of patient-controlled analgesia devices is effective for improved narcotic delivery. However, treatment of pain is one of the most daunting tasks that requires a comprehensive team strategy.[5] It is unfortunate that successful pain control is often hampered by misperceptions of care providers about the cause of the pain and fear of addiction.[5]

BLOOD TRANSFUSION IN SCD

Although controversial, pre-operative blood transfusion in SCD patients undergoing major surgical procedures remains a key component of the comprehensive management as it reduces the peri-operative risks associated with surgery and anaesthesia.[12] It is also an effective treatment for many serious complications, but should be considered in consultation with a haematologist. Transfusion aims to increase the oxygen carrying capacity of blood by increasing haemoglobin concentration and decreasing the haemoglobin-S level. However, increasing the haemoglobin to over 11 g/dl increases viscosity and thus may cause complications. The exchange transfusion results in little iron gain and decreases the concentration of haemoglobin-S while keeping the blood viscosity unchanged. Therefore, it is implemented when the haemoglobin concentration is high, and simple top-up transfusion is given when the haemoglobin is < 9 g/dl.[12]

Key point 5

- Blood transfusion therapy remains a key component of the comprehensive management as it reduces the peri-operative risks associated with surgery and anaesthesia.

Some authors believe that the low haemoglobin level (6–9 g/dl) is well tolerated, partly because of a low oxygen affinity of haemoglobin-S within the red cells, which causes a marked shift in the oxygen dissociation curve. This explains why SCD patients at their steady low haemoglobin level rarely show classic symptoms of anaemia and may fail to benefit clinically from blood transfusions intended to improve oxygen delivery.[12] Therefore, it is important that patients undergo transfusion only when clearly indicated, such as in ACS, splenic sequestration crisis, and aplastic crisis. Patients with aggressive disease who are undergoing major surgery may also receive pre-operative exchange transfusion. However, steady state anaemia and minor surgery should not be treated with transfusions.[12]

Various pre-operative regimens have been suggested to correct the anaemia, ranging from conservative (correcting the anaemia by simple top-up transfusion irrespective of haemoglobin-S concentration) to more aggressive regimens.[13] The exchange transfusion (an aggressive regimen) aims to reduce haemoglobin-S to < 35%; a level at which the sickle cell crises is unlikely to occur, without a rise in haematocrit or blood viscosity. This is a problem that commonly occurs with simple blood transfusion and is best achieved by using modern cell separators, such as an automated red cell exchange, which is safe and rapid when compared to manual exchange procedures.

Key point 6

- Exchange transfusion is implemented when the haemoglobin-S is high, while simple top-up transfusion is used when the haemoglobin is lower than 9 g/dl.

Recent randomised trials have shown the conservative transfusion regimen to be as effective as an aggressive one in decreasing peri-operative complications in SCD patients and is associated with only half as many transfusion-associated complications.[13–16] Also, comparison of the two regimens has shown no differences in peri-operative complications. In the author's unit, experience with blood transfusion in SCD patients undergoing surgery demonstrated less morbidity in patients receiving exchange transfusion without any transfusion-related complications.[17] Nonetheless, based on randomised trials, the author advocates conservative regimens for patients undergoing minor surgical procedures. Exchange transfusion is reserved for those undergoing major surgery especially in the presence of severe disease, systemic complications or very high haemoglobin-S concentration, otherwise simple transfusion is sufficient.

GENERAL SURGICAL MANIFESTATIONS OF SCD

ABDOMINAL PAIN IN SCD

Abdominal pain is common during sickle cell crises. It represents a diagnostic challenge as it mimics many surgical emergencies. Careful evaluation of each patient, based on history, clinical examination, laboratory and radiological

---

Key point 7

- Abdominal pain in SCD represents a diagnostic challenge as it mimics many surgical emergencies. Careful evaluation of each patient is essential to avoid unnecessary surgical intervention.

Table 1 Differential diagnosis of abdominal pain in sickle cell disease

Splenic causes	
	Acute splenic sequestration crisis
	Splenic infarction
	Splenic abscess
Hepatobiliary causes	
	Biliary colic
	Common bile duct stones/polyp
	Acute cholecystitis
	Hepatic crisis
	Hepatitis
	Liver abscess
Other surgical conditions	
	Acute appendicitis
	Acute pancreatitis
	Peptic ulcer disease
	Ischaemic colitis
Other causes	
	Vaso-occlusive crisis
	Acute chest syndrome
	Bone marrow infarction of vertebral bodies
	Nerve root entrapment
	Avascular necrosis
	Vertebral collapse
	Chronic arthritis
	Enlarged mesenteric lymph nodes
	Enlarged retroperitoneal lymph nodes

investigations is essential to avoid unnecessary surgical intervention with its inherent risks. The pain can be attributed to marrow infarction of the vertebral bodies with subsequent pressure on nerve roots or to enlarged mesenteric and retroperitoneal lymph nodes. Other common causes of abdominal pain in SCD are shown in Table 1. Acute pain is usually caused by VOCs, ACS, and other serious complications, while chronic pain often results from orthopaedic problems, such as avascular necrosis, vertebral collapse, or chronic arthritis.[12] It must be emphasised that acute pain often requires hospital admission for parenteral opioids and hydration.

SPLENIC COMPLICATIONS

Due to repeated splenic infarction, the spleen undergoes fibrosis and often becomes a nodule (autosplenectomy). Patients with high haemoglobin-F or thalassaemia, however, will have a persistently enlarged spleen, which is often affected with repeated acute sequestration crises or infection of an infarcted area with abscess formation. Splenectomy in SCD is reserved for patients with recurrent acute splenic sequestration crises (ASSCs), troublesome hypersplenism associated with pancytopenia (anaemia, neutropenia and thrombocytopenia), splenic abscess and less commonly, persistent massive splenomegaly.

Acute splenic sequestration crisis
Acute splenic sequestration crisis (ASSC) is a life-threatening complication which is rare in adults due to progressive splenic fibrosis.[18] The diagnosis is a clinical one based on sudden and massive enlargement of the spleen, which is

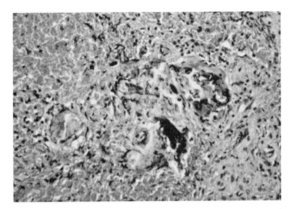

Fig. 1 Microscopic view of the spleen in a case of sickle cell disease with splenic infarction showing haemosedrin deposition (magnification x40).

associated with a rapid fall in haemoglobin and haematocrit due to the extensive pooling of blood.[18] The exact pathogenesis is unknown. However, a triggering factor is splenic outflow venous obstruction that leads to sequestration of red cells and platelets.[18] Radiologically, focal hypo-echogenic areas consistent with haemorrhage or infarction are seen on ultrasonography. Histologically, sinusoids are packed with sickled erythrocytes, and haemosedrin granules are scattered throughout the spleen (Fig. 1). Although minor crises may resolve spontaneously, the majority will require whole-blood transfusion. Splenectomy is reserved for patients with recurrent episodes of ASSC or who may develop allo-antibodies which may hamper future transfusions.[18]

Splenic abscess

SCD patients are at risk of developing splenic sepsis.[19] Splenic abscess occurs secondary to infection of splenic infarcts. About 12% of splenic abscesses occur in SCD patients but the exact incidence is unknown. Predisposing factors include repeated splenic infarctions as shown in Figure 2, especially in the

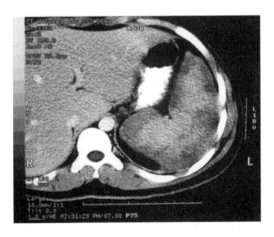

Fig. 2 Computerised tomography showing massively enlarged spleen in sickle cell disease patient with splenic infarction.

presence of splenomegaly and exposure to systemic bacterial infection as a result of hyposplenism.[19] The pus culture may be negative as patients may be on broad-spectrum antibiotics prior to laparotomy. However, *Streptococcus milleri* and other bacteria such as *Streptococci* spp., *Staphylococci* spp. and *Salmonella* spp. have been isolated.[19]

Typical presentation is development of left upper quadrant abdominal pain, fever with palpable tender spleen and neutrophil leukocytosis. Chest X-ray may reveal an elevated left hemidiaphragm and pleural effusion in 70% of cases.[19,20] Ultrasonography and computerised tomography (Fig. 2) are crucial in the diagnosis and can be employed for guided percutaneous drainage.[21] Definitive treatment is by splenectomy (open or laparoscopic).[19,20] However, percutaneous drainage is an attractive option in SCD and should be tried first to avoid the high morbidity associated with surgical intervention and to avoid splenectomy with its attendant risks such as post-splenectomy overwhelming sepsis.[20]

HEPATOBILIARY COMPLICATIONS

Cholelithiasis

SCD patients are at high risk of developing pigment gallstones due to chronic haemolysis. The incidence varies from one population to another and increases with age.[21,22] The prevalence in patients with haemoglobin-S increases to 75% at the age of 30 years and 85% by the age of 33 years.[21] Gallstones may be asymptomatic or may present with repeated attacks of biliary colic, cholecystitis or pancreatitis.[21,22] Intermittent epigastric pain, not always related to fatty meals, is a common presenting symptom in younger patients and typical biliary pain occurs in 68% of adults with gallstones.[22] In patients undergoing laparoscopic cholecystectomy and who have splenomegaly, the position of the spleen should be marked pre-operatively on the abdominal wall to avoid its injury during the insertion of Veress needle and the blind introduction of the first trocar. The small abdominal size in many SCD patients may cause some technical difficulties owing to crowdedness of the instruments.

Asymptomatic gallstones in SCD

The presence of gallstones causes diagnostic confusion in patients presenting with abdominal sickle cell crises. Therefore, prophylactic cholecystectomy in SCD patients with asymptomatic gallstones is advocated to avoid future stone-related complications and diagnostic confusion.[23] With the introduction of laparoscopic cholecystectomy, more SCD adults and children with asymptomatic stones are being referred to surgeons for laparoscopic cholecystectomy.[23-25] Moreover, paediatricians are screening their patients for

Key point 8

- Prophylactic cholecystectomy in SCD patients with asymptomatic gallstones is advocated to avoid future stone-related complications and diagnostic confusion.

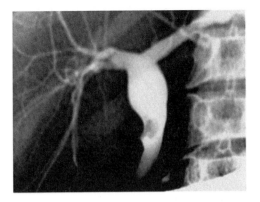

Fig. 3 Endoscopic retrograde cholangiopancreatography of a cholecystectomised sickle cell patient who presented with upper abdominal pain and obstructive jaundice. A pigment polyp at the cystic duct stump was excised surgically after failure of endoscopic excision.

gallstones and refer them for laparoscopic cholecystectomy before symptoms develop.[25] In the laparoscopic era, while surgery should be avoided during VOCs, laparoscopic cholecystectomy for acute cholecystitis is appropriate.[5,26]

Choledocholithiasis

In a review of several series, Schubert[27] estimated choledocholithiasis to occur in 14% of patients with gallstones and that 18% of patients undergoing cholecystectomy had choledocholithiasis. The standard teaching is to exclude choledocholithiasis in any patient with dilated biliary tree on ultrasonography by performing endoscopic retrograde cholangiopancreatography (ERCP). Endoscopic sphincterotomy is performed to clear the common bile duct (CBD) prior to laparoscopic cholecystectomy to avoid CBD exploration. Apart from dilated CBD on ultrasonography, other factors such as raised total bilirubin of > 5 mg/dl, elevated alkaline phosphatase, and recent history of pancreatitis either singly or in combination should raise the suspicion of choledocholithiasis.[28] It may be worth advocating routine endoscopic papillotomy in patients undergoing ERCP before laparoscopic cholecystectomy even if the CBD is found free of stones, but this needs further evaluation. Another cause of obstructive jaundice in SCD is a 'pigment' polyp in the CBD (Fig. 3) which may require duct exploration if endoscopic removal fails.[29]

GASTROINTESTINAL MANIFESTATIONS

Peptic ulceration

It is estimated that one-third of SCD patients with chronic recurrent epigastric pain have endoscopic evidence of peptic ulcer with predominance of duodenal (27%) over gastric (8%) ulcers.[30,31] Peptic ulcer pain may be attributed to abdominal pain crisis. The available evidence to determine whether peptic ulcer is more common than in the general population is insufficient and further studies are needed. However, despite the depressive nature of SCD, there is no evidence of an increased incidence of stress ulceration in this population. The aetiology of peptic ulcer is attributed to decreased mucosal resistance as a result of repeated ischaemic infarcts secondary to sickling crises.[32] As there is some vascular impairment, ulcer healing is often impaired[30,31] and the rate of complications such as stenosis and haemorrhage is high.[30–32] Recommended management includes repeat gastroscopy after 6–8 weeks of intensive medical treatment to monitor the ulcer size and the response to medical therapy. The surgical option should be offered early for ulcers showing poor healing as mortality associated with complications is high.[31,32] *Helicobacter pylori* is prevalent in endemic areas of non-industrialised countries, but data on the prevalence of *H. pylori* in SCD are lacking and a study is warranted.

Ischaemic colitis

Ischaemic colitis may occur in young SCD patients due to massive intravascular sickling. The exact pathophysiology is unknown, but cytokines such as tumour necrosis factor alpha (TNF-α) and interleukin-1 (IL-1) may play an important role. It has been suggested that sickling crisis represents a 'pre-shock' state with resultant vascular spasm, mesenteric arterial thrombosis and subsequent vascular necrosis.[33] However, ischaemia of the colon is fortunately rare due to the presence of an extensive collateral circulation in the mesentery and in the bowel wall, and to the low percentage of oxygen extracted by the bowel. Nevertheless, this diagnosis should be considered in any patient with sickling crisis who develops severe abdominal pain, rectal bleeding and signs of peritonism. High fever, marked leukocytosis and generalised peritoneal signs suggest bowel infarction and warrants urgent laparotomy.[33] Initial management includes nasogastric decompression, broad-spectrum antibiotics and haemodynamic support including exchange transfusion. Close and repeated clinical examination is essential before proceeding to surgical exploration and resection of the ischaemic bowel.[33]

LEG ULCERS

Leg ulcers are common in SCD; it is estimated that 8–10% of patients will develop leg ulceration.[33] The incidence is lower in patients with high haemoglobin-F due to its protective role. The ulcers occur spontaneously or as a result of local trauma with subsequent infection and skin necrosis but no specific organisms have been incriminated. Other contributing factors such as vessel occlusion by sickled cells, increased venous pressure and decreased oxygen carrying capacity with resultant tissue hypoxia have been implicated.[34] The majority of ulcers are located at the lower third of the leg above the ankle, less commonly on the dorsum and rarely on the sole of the foot.[34] Malignant changes have not been described in chronic ulcers associated with SCD. The ulcer is treated conservatively by keeping it clean by regular daily dressings with a mild antiseptic. Bed rest is essential and thick slough may require debridement at the bedside with analgesia, sedation and local anaesthesia. Local therapy such as soaks, salves, gel boots, topical zinc, topical steroids and topical antibiotics have been tried singly or in combination with variable results. The rate of healing can be increased by prolonged administration of zinc sulphate tablets without reported side effects.[35] Surgical procedures such as split skin and full-thickness grafts require general anaesthesia, leave unsightly scars and the results have been disappointing with a high recurrence rate of 52%. The immediate and long-term results of pinch grafting are promising; this has the advantage of being a minor procedure that can be performed under local anaesthesia and repeated as necessary. Aggressive forms of treatments with blood transfusion with its risks and complications and skin grafting are reserved for non-healing ulcers with a diameter of more than 8 cm. Methods to raise levels of haemoglobin-F such as hydroxyurea and recombinant human erythropoietin[36] can induce rapid healing, possibly by improving local oxygen delivery and nutrition or by production of other proteins which act as growth factors to promote ulcer healing. However, further studies are needed to determine its optimal dose and the mechanism of action.

NEW PREVENTIVE THERAPY

The new preventive therapy aims at reducing the frequency and severity of sickle cell crises by increasing haemoglobin-F synthesis. Hydroxurea, which is commonly prescribed, is a ribonuclease reductase inhibitor that stimulates myelosuppressive-induced haemoglobin-F synthesis, thus improving red-cell survival and decreasing SCD complications.[37–39] Its short-term use is safe but toxicity, mainly related to cytopenias, may occur and thus patients must be carefully monitored. Also, 40% of treated patients do not respond or have progressive organ failure.[38] Short-chain fatty acids (*e.g.* valproic acid) correct anaemia and work by affecting globin gene-expression, possibly by inhibition of histone deacetylases.[38] 5-Azacytidine is another haemoglobin-F modulator which increases γ-gene expression, but it is tumorigenic. A safer azacytidine analogue, decitabine, is now available. It increases total haemoglobin and haemoglobin-F in patients resistant to hydroxyurea.[40,41] Inhaled nitric oxide (NO) is a potent vasodilator with anti-sickling activity which is also being used with success to slow the sickling process.[39] In SCD patients, L-arginine, the NO precursor, levels are low and thus arginine supplementation appears to correct the NO deficiency and improve pulmonary hypertension.[40,41] NO or arginine supplementation may be synergistic when used with hydroxyurea.

Key point 9

- New preventive therapies such as hydroxurea aim at reducing the number and severity of sickle cell crises by increasing the synthesis of fetal haemoglobin (haemoglobin-F).

Other therapies include two new drugs that showed promise in decreasing sickling – poloxamer 188 and fructose 1-6 diphosphate. They may help to improve the anaesthetic course, reduce postoperative complications, and shorten hospital stays of SCD patients.[38,41] Bone marrow transplantation in children is curative in some patients and is now accepted therapy for symptomatic children.[42] However, progress in gene therapy has been slow due to inadequate gene transfer and low gene-expression.[38,41]

GENETIC COUNSELLING

Genetic counselling is beneficial to all SCD patients, especially couples whose haemoglobin genotypes imply they could have offspring with a clinically

Key point 10

- Genetic counselling is beneficial to all SCD patients.

significant haemoglobinopathy. Ideally, patients should be identified at birth as part of a screening programme and referred for periodic evaluations.[43,44] Parents of newborn infants with SCD should receive genetic counselling and support. They are taught to assess pain, fever, respiratory distress, splenomegaly, and jaundice. It is, also important to provide preconception genetic counselling for women of child-bearing age with SCD.[44]

CONCLUSIONS

Sickle cell disease patients present with various surgical manifestations posing a formidable diagnostic challenge. Patients requiring surgical intervention need a comprehensive management plan including pre-operative blood transfusion, special peri-operative care and effective postoperative analgesia. It is hoped that the increasing awareness of the surgical manifestations of SCD, the introduction of minimally invasive techniques and the new preventive therapies will greatly reduce the high mortality and morbidity associated with surgery in this high-risk population. Furthermore, the introduction of modern screening programmes and counselling will help to reduce the prevalence of sickle cell disease.

Key points for clinical practice

- Greater population mobility in recent years makes recognition of the disease and its various surgical manifestations of paramount importance in clinical practice.

- The clinical problems of sickle cell disease are related to the high level of sickle haemoglobin (haemoglobin-S).

- Sepsis secondary to infection is the most common precipitating factor for sickle cell crisis and the leading cause of death.

- General anaesthesia and surgical trauma add additional risk of complications.

- Blood transfusion therapy remains a key component of the comprehensive management as it reduces the peri-operative risks associated with surgery and anaesthesia.

- Exchange transfusion is implemented when the haemoglobin-S is high, while simple top-up transfusion is used when the haemoglobin is lower than 9 g/dl.

- Abdominal pain in SCD represents a diagnostic challenge as it mimics many surgical emergencies. Careful evaluation of each patient is essential to avoid unnecessary surgical intervention.

Key points for clinical practice *(continued)*

- Prophylactic cholecystectomy in SCD patients with asymptomatic gallstones is advocated to avoid future stone-related complications and diagnostic confusion.

- New preventive therapies such as hydroxurea aim at reducing the number and severity of sickle cell crises by increasing the synthesis of fetal haemoglobin (haemoglobin-F).

- Genetic counselling is beneficial to all SCD patients..

References

1. Herrick JB. Peculiar elongated and sickle-shaped corpuscles in a case of severe anaemia. *Arch Intern Med* 1910; **6**: 517–521.
2. Mason VR. Sickle cell anemia. *JAMA* 1922; **79**: 1318–1320.
3. Beet EA. The genetics of sickle cell trait in a Bantu tribe. *Ann Eur Genet* 1949; **14**: 279–282.
4. Meshikhes A-WN. Sickle cell disease and the general surgeon. *J R Coll Surg Edinb* 1998; **43**: 73–79.
5. Claster S, Vichinsky EP. Managing sickle cell disease. *BMJ* 2003; **327**: 1151–1155.
6. Balasubramaniam J, Phelan I, Bain BJ. Evaluation of a new screening test for sickle cell haemoglobin. *Clin Lab Haematol* 2001; **23**: 379–383.
7. Frietsch T, Ewen I, Waschke KF. Anaesthetic care for sickle cell disease. *Eur J Anaesthesiol* 2001; **18**: 137–150.
8. Lessin IS, Kurantsin-Mills J, Klug PP, Weems HB. Determination of rheologically optimal mixtures of AA and SS erythrocytes for transfusion. *Prog Clin Biol Res* 1978; **20**: 123–137.
. Meshikhes A-WN. Thromboprophylaxis in laparoscopic abdominal surgery. *Ann Coll Surg HK* 2003; **7**: 52–54.
10. Meshikhes A-WN, Al-Abkari, HA, Al-Faraj AA, Al-Dhurais SA, Al-Saif O. Safety of laparoscopic cholecystectomy in sickle cell disease: an update. *Ann Saudi Med* 1998; **18**: 12–14.
11. Delatte SJ, Hebra A, Tagge EP, Jackson S, Jacques K, Othersen Jr HB. Acute chest syndrome in the postoperative sickle cell patient. *J Pediatr Surg* 1999; **34**: 188–191.
12. Serjeant GR. The emerging understanding of sickle cell disease. *Br J Haematol* 2001; **112**: 3–18.
13. Vichinsky EP, Heberkern CM, Neumayrl L *et al*. A comparison of conservative and aggressive transfusion regimens in the peri-operative management of sickle cell disease. *N Engl J Med* 1995; **27**: 206–213.
14. Surgery and anesthesia. In: Charache S, Lubin B, Reid CD. (eds) *Management and Therapy of Sickle Cell Disease*. Washington, DC: National Institutes of Health. 1992; 49–50.
15. Lawson SE, Oakley S, Smith NA, Bareford D. Exchange blood transfusion in sickle cell disease. *Clin Lab Haematol* 1999; **21**: 99–102.
16. Haberkern CM, Neumayr LD, Orringer EP *et al*. Cholecystectomy in sickle cell anemia patients: perioperative outcome of 364 cases from the National Preoperative Transfusion Study. *Blood* 1997; **89**: 1533–1542.
17. Meshikhes A-WN, Al-Abkari HA, Al-Faraj AA. Comparison of three preoperative blood transfusion regimens in sickle cell patients undergoing laparoscopic cholecystectomy. *J Irish Coll Phys Surg* 1999; **28**: 200–202.
18. Solanki DL, Kletter GG, Castro O. Acute splenic sequestration crises in adults with sickle cell disease. *Am J Med* 1986; **80**: 985–990.
19. Cavenagh JD, Joseph AEA, Dilly S, Bevan DR. Splenic sepsis in sickle cell disease. *Br J Haematol* 1994; **86**: 187–189.
20. Gleich S, Wolin DA, Rerbsman R. A review of percutaneous drainage of splenic abscess. *Surg Gynecol Obstet* 1988; **167**: 211–216.

21. Bond LR, Hatry SR, Horn MEC, Dick M, Meire HB, Bellingham AJ. Gall stones in sickle cell disease in the United Kingdom. *BMJ* l987; **295**: 234–236.
22. McCall W, Desai P, Serjeant BE, Serjcanr GR. Cholelithiasis in Jamaican patients with homozygous sickle cell disease. *Am J Hematol* 1977; **3**: 15–21.
23. Meshikhes A-W. Asymptomatic gallstones in the laparoscopic era. *J R Coll Surg Edinb* 2002; **47**: 742–748.
24. Meshikhes A-WN. Laparoscopic cholecystectomy in patients with sickle cell disease [editorial]. *J Ir Coll Phys Surg* 1995; **24**: 91–92.
25. Ware RE, Kinney TR, Casey IR, Pappas TN, Meyers WC. Laparoscopic cholecystectomy in young patients with sickle haemoglobinopathies. *J Paediatr* 1992; **120**: 58–61.
26. Meshikhes A-WN, Al-Dhurais SA, Al-Jamaa AR, Al-Faraj AA, Al-Khatir AS, Al-Abkari H. Laparoscopic cholecystectomy in patients with sickle cell disease. *J R Coll Surg Edin* 1995; **40**: 383–385.
27. Schubert YE. Hepatobiliary system in sickle cell disease. *Gastroenterology* 1986; **90**: 2013–2021.
28. Al-Salem AH, Nourallah H. Sequential endoscopic/laparoscopic management of cholelithiasis and choledocholithiasis in children who have sickle cell disease. *J Pediatr Surg* 1997; **32**: 1432–1435.
29. Meshikhes A-WN, Al-Talak FT, Al Faraj AA, Al Momen SA. Pigment polyp in the common bile duct. *Saudi Med J* 2003; **24**: 776–777.
30. Lee MG, Thirumalai CHR, Terry SI, Setjeant GR. Endoscopic and gastric acid studies in homozygous sickle cell disease and upper abdominal pain. *Gut* 1989; **30**: 569–572.
31. Serjeant BE, May H, Patrick A, Slifer ED. Duodenal ulceration in sickle cell anaemia. *Trans R Soc Trop Med Hyg* 1973; **67**: 59.
32. Rao S, Royal JE, Conard Jr HA, Harris V, Ahuja I. Duodenal ulcer in sickle cell anaemia. *J Pediatr Gastroenterol Nutr* 1990; **10**: 117–120.
33. Williams LF, Wistenberg J. Ischaemic colitis: a useful clinical diagnosis, but is it ischaemic? *Ann Surg* 1975; **182**: 439–448.
34. Koshy M, Entsuah R, Koranda A *et al*. Leg ulcers in patients with sickle cell disease. *Blood* 1989; **74**: 1403–1408.
35. Serjeant GR, Galloway RE, Gueri M. Oral zinc sulphate in sickle cell ulcers. *Lancet* 1970; **2**: 891–893.
36. Al-Momen A-KM. Recombinant human erythropoietin induced rapid healing of chronic leg ulcer in a patient with sickle cell disease. *Acta Haematol* 1991; **86**: 46–48.
37. Atweh GF, Loukopoulos D. Pharmacological induction of fetal hemoglobin in sickle cell disease and beta-thalassemia. *Semin Hematol* 2001; **38**: 367–373.
38. Vichinsky EP. New therapies in sickle cell disease. *Lancet* 2002; **360**: 629–631.
39. Koshy M, Dorn L, Bressler L *et al*. 2-Deoxy 5-azacytidine and fetal hemoglobin induction in sickle cell anemia. *Blood* 2000; **96**: 2379–2384.
40. Morris CR, Kuypers FA, Larkin S *et al*. Arginine therapy: a novel strategy to induce nitric oxide production in sickle cell disease. *Br J Haematol* 2000; **111**: 498–500.
41. Dix HM. New advances in the treatment of sickle cell disease: focus on perioperative significance. *AANA J* 2001; **69**: 281–286.
42. Walters MC, Storb R, Patience M *et al*. Impact of bone marrow transplantation for symptomatic sickle cell disease: an interim report. Multicenter investigation of bone marrow transplantation for sickle cell disease. *Blood* 2000; **95**: 1918–1924.
43. Kmietowicz Z. Screening for sickle cell disease and thalassaemia: saving lives. *BMJ* 2004; **329**: 69.
44. Okpala I, Thomas V, Westerdale N *et al*. The comprehensive care of sickle cell disease. *Eur J Haematol* 2002; **68**:157–162.

Adarsh Kumar   John H. Scholefield
Jens Andersen   Nicholas C. Armitage

5

Fast-track surgery

Fast-track surgery has evolved as a result of co-ordinated effort to combine recent evidence-based advances in the modern care of surgical patients.[1] Fast-track surgery, also referred to as multimodal rehabilitation or enhanced recovery after surgery (ERAS) is a multimodal comprehensive programme aimed at enhancing postoperative recovery and outcome.[2,3] Kehlet and colleagues popularised this concept and have demonstrated planned discharge after 48 h in patients undergoing elective open colonic surgery for malignant and benign diseases.[4,5] Subsequently, several groups around the world confirmed the benefits of this combined anaesthetic and surgical approach for peri-operative care and demonstrated reduced hospitalisation, potential complications and cost.[6–9] Two prospective, randomised, controlled trials[6,8] and several single-institute case series reports have confirmed the effectiveness and safety of this approach.[7,9,10] Similar results have been demonstrated in patients with significant co-morbidity undergoing more complex surgery.[7] Although most outcome data have been studied in context to elective colorectal surgery, a number of published series have reported the

Adarsh Kumar FRCS MS DM FRCS (for correspondence)
Senior Fellow in Laparoscopic Colorectal Surgery, University Department of Colorectal Surgery, The Queen Elizabeth Hospital, 28 Woodville Road, Woodville South 5011, Adelaide, Australia
E-mail: adarshkumar25@hotmail.com

John H. Scholefield ChM FRCS
Professor of Surgery, Section of Surgery, E Floor West Block, University Hospital, Nottingham NG7 2UH, UK

Jens Andersen MD
Consultant Surgeon and Head of Colorectal Surgery, Department of Surgical Gastroenterology, Hvidovre University Hospital, DK-2650 Hvidovre, Denmark

Nicholas C. Armitage DM FRCS
Consultant Surgeon, Section of Surgery, E Floor West Block, University Hospital, Nottingham NG7 2UH, UK

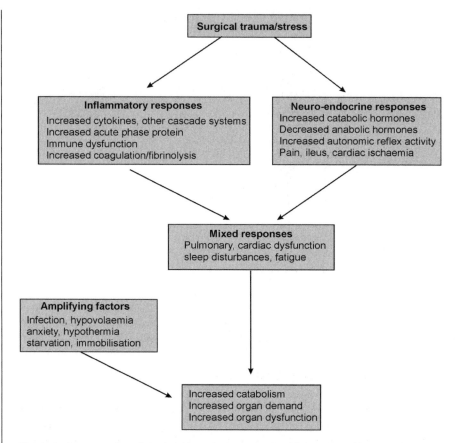

Fig. 1 Mediators and modulators of catabolic pathways after surgery.[14]

benefits of fast-track surgery in other specialities.[3] Enhanced convalescence recovery and reduced hospital stay have been achieved in patients undergoing pulmonary resection, abdominal aortic aneurysm surgery and hip operation.[11–13]

The main thrust of this integrated approach is to reduce psychological and physiological stresses associated with operations thereby alleviating tissue catabolism and subsequent organ dysfunction.[1,14] Stress response in surgical illness, as illustrated in Figure 1, is mediated through neuro-endocrine,

Key points 1 & 2

- Fast-track surgery is a multimodal, evidence-based compre-hensive programme aimed at enhancing postoperative recovery and outcome by attenuating stress-related organ dysfunction.

- It is important to understand that the discharge criteria (mobile patient, pain-free on oral analgesia, complete recovery of gut and bladder functions) in fast-track surgery remain unaltered but achieved sooner.

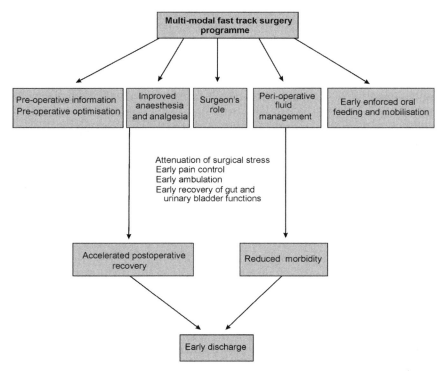

Fig. 2 Multimodal concept of fast-track surgery.[2]

metabolic, and inflammatory pathways.[14] Various stress-reduction methods incorporated into fast-track surgery include pre-operative patient education and optimisation, improved anaesthesia and epidural analgesia, adoption of modern surgical principles, optimised dynamic pain relief, and enforced early ambulation and oral nutrition support.[2,14] Postoperative organ dysfunction appears significantly attenuated, as demonstrated in fast-track programme studies evaluating pulmonary function, ileus, fatigue, the cardiovascular response to exercise, preservation of body composition and generation of muscle force.[8,14–16]

It is important to understand that discharge criteria with fast-track surgery are the same as those of conventional care, but achieved sooner under the fast-track system.[1] Postoperative pain control, ambulation and, complete recovery of gut and urinary bladder functions are essential prerequisites in planning discharge from hospital. These goals can be achieved early with the application of fast-track surgery principles (Fig. 2) to combat the profound changes in endocrine, metabolic, and pulmonary function seen in surgical illness.[2,14]

COMPONENTS OF FAST-TRACK SURGICAL CARE

PRE-OPTIMISATION AND PRE-OPERATIVE PATIENT EDUCATION

Postoperative morbidity and prolonged recovery is related to pre-operative co-morbidity.[17] Therefore, pre-operative evaluation and optimisation of organ dysfunction should be instituted in all patients to reduce morbidity and mortality.[14] Appropriate guidelines are available for optimisation of patients with cardiac disease, chronic pulmonary disease, diabetes mellitus and various other disorders.[18,19] Patients with history of alcohol abuse even in the absence of alcohol-related organ dysfunction are more prone to increased postoperative morbidity and prolonged recovery[20] and benefit from abstinence of 4 weeks in the pre-operative period.[21] Similarly, cessation of smoking 2 months prior to surgery has resulted in better outcome[22] as smoking is known to reduce phagocytic and microbicidal activity of lung macrophages.[23] Pre-operative nutritional support in severely malnourished patients (> 15% weight loss) has been shown to reduce postoperative morbidity and enhance recovery.[24] A recent multicentre, randomised trial from the UK[25] evaluated the effects of pre- and postoperative oral nutritional supplements (drink containing 1.5 kcal/ml and 0.05 g protein/ml) on clinical course and cost effectiveness in patients undergoing colorectal surgery. Pre-operative oral nutritional supplementation started before hospital admission diminished the degree of weight loss and incidence of minor complications and was cost effective.[25] Pre-operative evaluation and supplementation of micronutrients in selected group of patients (*e.g.* the elderly and Crohn's patients) may be beneficial.[14] Pre-operative intake of a carbohydrate drink has been shown to reduce postoperative, stress-related insulin resistance,[26] an independent predictor of duration of postoperative hospital stay.[27] The clinical significance of stress-related insulin resistance is further illustrated by a trial in which intensive treatment of hyperglycaemia with insulin infusion significantly reduced morbidity and mortality rates in surgical patients in intensive care.[28]

Psychological preparation of a patient undergoing surgery can play a major role in modifying the individual's response to the operative experience.[14] Carefully presented information from surgeons, anaesthetists, and nurses about surgical procedures, anticipated sensory experiences, and analgesic treatment has been shown to aid coping, less pre-operative anxiety and reduced postoperative pain experience and the need for analgesia.[29,30] Reduction of convalescence period is also highly dependent on pre-operative advice from the surgeon.[31] Short convalescence recommendations are followed by enhanced postoperative recovery and shortened hospital stay.[31]

IMPROVED ANAESTHESIA AND ANALGESIA

Modern anaesthetic care has greatly contributed to reducing surgical stress responses.[2] Premedication therapy reduces anxiety, intra-operative analgesic requirement, smooth recovery from anaesthesia, and reduced postoperative nausea and vomiting. New, short-acting anaesthetic agents that allow quick recovery of vital organ functions and provide stress-reducing effects to prevent organ dysfunction after major operations have contributed to the success of the fast-track surgery programme.[2] Proprofol anaesthesia exerts significant anti-nausea and vomiting effects, as do ondansetron or other similar drugs.[14] The incidence of postoperative nausea and vomiting is also reduced by the omission of nitrous oxide.[32] Prevention of intra-operative hypothermia reduces cardiac morbidity, bleeding, and septic complications due to less attenuation of the immune system.[33] Adequate tissue perfusion and oxygenation during surgery are important to attenuate stress response; a high inspired fraction of oxygen (80%) has been shown to reduce the risk of wound infection after colorectal surgery compared with 30% oxygen.[34] Correction of early postoperative anaesthesia-related hypoxaemia may also reduce nausea and vomiting, reduce tachycardia, and cerebral dysfunction.[14] A single dose of glucocorticoids has been shown to reduce postoperative nausea, vomiting, pain, and pulmonary dysfunction without side effects.[35] Administration of bbb-blockers to reduce sympathetic stimulation of the heart has improved cardiac outcome in several randomised trials; therefore, its routine use has been recommended in patients at cardiac risk.[36] A recent study concluded that a long-acting bbb-blocker (atenolol) as compared to a short-acting bbb-blocker (metoprolol) was more effective in reducing peri-operative cardiac morbidity in elderly patients undergoing elective non-cardiac surgery.[37] bbb-Blockers might also have beneficial metabolic effects, since they reduce injury-induced catabolism in patients with burns.[38] The use of anabolic agents such as growth hormone and insulin has been shown to reduce catabolism and promote recovery.[3] Published evidence suggests that an increased incidence of cerebrovascular complications may occur in the postoperative period with cessation of chronically used medications after operation;[39] therefore, these drugs should be continued postoperatively. The concept of procedure-specific and minimally invasive anaesthesia involving short-acting anaesthetic agents, neuromuscular blocking agents only if necessary, minimal airway handling, and invasive monitoring may further contribute to reduce stress and enhance recovery.[2]

Analgesia

Effective peri-operative pain control has revolutionised the care of surgical patients. Optimum pain treatment reduces anxiety, provides subjective comfort, helps to blunt autonomic and somatic reflex responses and thus restore organ functions. It also enables early oral intake and mobilisation, thereby improving postoperative recovery and outcome.[2] A combination of pre-, intra- and postoperative measures to control pain seems to be an effective approach. The concept of pre-emptive analgesia to prevent pain resulting in neurophysiological and biochemical consequences may be preferable to treatment of pain when these consequences are already established.[40] Pre-emptive analgesia also reduces the analgesic requirement intra-operatively and contributes to pain-free emergence from anaesthesia. The concept of multimodal or balanced analgesia to treat postoperative pain takes advantage of the additive or synergistic effects by combinations of different analgesic agents (opioids, local anaesthetics, NSAIDs, COX-2 inhibitors, paracetamol) or techniques (peripheral nerve blocks, central neuraxial block and patient-controlled analgesia) and provides reduction of side-effects owing to the lower doses of the individual drugs.[41] The combinations of epidural local anaesthetic plus opioids, opioids and NSAIDs, and paracetamol and NSAIDs have been shown to improve analgesia in several randomised trials.[41,42] Peripheral nerve blocks provide excellent pain relief after several procedures and evidence suggests that continuous infusion of local anaesthetics for peripheral nerve blocks is effective and safe.[43]

Epidural analgesia (a combination of local anaesthetics and low-dose opioids) has added a new dimension to the enhanced recovery programme by attenuating neuro-endocrine stress responses, effective pain relief and, ileus-reducing effect.[14] The inhibitory effects on catabolic responses are more pronounced when epidural anaesthesia is used as a continuous technique for up to 48 h and for procedures performed on the lower body to provide a near-total afferent neural blockade.[44] Meta-analyses of randomised trials comparing use of central blockade (spinal or epidural anaesthesia) with or without general anaesthesia versus general anaesthesia alone demonstrated significant reduction in postoperative mortality and morbidity including myocardial infarction, pneumonia, thrombo-embolic complications, acute renal failure, and bleeding and transfusion requirement.[45] Another, large, multicentre, randomised, controlled study evaluated the safety and benefits of epidural block as compared to other analgesic regimens with general anaesthesia in 915 high-risk patients undergoing major abdominal surgery.[46] The authors demonstrated that epidural analgesia was safe and resulted in better pain relief during the first 3 postoperative days and reduced pulmonary morbidity compared to other analgesic techniques. Introduction of an acute pain team service routinely is a promising step in the effective management of postoperative pain.[47] Therefore, implementation of balanced analgesic protocols including continuous low-dose epidural block postoperatively and integration of an acute pain team service are prerequisites for the effective pain treatment to hasten recovery in fast-track surgery.

Surgeon's role

The surgeon has an important role to play in reducing stress to enhance recovery in surgical illness.[2] This begins in the out-patient clinic with extensive pre-operative teaching detailing projected length of stay and return of bowel function.[9] Patient and procedure selections have a significant impact on reducing postoperative morbidity and improving outcome.[2] Routine bowel preparation in elective colorectal surgery does not influence anastomotic leak rates or reduce septic complications and has been associated with increased morbidity and cost.[48] The choice of incisions could have implications for postoperative pain and organ function. Abdominal transverse incisions including only a few nerve segments result in reduced pain and pulmonary dysfunction compared with longitudinal incisions.[49] The blockade of afferent neural stimuli from the surgical area by infiltration anaesthesia and peripheral nerve blocks reduces endocrine-metabolic response but not inflammation.[50] The metabolic blocking effect of local anaesthetics is further enhanced if the block is maintained postoperatively for pain treatment.[50]

Tubes and drains

The routine use of nasogastric tubes, drains and catheters imposes restrictions on early oral intake and mobilisation and, therefore, prolongs recovery.[14] A meta-analysis of several randomised trials has suggested the routine use of nasogastric tubes after elective abdominal surgery is unnecessary and may contribute to pulmonary complications.[51] Another recent meta-analysis concluded that routine nasogastric decompression after abdominal surgery did not hasten the return of bowel function, reduce risk of anastomotic leakage or improve patient comfort and hospital stay.[52] The authors suggested that routine nasogastric decompression should be abandoned in favour of selective use of nasogastric tube. Similarly, routine use of drains does not improve outcome.[53,54] It has been suggested that, after low rectal operations, urinary bladder drainage should be limited to about 3 days and to 1 day after other types of colonic surgery.[55,56] The use of low-dose thoracic epidural bupivacaine–opioid administration for postoperative pain relief should not be an indication for bladder drainage beyond 24 h, despite continuous epidural analgesia.[56]

Complications

Anastomotic and wound-related morbidity and sepsis lead to further deterioration in stress response and organ dysfunction and this highlights the importance of precise dissection along appropriate tissue planes, to minimise trauma, meticulous haemostasis and prevention of septic complications.[14] Specialist approach and experience reduce the surgical variability resulting in improved outcome. In a fast-track programme study,[6] further reduction in hospital stay and improved outcome was observed with increasing experience of the surgeon.

Surgical access

The minimally invasive approach has not resulted in a significant reduction of classical endocrine metabolic responses but has reduced various inflammatory responses.[57] However, the laparoscopic route is increasingly being used to tackle various colorectal and other intra-abdominal pathologies as patients seems to have better pulmonary function, less bleeding, less attenuation of the immune system, early resolution of ileus and low morbidity related to wounds and adhesion formation.[58] Data from COST and CLASICC trials have demonstrated reduced morbidity and reported less pain and shorter hospital stay with the laparoscopic route in colorectal surgery.[59,60] Similarly, a randomised controlled trial from Barcelona[61] confirmed these observations and additionally showed survival benefit for Dukes' C colon cancer patients undergoing laparoscopic surgery probably due to better preservation of the immune system and 'no touch' technique seen with the laparoscopic approach. However, a critical review of randomised trials comparing open and laparoscopic procedures indicates that traditional care regimens have rarely been revised in the open treatment groups, but have been modified in the laparoscopic group, thereby favouring the expected improved outcome after minimally invasive surgery.[14] Therefore, it has been argued that such studies, in which hospital stay and convalescence were utilised as end points, may merely reflect traditions of peri-operative care associated with open procedures rather than differences between open and laparoscopic procedures.[57] A recently published trial evaluated the functional recovery of various organ systems after open versus laparoscopic colonic resection where both groups received a peri-operative care adjusted to fast-track surgery principles in a randomised-observer and patient-blinded fashion, and with planned discharge after 48 h.[15] Early functional recovery and median hospital stay of 2 days were found to be similar in both groups, indicating benefits of a multimodal rehabilitation regimen rather than surgical route.[15] Further large-scale studies are required to validate this observation and, more importantly, to evaluate potential differences in mortality with open and laparoscopic approaches. Despite a small benefit for postoperative analgesic requirement and hospital stay, laparoscopic colorectal procedures will continue to be performed in the future due to increasing patient awareness and improvement in technology.[62] The long-term data from on-going trials in laparoscopic colorectal surgery[59,60,63] may confirm previous observations of survival benefit with the laparoscopic approach,[61] and this would further increase consumer pressure, with a high demand for laparoscopic colorectal surgery.

Fluid management

Appropriate peri-operative fluid therapy is a vital component of fast-track surgery and greatly influences the postoperative recovery and outcome.[64] Patients should be allowed oral liquid until 2 h prior to operation as prolonged pre-operative starvation is unnecessary and may contribute to increased morbidity.[64] The replacement of appropriate amounts of fluid to correct pre-existing dehydration in some cases has an important role in pre-optimisation of cardiovascular function.[2] Similarly, aggressive intra-operative fluid therapy should be avoided as it may result in further deterioration of organ function postoperatively and delay recovery.[14] Postoperative fluid management has varied from 'wet' to 'dry' regimens, but evidence-based, procedure-specific regimens for fluid administration are not available.[64] For minor procedures, pre-operative and intra-operative administration of 1–1.5 l of fluid is important to enhance recovery by compensating for pre-operative dehydration.[2] In major operations, administration of excess fluid can increase cardiac and pulmonary complications, impair wound healing due to poor oxygenation, prolonged duration of ileus, and probably contributes to thrombo-embolic complications.[64,65] Excess fluid administration accentuates the water and sodium conserving effect of surgical stress response, and may increase the risk of electrolyte disturbances such as hyponatraemia and metabolic acidosis.[64,66] In contrast, a 'dry' regimen in pulmonary surgery resulting in reduced pulmonary morbidity supports the safety of a 'dry' regimen in high-risk patients undergoing major operations.[64] A 'dry' regimen (< 2 L) when compared with a 'wet' regimen (> 3 l) does not influence urine output in the early postoperative period or result in elevation of blood urea levels above normal values.[65] A randomised, controlled trial[65] evaluated the effect of salt and water balance on recovery of gastrointestinal function after elective colonic surgery. In this study, a 'wet' regimen sufficient to cause a 3-kg weight gain after surgery delayed return of gastrointestinal function and prolonged hospital stay. It has been suggested that excess fluid therapy to treat hypotension associated with regional anaesthesia should be avoided and managed by sympathomimetics instead.[64]

Postoperative ileus and early enforced oral feeding

Every effort should be made to achieve early resolution of postoperative ileus as it contributes to abdominal discomfort, nausea and vomiting, pulmonary complications, and delay in oral intake.[67] The pathogenesis of postoperative ileus includes inhibitory sympathetic reflexes initiated from the site of injury, local intestinal inflammatory response, opioids, and excess fluid therapy.[65,68] A combined surgical and anaesthetic approach can help to alleviate ileus by provision of opioid-reduced analgesia, continuous epidural local anaesthetic analgesia and appropriate peri-operative fluid therapy.[2] The ileus-reducing effect of continuous thoracic epidural local anaesthetic with or without small doses of opioids has not been observed after lumbar epidural local analgesia or epidural opioid analgesia.[69] The minimal invasive approach alone has been shown to reduce duration of ileus.[68] Similarly, stimulatory effects of early oral feeding and use of laxatives may contribute to early normalisation of gastrointestinal function after surgery.[70] Basse et al.[67] demonstrated an early normalisation of gastrointestinal motility after open colonic resection with a multimodal rehabilitation programme involving epidural analgesia, early oral nutrition and mobilisation and laxative.

Early oral feeding within 24 h after gastrointestinal surgery is well-tolerated, safe and plays an important role to enhance recovery and outcome.[71] Several experimental and clinical studies have demonstrated that early enteral nutrition reduces gut permeability (and presumed bacterial translocation) and may reduce septic complications and improve outcome.[72] Experimental data also suggest that early enteral feeding increases anastomotic collagen deposition and strength and is associated with an improvement in wound healing.[73] A recently published trial[74] confirmed a significant improvement in postoperative insulin resistance and nitrogen losses with early feeding, which has been shown to reduce hospital stay.[27] In a meta-analysis,[71] early enteral feeding reduced the risk of any type of infection and the mean length of stay in hospital. Risk reductions were also seen for anastomotic dehiscence and mortality but these failed to reach statistical significance.[71] However, a beneficial effect of specific nutrient pharmacotherapy using immune-enhancing nutrients on outcome remains controversial and needs further evaluation.[14] It has been suggested that early oral feeding may also impose a stimulatory effect on postoperative gut function.[67,70] On the other hand, restrictions on oral intake after major operations contributes to catabolism, with loss of muscle mass and weight, thereby increasing postoperative fatigue and delaying recovery.[14] Prolonged nutritional therapy for 10–16 weeks after discharge has no major benefit except in depleted patients.[14]

Aggressive early mobilisation

Traditional postoperative care includes bed rest, which is undesirable because it increases muscle loss and weakness, impairs pulmonary function and tissue oxygenation and pre-disposes to thrombo-embolic and pulmonary complications and orthostatic intolerance.[75] Conversely, increased activity and ambulation may reduce cardiac, respiratory, fluid shift, bone and joint changes of bed rest to which surgical patients are predisposed.[75] Although postoperative ambulation alone does not prevent ileus,[76] it contributes to early resolution of ileus in combination with other measures such as epidural analgesia, early oral nutrition, and laxatives.[67] Loss of muscle tissue and function and de-conditioning of cardiovascular response to exercise as a result of bed rest, all contribute to postoperative fatigue resulting in a long convalescence period.[2] Therefore, every effort should be made to enforce postoperative mobilisation, which is possible with effective pain relief and active involvement of nurses and physiotherapists.[2] Fatigue may also be reduced by combined inhibition of the catabolic response with neural blockade techniques and early nutrition. Other factors contributing to postoperative

Key point 3

- The modern concepts of patient education, pre-optimisation, improved anaesthesia, analgesia and surgical techniques and better understanding of peri-operative care principles with enforced early oral feeding and ambulation have led to the success of fast-track surgery.

fatigue are distorted sleep due to noise and drugs (opioids, benzodiazepine), and inflammatory response.[14]

BENEFITS AND SAFETY

Adoption of stress reduction therapy has greatly shortened length of convalescence recovery, reduced hospitalisation and complications and has contributed to improved operative outcome.[3] The fast-track surgery programme has achieved a planned discharge 48 h after open surgery, with a median length of stay of 2 days and a mean of 4 days.[4,10] Although most outcome data have been studied in relation to elective colorectal surgery, postoperative hospital stay has been reduced to 2–4 days after aortic aneurysm repair,[12] and 1–2 days after hip operation[11] and pulmonary resection.[2] Table 1 shows length of stay with fast-track surgery in other specialities.[3] Reduced hospital stay would increase the availability of resources for other patients but it would be inappropriate if it were associated with an increased risk of complications or a reduction in patient satisfaction.[6] Two randomised controlled trials[6,8] and several single institute case series reports have demonstrated reduction in postoperative organ dysfunction and morbidity with multimodal rehabilitation programmes.[7,9,10] Such a reduction in complications combined with a decreased stay in hospital should reduce costs.[1] Stephen and Berger[9] demonstrated that the average cost per patient on multimodal rehabilitation (taking into account the cost of re-admissions) was significantly less than the average cost per patient not on the fast-track surgery programme. Patient satisfaction and quality of life appear similar to those associated with conventional care.[6]

Table 1 Length of stay with fast-track surgery[3]

Type of procedure	Length of stay
Inguinal hernia repair	Ambulatory surgery
Laparoscopic cholecystectomy	Ambulatory surgery
Mastectomy	< 1 day
Adrenalectomy	< 1 day
Donor nephrectomy	< 1 day
Lung resection	1–2 days
Radical prostatectomy	1–2 days
Colectomy	2–3 days
Abdominal aortic aneurysmectomy	3 days

> ## Key point 4
>
> - Published evidence confirms the benefits of fast-track surgery including reduced hospitalisation, low morbidity, cost-effectiveness, patient satisfaction and safety, with very low re-admission rates.

Safety is an important issue and the main concern for many physicians who remain sceptical to such an approach in surgical illness. Published evidence has not shown increased morbidity or mortality with the fast-track approach.[2,6,12] It has been suggested that the support of family and friends is essential for an early and safe transition from hospital to home.[1] Early re-admission has not been a problem in many studies,[2,6,8,9,12] although in one study a re-admission rate of 20% was observed.[16] The available data from fast-track surgery have not shown an increase in use of health services after discharge.[14] Concern has also been expressed about the potential increased risk of severe complications such as pulmonary thrombo-embolism, anastomotic breakdown, and wound-related problems in the home after discharge, but there is no evidence so far that this is a greater problem than with traditional practice.[1] However, to ensure smooth transfer of the patient from the hospital to the home environment, discharge planning, pre-operative information and socio-economic circumstances must be taken into consideration.

IMPLEMENTATION

Organisation and team delivery with strict attention to protocols are vital for the successful implementation of a fast-track surgery programme. A team of motivated individuals must be created to formulate a plan and work together: this involves anaesthetists, surgeons, nurses and physiotherapists. It is useful for team members to visit another institution with an active fast-track programme in place. All team members must understand that each step in care under a fast-track surgery programme is crucial and a collaborative approach must be established to obtain a successful recovery programme. In this context, patient education and pre-operative optimisation of organ function are essential. Defined protocols and care pathways including an outline of postoperative nursing care are needed to reduce variability in peri-operative care and to improve the outcome (Table 2). An example is standardisation of approach to epidural-induced hypotension, where initial resistance to fluid challenge (500 ml colloid) should be treated with drug therapy to avoid fluid overload and its harmful effects. During the postoperative recovery period, doctors, nurses, and the physiotherapist need to follow the pathway to ensure timely removal of tubes and drains, appropriate diet advancement, and aggressive early mobilisation. These protocols should also include sections where the occurrence of events, which could preclude early recovery and discharge, are recorded to facilitate interpretation of the protocols and to provide information for future areas that need development.[2] There is also a need to optimise peri-operative pain management and to integrate acute pain services into peri-operative rehabilitation, since the overall effects of acute pain

Table 2 Main features of the practical care pathway for fast-track surgery

- Pre-operative counselling and optimisation
- Epidural catheter
- General anaesthesia
- No bowel preparation
- Transverse or curved incision
- Continuous epidural analgesia (2 days)
- Breakthrough pain managed actively
- Food – protein drink (~60–80 g protein/day and solid food
- Mobilisation – well-defined nursing care programme (day of surgery, 2 h; postoperative days 1–3, 8 h)
- Bowel function – day of surgery start laxative and prokinetic agent
- Postoperative day 1 – remove bladder catheter in the morning
- Postoperative day 2 – remove the epidural catheter in the morning
- Postoperative day 3 – discharge after lunch

services on postoperative outcome have previously been rather restricted.[77] It is also important to involve a member of the hospital's administrative staff to facilitate and evaluate facilities and resource utilisation. Finally, an analysis of outcome is essential to success and a database should be maintained to aid this assessment. It has been proposed that anaesthetists should take a lead role in studying the impact of post-discharge symptoms and advocate best care even if it requires involvement beyond the traditional period.[78]

Key points 5 & 6

- Organisation and team delivery with strict attention to the protocols are vital to the success of a fast-track surgery programme.
- An analysis of outcome is essential to success and a database should be maintained to aid this assessment.

Fast-track surgery combines recent evidence-based advances and other new developments to combat psychological and physiological stresses to enhance postoperative recovery and outcome. As this approach becomes disseminated and is seen to be successful, it is likely that future patients will increasingly demand this style of care much as there was patient-led demand for minimal invasive surgery. Innovative approaches such as pharmacological manipulation with steroids, bbb-blockers, cytokine antagonists and anabolic agents may be incorporated into fast-track surgery to reduce stress in surgical illness and prevent associated organ dysfunction. However, future studies should also address the potential problems of stress-modifying techniques associated with special situations such as hypothermia, haemorrhage and hypovolaemia, hypoglycaemia and inflammation. Further research into peri-operative care principles such as fluid management, pain control and nutrition may allow application of a fast-track surgery programme to patients in the emergency situation and with profound disordered physiology as seen in trauma victims and those with severe sepsis. There is also a need for a large and sophisticated economic analysis if fast-track surgery is to be understood within the context of other healthcare expenditure, as there is a risk of transference of cost from the hospital to the post-discharge environment.

Further advances in technology and developments in the field of anaesthesia such as minimal invasive and procedure-specific anaesthesia may bring new perspectives to the application of a fast-track surgery programme to severely, medically-compromised patients. Future fast-track surgery may evolve into a new speciality as 'peri-operative medicine', which would allow major operations in a pain- and risk-free ambulatory or semi-ambulatory setting. However, a large clinical trial of several factors against each other and controls is needed to clarify the relative importance of various components in achieving early recovery under a fast-track surgery programme.

Key points for clinical practice

- Fast-track surgery is a multimodal, evidence-based comprehensive programme aimed at enhancing postoperative recovery and outcome by attenuating stress-related organ dysfunction.

- It is important to understand that the discharge criteria (mobile patient, pain-free on oral analgesia, complete recovery of gut and bladder functions) in fast-track surgery remain unaltered but achieved sooner.

- The modern concepts of patient education, pre-optimisation, improved anaesthesia, analgesia and surgical techniques and better understanding of peri-operative care principles with enforced early oral feeding and ambulation have led to the success of fast-track surgery.

- Published evidence confirms the benefits of fast-track surgery including reduced hospitalisation, low morbidity, cost-effectiveness, patient satisfaction and safety, with very low re-admission rates.

- Organisation and team delivery with strict attention to the protocols are vital to the success of a fast-track surgery programme.

- An analysis of outcome is essential to success and a database should be maintained to aid this assessment.

ACKNOWLEDGEMENTS

The corresponding author would like to thank Dr J Andersen, Head of the Colorectal Surgery Department at Hvidovre University Hospital, Copenhagen, Denmark for an invitation to visit the unit to study the practical aspects of fast-track surgery. Thanks also to Mr J.P. Williams, Consultant Colorectal Surgeon at University Hospital, Nottingham, UK for his strong support.

References

1. Kehlet H, Wilmore DW. Fast-track surgery. *Br J Surg* 2005; **92**: 3–4.
2. Kehlet H, Dahl JB. Anaesthesia, surgery, and challenges in post-operative recovery. *Lancet* 2003; **362**: 1921–1928.
3. Wilmore DW. From Cuthbertson to fast-track surgery: 70 years of progress in reducing stress in surgical patients. *Ann Surg* 2002; **236**: 643–648.
4. Kehlet H, Mogensen T. Hospital stay of 2 days after open sigmoidectomy with a multimodal rehabilitation programme. *Br J Surg* 1999; **86**: 227–230.
5. Basse L, Jakobsen DH, Billesbolle P, Werner M, Kehlet H. A clinical pathway to accelerated recovery. *Ann Surg* 2000; **232**: 51–57.
6. Delaney CP, Zutshi M, Senagor AJ, Remzi FM, Hammel J, Fazio VW. Prospective, randomised, controlled trial between a pathway of controlled rehabilitation with early ambulation and diet and traditional postoperative care after laparotomy and intestinal resection. *Dis Colon Rectum* 2003; **46**: 851–859.
7. Delaney CP, Fazio VW, Senagor AJ, Robinson B, Halverson A, Remzi FM. Fast track postoperative management for patients with high comorbidity undergoing complex abdominal and pelvic colorectal surgery. *Br J Surg* 2001; **88**: 1533–1538.
8. Anderson ADG, McNaught CE, McFie J, Tring I, Barker P, Mitchell CJ. Randomised clinical trial of multimodal optimisation and standard preoperative surgical care. *Br J Surg* 2003; **90**: 1497–1504.
9. Stephen AE, Berger DL. Shortened length of stay and hospital cost reduction with implementation of an accelerated clinical care pathway after elective colon resection. *Surgery* 2003; **133**: 277–282.
10. Andersen J, Kehlet H. Fast track open ileo-colic resections for Crohn's disease. *Colorectal Dis* 2005; **7**: 1–4.
11. Berry DJ, Berger RJ, Callaghan JJ *et al*. Minimal invasive total hip arthroplasty. Development, early results and a critical analysis. *J Bone Joint Surg Am* 2003; **85**: 2235–2246.
12. Brustia P, Renghi A, Gramaglia L *et al*. Mini-invasive abdominal aortic surgery. Early recovery and reduced hospitalisation after multidisciplinary approach. *J Cardiovasc Surg* 2003; **44**: 629–635.
13. Bohmer RM, Newell J, Torchiana DF. The effect of decreasing length of stay on discharge destination and readmission after coronary bypass operation. *Surgery* 2002; **132**: 10–15.
14. Kehlet H, Wilmore DW. Multimodal strategies to improve surgical outcome. *Am J Surg* 2002; **183**: 630–641.
15. Basse L, Jakobsen DH, Bardram L *et al*. Functional recovery after open versus laparoscopic colon resection. A randomised blinded study. *Ann Surg* 2005; **241**: 416–423.
16. Basse L, Thorbol JE, Lossl K, Kehlet H. Colonic surgery with accelerated rehabilitation or conventional care. *Dis Colon Rectum* 2004; **47**: 271–278.
17. Gracia-Miguel FJ, Serrano-Aguilar PG, Lopez-Bastida. Preoperative assessment. *Lancet* 2003; **362**: 1749–1757.
18. Mangano DT, Goldman L. Preoperative assessment of patients with known or suspected coronary disease. *N Engl J Med* 1995; **333**: 1750–1756.
19. Doyle RL. Assessment and modifying risk of postoperative pulmonary complications. *Chest* 1999; **115**: 77S–81S.
20. Tonnesen H, Kehlet H. Preoperative alcoholism and postoperative morbidity. *Br J Surg* 1999; **86**: 867–874.
21. Tonnesen H, Rosenberg J, Nielsen HJ *et al*. Effect of preoperative abstinence on poor postoperative outcome in alcohol misusers: a randomised controlled trial. *BMJ* 1999; **318**: 1311–1316.
22. Jackson CV. Preoperative pulmonary evaluation. *Arch Intern Med* 1988; **148**: 2120–2127.
23. Kotani H, Hashimoto H, Sessler DH *et al*. Smoking decreases alveolar macrophage function during anaesthetic and surgery. *Anaesthesiology* 2000; **2**: 1268–1277.
24. Veterans' Affair Total Parenteral Nutrition Study Group. Perioperative total parenteral nutrition in surgical patients. *N Engl J Med* 1991; **325**: 525–532.
25. Smedley F, Bowling T, James M *et al*. Randomised clinical trial of the effects of pre-operative and post-operative oral nutritional supplements on clinical course and cost of care. *Br J Surg* 2004; **91**: 983–990.

26. Nygren J, Soop M, Thorell A *et al*. Preoperative oral carbohydrates and postoperative insulin resistance. *Clin Nutr* 1999; **18**: 117–120.

27. Thorell A, Nygren J, Ljungqvist O. Insulin resistance: a marker of surgical stress. *Curr Opin Clin Nutr Metab Care* 1999; **2**: 69–78.

28. Van den Berghe G, Wouters P, Weekers F *et al*. *N Engl J Med* 2001; **345**: 1359–1367.

29. Egbert LD, Bant GE, Welch CE *et al*. Reduction of postoperative pain by encouragement and instruction of patient. *N Engl J Med* 1964; **207**: 824–827.

30. Daltroy LH, Morlino CI Eaton HM *et al*. Preoperative education for total hip and knee replacement patients. *Arthritis Care Res* 1998; **11**: 469–478.

31. Bisgaard T, Klarskov B, Rosenberg J, Kehlet H. Factors determining convalescence after uncomplicated laparoscopic cholecystectomy. *Arch Surg* 2001; **136**: 917–921.

32. Tramer MR, Moore RA, McQuay H. Omitting nitrous oxide in general anaesthesia: meta-analyses of intraoperative awareness emesis in randomised controlled trials. *Br J Anaesth* 1996; **76**: 186–193.

33. Sessler DI. Mild perioperative hypothermia. *N Engl J Med* 1997; **336**: 1730–1737.

34. Greif R, Akca O, Horn EP *et al*. Supplemental perioperative oxygen to reduce the incidence of surgical-wound infection. *N Engl J Med* 2000; **342**: 161–167.

35. Holte K, Kehlet H. Perioperative single-dose glucocorticoid administration – pathophysiological effect in clinical implications. *J Am Coll Surg* 2002; **195**: 694–711.

36. Auerbach AD, Goldman L. Beta-blockers and reduction of cardiac events in non-cardiac surgery. *JAMA* 2002; **287**: 1435–1444.

37. Redelmeier DA, Scales DC, Kopp A. Beta blockers for elective surgery in elderly patients: population based retrospective cohort study. *BMJ* 2005; **331**: 932–934.

38. Hart DW, Wolfe SE, Chinks DL *et al*. Beta-blockade and growth hormone after burn. *Ann Surg* 2002; **236**: 450–457.

39. Noble DW, Kehlet H. Risks of interrupting drug treatment before surgery. *BMJ* 2000; **321**: 719–720.

40. Carr DB, Goudas LC. Acute pain. *Lancet* 1999; **353**: 2051–2058.

41. Kehlet H, Werner M, Perkins F. Balanced analgesia: what are its advantages in postoperative pain? *Drugs* 1999; **58**: 793–797.

42. Jin F, Chung F. Multimodal analgesia for postoperative pain control. *J Clin Anaesth* 2001; **13**: 524–539.

43. Ilfeld B, Morey T, Enneking F. Continuous infraclavicular brachial plexus block for postoperative pain control at home: a randomised double blinded placebo controlled study. *Anaesthesiology* 2002; **96**: 1297–1302.

44. Ballantyne JC, Carr DB, DeFerranti S *et al*. The comparative effect of postoperative analgesic therapies on pulmonary outcome: cumulative meta-analyses of randomised controlled trials. *Anesth Analg* 1998; **86**: 598–612.

45. Rogers A, Walker N, Schug S *et al*. Reduction of postoperative mortality and morbidity with epidural or spinal anaesthesia: results from an overview of randomised trials. *BMJ* 2000; **321**: 1493–1504.

46. Rigg JRA, Jamrozik K, Myles PS *et al*. Epidural anaesthesia and analgesia and outcome of major surgery: a randomised trial. *Lancet* 2002; **359**: 1276–1282.

47. Kehlet H, Holte K. Effect of postoperative analgesia on surgical outcome. *Br J Anaesth* 2001; **87**: 62–72.

48. Slim K, Vicant E, Panis Y, Chipponi J. Meta-analyses of randomised clinical trials of colorectal surgery with or without mechanical bowel preparation. *Br J Surg* 2004; **91**: 1125–1130.

49. Grantcharov TP, Rosenberg J. Vertical compared with transverse incisions in abdominal surgery. *Eur J Surg* 2001; **167**: 260–267.

50. Kehlet H. Modification to responses to surgery by neural blockade: clinical implications. In: Cousins MJ, Bridenbaugh PO. (eds) *Neural Blockade in Clinical Anesthesia and Management of Pain*. Philadelphia, PA: Lippincott, 1998; 129–175.

51. Cheatham ML, Chapmann WC, Key SP *et al*. A meta-analysis of selective versus routine nasogastric decompression after elective laparotomy. *Ann Surg* 1995; **221**: 469–476.

52. Nelson R, Tse B, Edwards S. Systematic review of prophylactic nasogastric decompression after abdominal operations. *Br J Surg* 2005; **92**: 673–680.

53. Hoffman J, Lorentzen M. Drainage after cholecystectomy. *Br J Surg* 1985; **72**: 423–427.

54. Merad F, Yahchouchi E, Hay JM *et al*. Prophylactic abdominal drainage after elective colonic resection and suprapromonitory anastomosis: a multicentre study controlled by randomisation. *Arch Surg* 1998; **133**: 309–314.

55. Benoist S, Panis Y, Denet C *et al*. Optimal duration of urinary drainage after rectal resection: a randomised controlled trial. *Surgery* 1999; **125**: 135–141.

56. Basse L, Werner M, Kehlet H. Is urinary drainage necessary during continuous epidural analgesia after colonic resection? *Reg Anaesth Pain Med* 2000; **25**: 498–501.

57. Kehlet H. Surgical stress response: does endoscopic surgery confer an advantage? *World J Surg* 1999; **23**: 801–807.

58. Gandy CP, Kipling RM, Kennedy RH. Laparoscopic colorectal surgery. *Rec Adv Surg* 2004; **27**. 123–136.

59. Clinical Outcome of Surgical Therapy Study Group. A comparison of laparoscopically assisted and open colectomy for colon cancer. *N Engl J Med* 2004; **350**: 2050–2059.

60. Guillou P, Quirke P, Monson J *et al*. CLASICC trial: conversion versus laparoscopic assisted surgery in colorectal cancer. Tripartite Colorectal Meeting, Melbourne, 2002.

61. Lacey AM, Garcia-Valdecasas JC, Delgado S *et al*. Laparoscopic assisted colectomy versus open colectomy for treatment of non-metastatic colon cancer: a randomised trial. *Lancet* 2002; **359**: 2224–2229.

62. Motson RW. Laparoscopic surgery for colorectal cancer. *Br J Surg* 2005; **92**: 519–520.

63. Hazebroek EJ, Color Study Group. COLOR: a randomised clinical trial comparing laparoscopic and open resection for colon cancer. *Surg Endosc* 2002: **16**: 949–953.

64. Holte K, Sharrock NE, Kehlet H. Pathophysiology and clinical implications of perioperative fluid excess. *Br J Anaesth* 2002; **89**: 622–632.

65. Lobo DN, Bostock KA, Neal KR *et al*. Effect of salt and water balance on recovery of gastrointestinal function after elective colonic resection: a randomised controlled trial. *Lancet* 2002; **359**: 1812–1818.

66. Scheinhraber S, Rehm M, Sehmisch C *et al*. Rapid saline infusion produces hyperchloremic acidosis in patients undergoing gynecologic surgery. *Anesthesiology* 1999; **90**: 1265–1270.

67. Basse L, Madsen JL, Kehlet H. Normal gastrointestinal transit after colonic resection using epidural analgesia, enforced oral nutrition and laxative. *Br J Surg* 2001: **88**: 1498–1500.

68. Holte K, Kehlet H. Postoperative ileus. Progress towards effective management. *Drugs* 2002; **62**: 2603–2615.

69. Holte K, Kehlet H. Postoperative ileus: a preventable event. *Br J Surg* 2000; **87**: 1480–1493.

70. Kraus K, Fanning J. Prospective trial of early feeding and bowel stimulation after radical hysterectomy. *Am J Obstet Gynecol* 2000; **182**: 996–998.

71. Lewis JS, Egger M, Sylvester PA, Thomas S. Early enteral feeding versus nil by mouth after gastrointestinal surgery: systematic review and meta-analyses of controlled trials. *BMJ* 2001; **323**: 773–776.

72. Moore FA, Feliciano DV, Andrassy RJ *et al*. Early enteral feedings, compared with parenteral, reduces postoperative septic complications. The results of meta-analyses. *Ann Surg* 1992; **216**: 172–183.

73. Schroeder D, Gillanders L, Mahr K, Hill GL. Effects of immediate postoperative enteral nutrition on body composition, muscle function, and wound healing. *J Parenter Enteral Nutr* 1991; **15**: 376–383.

74. Soop M, Carlson GL, Hopkinson J *et al*. Randomised clinical trial of immediate enteral nutrition on metabolic responses to major colorectal surgery in an enhanced recovery protocol. *Br J Surg* 2004; **91**: 1138–1145.

75. Harper CM, Lyles YM. Physiology and complications of bed rest. *J Am Geriatr Soc* 1988; **36**: 1047–1054.

76. Waldenhausen JH, Schirmer BD. The effect of ambulation on recovery from postoperative ileus. *Ann Surg* 1990; **212**: 671–677.

77. Werner MU, Soholm L, Rotboll-Nielsen P, Kehlet H. Does an acute pain service improve postoperative outcome? *Anesth Analg* 2002; **95**: 1361–1372.

78. Miller RD. The place of research and the role of academic anaesthetists in anaesthetic departments. *Best Pract Res Clin Anaesthesiol* 2002; **16**: 353–370.

Mohammad Abu Hilal David J. Breen

6

Radiofrequency thermal ablation in the treatment of malignant tumours

In 1868, the French scientist Jaques Arsen D'Arsonval described the basic principle of radiofrequency ablation (RFA) demonstrating that an alternating electric current greater than 10 kHz could pass through living tissue without neuromuscular effect.[1] However, it was only in the late 1980s that new radiofrequency technology was developed which enabled ablation deep within the body tissues,[2] the main difference being the ability to disperse relatively mild radiofrequency energy (current flux densities) around the uninsulated probe tip within perfused tissue to produce larger volumes of ablated tissue. This deep thermal injury was first demonstrated in the liver by Rossi *et al.*[3] who proved that a thermal injury could be induced by an alternating and localized 480-kHz current in pig liver.

Since then, more studies have proved the utility and essential efficacy of RFA in treating discrete tumours in humans. Many different ablation systems have been explored, including monopolar, bipolar and multipolar electrodes, cooled-tip electrodes and expandable electrodes with multiple tines,[4-6] with the aim of improving local thermal efficacy and, thereby, oncological results.

In the last decade, this technique has been increasingly used as an alternative, or as an adjunct or bridge, to surgery and/or transplant in the treatment of liver tumours. More recently, RFA has confirmed its usefulness in the treatment of renal, adrenal, lung and other focal cancers.

This chapter will discuss the mechanism, technique, indications, and results in the most frequently treated tumours, especially in primary and metastatic liver tumours.

Mohammad Abu Hilal MD (for correspondence)
Specialist Registrar in General Surgery, Department of Surgery, University Surgical Unit, Southampton University Hospitals, Southampton SO16 6YD, UK. E-mail:abu_hlal@yahoo.com

David J. Breen MRCP FRCR
Consultant Abdominal Radiologist, Department of Radiology, Southampton University Hospitals, Southampton SO16 6YD, UK

RADIOFREQUENCY ENERGY

Radiofrequency ablation works by converting electromagnetic energy into thermal injury within the target tissue. The passage of an alternating, high-frequency, electric current around the tip of a specialised probe to a large grounding pad through tissue causes focused heat production around the uninsulated probe tip,[7] as a result of ionic agitation as charged ions follow the alternating polarity resulting in frictional heating which diffuses by conduction into the surrounding tissue. The probe itself dose not release heat and local tissue heating depends on the thermal conductivity of the tissue and the distance from the probe.[8,9] Dependent on time and tissue perfusion, coagulative necrosis occurs when the tissue is heated to a temperature

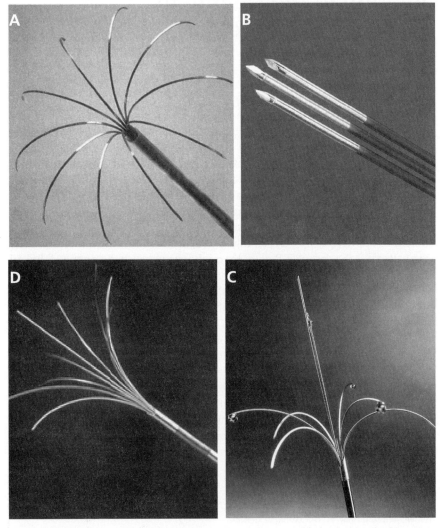

Fig. 1 Radiofrequency electrodes (clockwise from the top left). (A) 'Umbrella-shaped expansible RF electrode from Boston Scientific. This works to an impedence-regulated algorithm. (B) The 'cluster' electrode from Tyco Healthcare again working to an impedence algorithm. (C) The expansible multi-tined RF electrode 'starburst XL' from RITA Medical Systems working to a temperature-based algorithm. (D) The expanding perfused 'Xli' probe again from RITA.

greater than 60°C.[10] Heating to higher temperatures results in damage to cellular membrane, nucleus and to the whole cellular architecture. Tissue inhomogeneity, such as the presence of cysts or calcification within the tumour, can affect uniform tissue heating compromising the efficacy of the thermal ablation. The treatment can also be compromised by the presence of larger vessels (≥ 3 mm) adjacent to the targeted area which causes cooling of the perivascular parenchyma, possibly resulting in sparing of tumour which lies closely adjacent to such flowing vessels.

> ## Key point 1
> - Radiofrequency ablation works by converting electromagnetic energy into heat but its effectiveness is influenced by thermal conductivity and perfusion of the target tissue.

THE RADIOFREQUENCY DEVICE

Different instruments are currently available, with variations in electrodes and generators, but they all use the same basic principle. In our institution, we largely use a 150-W generator operating at 460 kHz manufactured by RITA Medical Systems (Mountain View, CA, USA).

The generator has a simple display with indicators for the continuous monitoring of the temperature, power and duration of the treatment. The device can be programmed to maintain a constant temperature by feedback variations in the delivered power. The current is automatically suspended when the impedance created by the treated tissue is more than 200 Ω. The system is connected to a needle electrode which has a movable hub that advances and retracts curved electrodes from its tip. Temperature detection is located at five points around the tips of the tine array. More recent modifications of these expandable probes enable perfusion of the tissue during treatment so as to improve tissue ionicity and, thereby, susceptibility to thermal ablation. The needle is 15–25 cm long and covered with a very thin layer of plastic material over its length except for the last 5 mm from where the curved electrodes exit (Fig. 1). The circuit is closed with large grounding pads positioned on the patient's skin distant from the treatment site (Fig. 2).

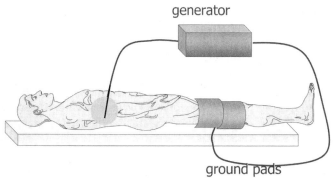

generator

ground pads

Fig. 2 The uninsulated probe top of the radiofrequency electrode forms part of a closed circuit with large area grounding pads usually placed on the patient's thighs in monopolar radiofrequency.

GUIDANCE TECHNIQUES AND APPLICATIONS

Radiofrequency thermal ablation can be performed via a percutaneous image-guided approach, laparoscopically or during open laparotomy. Improved treatment volumes have been achieved during these approaches by diminishing the overall tissue perfusion of the organ under treatment. Temporary occlusion of hepatic blood flow can be achieved by Pringle's manoeuvre at laparotomy and laparoscopy or percutaneous balloon occlusion of the hepatic artery, portal vein or hepatic vein.[6]

Percutaneous radiofrequency is the most frequently used method and can be performed under general anaesthesia or conscious sedation. It is most often performed under ultrasound guidance. However, the addition of computed tomography (CT) guidance provides more information about the position and proximity of adjacent temperature-sensitive organs. Mutiplanar assessment of probe position is essential and achievable with multislice CT or MRI.

For lung tumours, RFA is necessarily performed under CT guidance.

Surgical approaches are associated with increased morbidity, mortality and costs and they should be only used if the percutaneous approach is not possible, usually for lesions close to the bowel or in combination with laparotomy performed for the treatment of other lesions.

Key points 2 & 3

- Radiofrequency thermal ablation can be performed via a percutaneous approach, laparoscopically or during open laparotomy. The percutaneous approach offers lower mortality, morbidity and costs and should be used whenever possible.

- For liver and renal tumours, radiofrequency ablation is usually performed under ultrasound guidance. For lung tumours, the procedure is necessarily performed under computed tomography guidance.

PERCUTANEOUS RADIOFREQUENCY IN THE LIVER

Patient assessment

An out-patient assessment is performed a week before the procedure and available imaging is thoroughly reviewed. At this point, ultrasonography is performed to decide the feasibility, visibility and approach to the lesion. The patient is informed about the procedure, its risks and benefits, and consent is obtained. Baseline blood tests for platelet count, coagulation profile, liver function tests, and tumour markers are obtained as appropriate. Coagulopathy should be corrected prior to radiofrequency treatment, especially given the relatively large needle size and the possible need for multiple punctures. Conditions which may contra-indicate RFA (such as active acute infection or obstructive jaundice) should be excluded. Bilio-enteric anastomoses clearly increase the risk of liver abscess formation and represent a relative contra-indication[11] which may be obviated by post-procedural, broad-spectrum antibiotics.

Technique

Large grounding pads are placed on well-prepared skin to avoid local burning, usually on the patient's back or thigh, and connected to the generator. Patient positioning remains important to the percutaneous approach and often lumbar hyperextension or degrees of decubitus positioning can considerably facilitate the procedure. The skin is sterilised and local anaesthetic (1% lidocaine) is administered at the chosen site of needle insertion. The patient is then sedated usually with intravenous benzodiazepine and short-acting opiates, a small skin incision is made and the needle is carefully inserted under ultrasound guidance. For lesions < 3 cm in diameter, the expandable needle is positioned about one-third of the way into the tumour, and the hub is then opened to advance the curved needles under ultrasound control.

In the case of 'clustered' rigid needles (Tyco 'cool-tip' probe: Tyco Healthcare, Boulder, CO, USA), the exposed tips are simply placed across the lesion (usually 2.5–3 cm exposed tips). Multi-tined needle systems are inserted around the target at 15–20 mm intervals.

In a temperature-dependent treatment algorithm, the tines are advanced through the tumour in a step-wise fashion until a critical temperature threshold, usually ~100°C, has been reached. The whole volume target temperature is then maintained at around 100°C for 7–10 min. The whole procedure for the treatment of a 3-cm tumour takes around 15–20 min. At the end of the procedure, the lesion temperature is measured for ~20 s – the 'cool-down cycle' – and a temperature of 70°C or above is sought at this point. Probe withdrawal is with active heating of the needle tract – track ablation – so as to reduce the risk of bleeding or track seeding. The operator aims to make as few passes to the lesion as possible often carrying out staged ablations along the long axis of the tumour. Fit patients are usually discharged later the same day assuming normal post-procedural observations. Elderly patients or those who have complex treatments of larger tumours are discharged the following day.

> ## Key point 4
>
> - The ideal lesion for radiofrequency ablation using current technology is around 3 cm in diameter, not superficial and distant from large bowel and large vascular structures.

Radiological monitoring

During the radiofrequency heating process, there is considerable 'outgassing' and the resultant bubble formation causes significant obscuration of the target lesion. This gas formation has compromised intraprocedural determination of treatment adequacy by ultrasonography. It is our practice to treat more deeply set or less conspicuous lesions at the outset. More superficial lesions can be targeted later in the procedure. Alternatively, by waiting 5–8 min, there is considerable clearance of these microbubbles, improving visualisation for further treatments. If the procedure is being performed under CT guidance, intraprocedural, contrast-enhanced acquisitions can help to determine areas of subtotal treatment.

Current work suggests that magnetic resonance guidance with its multiplanar capability and techniques such as 'T1-thermometry' may be able to provide real-time temperature 'maps' and signal changes which could more effectively confirm treatment adequacy at the time of the procedure.[12,13]

Complications

All published data indicate a low mortality and complication rate for RFA. In a multicentre Italian experience of 2320 patients – about two-thirds hepatocellular carcinoma and one-third with colorectal metastases – there was a mortality of 0.25% (6/2320).[14] This reflects the safety of RFA bearing in mind the often problematic nature of the referred patients and the currently reported 1–4% mortality and 16–27% morbidity rate[15] of liver resection. In this study, the most frequent causes of mortality were faecal peritonitis due to colonic perforation and haemorrhage often from cirrhotic livers. Ablation of lesions near the hepatic flexure, especially in the presence of adhesions, may cause adjacent colonic injury and perforation several days following radiofrequency treatment.[16]

The same study reported a major complication rate for liver RFA of 2.1%. Bleeding, liver abscesses and, again, colonic perforation were the most frequently reported complications. Other, less-frequent complications were bilomas, biliary strictures, and haemothorax. To reduce the incidence of complications, caution should be used when treating lesions near the proximal bile ducts, large vessels, diaphragm and gut.

The central liver can be problematic in terms of treatment adequacy without causing biliary injury or leaving behind untreated residual tumour. Proximity to the diaphragm and gut can be problematic but techniques such as the installation of 5% dextrose under image guidance to displace adjacent temperature-sensitive viscera ('hydrodissection') have proved to be a useful adjunctive procedure.

Although radiofrequency appears to be a safe procedure, with low rates of mortality and morbidity, the indication should be always be discussed in multidisciplinary meetings and the procedure should be performed only following guidance and adequate training.

Key point 5

- Radiofrequency ablation in the liver is a safe technique with low mortality and morbidity rates, However, it should be only performed following adequate training.

Key point 6

- Caution should be taken when treating lesions near the proximal bile ducts, large vessels, diaphragm and gut to avoid possible complications such as bleeding, infection, bilomas, biliary strictures, haemothorax and colonic perforation due to heat transmission.

Radiological follow-up

As RFA is an *in situ* technique, considerable care must be taken with the post-procedural imaging and follow-up. The frequency of follow-up will be dependent on the underlying tumour biology of the treated disease. An initial post-procedural CT study is best carried out 1 week following the procedure as the area of thermal injury matures and appears more clearly defined at this stage. In the early weeks following the procedure, and frequently persisting for a few months, there is often partially increased attenuation within the treated area, felt to be related to degraded blood products. An initial unenhanced CT defines whether this is the case and ensures that the latter is not interpreted as viable enhancing disease. In the late arterial phase (30–40 s after intravenous contrast), there is often marginal enhancement around the thermal injury and frequently a subtended area of increased enhancement related to portal venular obstruction and possibly arterio-portal shunting (Fig. 3). None of these features should be misinterpreted as residual disease and tend to diminish over 4–6 weeks following the procedure.[17]

As regards RFA of colorectal metastases, CT scans are usually performed at 3, 6 and 12 months as more than 85% of recurrences are apparent within one year.[18] Depending on underlying tumour biology, CT is usually performed at 18 and 24 months and annually to 5 years. It is important to distinguish local recurrence from new, but perhaps closely related, disease. The late arterial phase is often best for appreciation of local disease recurrence. Locally recurrent colorectal disease often declares itself as an expanding radiofrequency lesion following ablation or as an eccentric nodular recurrence. Recurrent hepatocellular carcinoma on the other hand often declares itself with nodules of enhancing recurrent disease within the RFA lesion itself (Fig. 4).

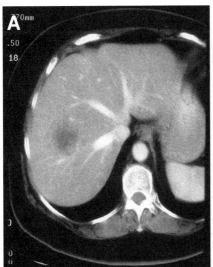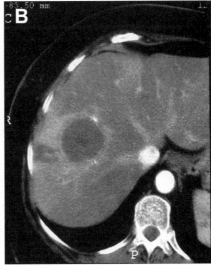

Fig. 3 (A) Right lobar colorectal metastasis prior to treatment on portal venous phase CT. (B) Arterial phase CT image following RFA demonstrates lesion ablation as shown by non-enhancement and brisk marginal enhancement at the penumbra of the treated lesion defining the thin rim of thermally-injured parenchyma. There is a subtended area of enhancement likely related to portal perfusion injury leading to arterioportal shunting.

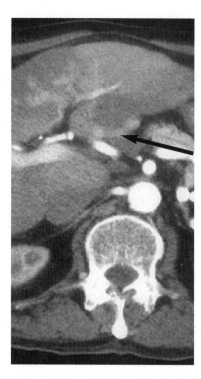

Fig. 4 A follow-up late arterial phase CT image at 6 months following RFA of a hepatoma at the posterior aspect of the left lobe of a cirrhotic liver. There is evidence of recurrent nodular enhancement at the posterior aspect of the treated lesion (arrow).

CLINICAL RESULTS OF LIVER RFA

Although radiofrequency ablation has been widely adopted, it still remains a relatively novel technique. Only recently, have large series and long-term results in the treatment of hepatocellular carcinoma, colorectal liver metastases and, to lesser extent, metastatic neuroendocrine disease been published.

The use of RFA in lung and renal cancers is more recent and long-term results are still awaited. Its role in pancreatic and breast lesions is still experimental and this remains a controversial application.

Hepatocellular carcinoma

Hepatocellular carcinoma (HCC) is one of the most commonly occurring cancers in the world.[19,20] Orthotopic liver transplantation (OLT) is the optimal treatment for paucinodular, small volume HCC in patients with favourable Child-Pugh A or B disease. This can increase 5-year survival up to 75–92%.[21–23]. However, the small donor pool and the current guidance – Milan criteria – restrict OLT to the small number of patients with solitary HCCs of a diameter less than 5 cm or three or fewer tumours with a maximum diameter of 3 cm.[23] Surgical resection is rarely feasible due to multifocality of the tumour, the grade of cirrhosis or poor synthetic liver reserve.[21,22] Furthermore, recurrence rate following resection is high.[24,25] Therefore, parenchymal-sparing alternative or complementary techniques such as RFA, percutaneous ethanol injection (PEI) and cryotherapy have evolved. RFA is able to destroy discrete nodular disease up to 4–5 cm in diameter with few complications.

Nodular hepatomas are optimally suited to RFA as they are often encapsulated, soft tumours surrounded by firm cirrhotic parenchyma which

Table 1 Clinical outcome in a randomised trial[30] of radiofrequency ablation (RFA), percutaneous ethanol injection (PEI) and percutaneous acetic acid injection (PAI) in patients with hepatocellular carcinomas ≤ 3 cm in diameter

	Local recurrence (at years)			Survival (at years)		
	1	2	3	1	2	3
RFA	10	14	14	93	81	74
PEI	16	34	34	88	66	51
PAI	14	31	31	90	67	53

increases the efficiency of the thermal ablation and, thereby, reduces the risk of local recurrence.[26] Buscarini *et al.*[27] reported complete necrosis following RFA on radiological assessment of 88 patients treated for 101 HCCs.[27] RFA was shown to be more effective than other local therapies in the treatment of unresectable liver lesions and in patients with poor liver function.[28] Compared to PEI, in a prospective, non-randomised study[29] that included 86 patients with 112 small HCCs (≤ 3 cm), the percentage of cases of complete necrosis was greater with radiofrequency (90% versus 80%); these results were obtained with lower average of sessions (1.2 versus 4.8) but a higher complication rate of 2% versus 0%. Recently, a randomised study from Taiwan[30] included 187 patients with HCCs of ≤ 3 cm and compared the outcome of three different percutaneous techniques – RFA, PEI and percutaneous acetic acid injection (PAI). RFA showed better results than PEI and PAI (Table 1). Major complications were reported for the RFA cases at 4.8%.

Although the role of RFA as an alternative treatment, when surgery is not possible, is established, its role as an alternative definitive treatment is not defined. Vivarelli *et al.*[31] retrospectively analysed their results in 158 non-randomised, cirrhotic patients, half treated surgically and half with RFA. As expected, mean hospital stay was higher following surgery (9 versus 1 day, respectively), surgery demonstrated better results in 1- and 3-year survival (83% and 65% versus 78% and 33%, respectively) and 1- and 3-year disease-free survival (79% and 50% versus 60% and 20%, respectively). The mortality for surgery was 3.8% but was not reported for RFA. The complication rate for each modality was not detailed.

Key point 7

- Radical surgical resection remains the best treatment for discrete, non-transplantable hepatocellular carcinomas in favourable patients. RFA plays an important role as an alternative treatment of primary liver lesions when surgery is not possible and has been shown to be more effective than other local therapies such as percutaneous ethanol injection and cryotherapy.

There is a real need for a large-scale, truly randomised trial to compare the results of both techniques; meanwhile, radical surgical resection remains the best treatment for discrete, non-transplantable HCC in favourable patients. It offers the best overall survival and disease-free survival with a low mortality of 5% or less in specialist centres.[32,33] RFA should be considered as the best available option when surgery is not feasible. However, the morbidity and mortality of liver resection in these difficult patients must be borne in mind and with probe development and adjuvant manoeuvres (such as chemo-embolisation and/or vascular occlusion), RFA may prove to be equally effective. The use of both treatments can be supported in specialist, multidisciplinary liver units where the choice of technique should be decided on a case-by-case basis.

Key point 8

- The nature of hepatocellular carcinoma lesions, often soft and encapsulated, surrounded by firm, cirrhotic parenchyma, helps to maintain heat within the lesion and increases the efficiency of the thermal ablation 'oven effect', thereby reducing the risk of local recurrence.

Colorectal liver metastases

Hepatic metastases from colorectal cancer represent an important health problem considering the incidence of the primary disease in the Western population. Patients with colorectal metastases suitable for surgical resection should, on current evidence, be offered surgery which, in this setting, can significantly improve the prognosis.[34] However, even using new adjuvant drugs such as oxaliplatin and irinotecan, the percentage of resectable patients is still only around 25–30%.[35,36] The majority of patients who undergo surgery will develop recurrent disease. In patients who are not suitable for surgical treatment due to co-morbidity, tumour location and inadequate parenchymal reserve or where there is recurrence after previous liver resection, the advent of image-guided ablation has been a significant step forward. It remains the case, however, that local recurrence following RFA varies from 10–40%[37,38] but is significantly lower for metastases less than 3 cm in diameter with currently available technology.

Colorectal cancer metastases tend to exhibit irregular, permeative tumour margins and occasionally microsatellites in the adjacent liver parenchyma. Hence, if the ablated area is only as large as or smaller than tumour size, local recurrence is likely to occur due to microscopic rests along the treated tumour edges. Therefore, a 'safety margin' of a least 5 mm should be obtained. The fibrotic nature of the colorectal metastases, their permeative margin and adjacent normal parenchyma, able to respond by vasodilatation to a hyperthermic stimulus, has compromised the efficacy of RFA in the treatment of larger colorectal metastases.

Intra-operative RFA plays an important role as a complement to surgical resection. It can enhance 'operability' in those patients with 'poorly' resectable tumours usually those with small, deep-set, contralateral lesions, found at pre-operative staging or on intra-operative assessment.

RFA has been compared to surgery to evaluate its potential role in resectable patients. In a non-randomised, retrospective study, Oshowo et al.[39] compared surgery and RFA in the treatment of 45 solitary colorectal liver metastases. Patients referred for RFA had been declined surgery because of extrahepatic disease, vessel contiguity and co-morbidity. The authors reported a similar median and 3-year survival for surgery and RFA of 41 months and 55.4% versus 37 months and 52.6%, respectively.[39]

More recently, the Houston group reported retrospective results in 418 non-randomised patients treated for colorectal cancer liver metastases; 190 patients were treated surgically, 101 with RFA + surgery, 57 had RFA only and, in 70 patients, chemotherapy was the only treatment.[40] The overall recurrence was most common after RFA 84% versus 64% RFA + resection versus 52% resection only ($P < 0.001$). Local recurrence was clearly higher after RFA 9% of patients versus 5% RFA + resection versus 2% resection only ($P = 0.02$). Survival at 4 years was 65% after resection versus 36% with RFA + resection and 22% following RFA only ($P < 0.0001$). The survival for 'unresectable' patients was greater when treated with RFA + resection or RFA than with chemotherapy only ($P = 0.0017$).

Therefore, RFA dose not appear to provide survival comparable to resection, but provides survival superior to other non-surgical treatments and should be always considered when surgery is not possible.

Key point 9

- RFA plays an important role in the treatment of non-resectable liver colorectal metastases and as a complement to surgical resection.

Key point 10

- The fibrotic nature of the colorectal liver metastases, surrounded by normal parenchyma may compromise the efficacy of RFA. Lesions > 3 cm in diameter are considered at significantly higher risk of local recurrence.

Neuroendocrine liver metastases

Neuroendocrine liver metastases account for almost 10% of all liver metastases.[41] Their distinct biological and clinical features render the management challenging but an on-going 'cytoreductive' approach is often worthwhile. Although neuroendocrine tumours (NETs) are slow-growing tumours and survival for as many as 41 years has been reported,[42] survival rates for patients with untreated liver metastases range from 19% to 38% at 5 years.[43] However, the quality of those survived years can be seriously compromised by endocrine syndromes and overall tumour burden.

Although surgical resection is considered the gold standard treatment, this is usually feasible in only 10% of cases[44] and most patients treated by resection with curative intent develop recurrence.[45] Repeated liver resection is rarely possible and, when feasible, carries mortality rates of up to 6%.[42]

RFA has been increasingly used alone or in combination with surgery in an attempt to improve quality of life in patients with NET liver metastases.[46]

Results have been promising in achieving destruction of numerous tumour foci with little morbidity,[47] thereby improving quality of life, survival and compounding the response to medical treatment.[48] Gillams *et al.*[49] reported their experience in a series of patients with liver metastases from NETs treated with RFA. Local control was achieved in 14 out of 19 patients (74%); the response was complete in 6 patients, partial in 7 patients and in one patient the disease was stable at a median follow-up of 21 months (range, 4–74 months). Relief or a reduction of hormone-related symptoms was achieved in 9 of 14 patients (69%) with secreting, symptomatic tumours. The median survival from the time of diagnosis of liver metastasis was 53 months. Hellman *et al.*[50] treated 43 liver neuroendocrine metastases in 21 patients (12 mid-gut carcinoids, 4 non-functional endocrine pancreatic tumours, 1 VIPoma, 1 glucagonoma, 1 gastrinoma, and 2 adrenal carcinoma). In these 21 patients, there was intention-to-cure in 14 by RFA alone or RFA plus surgery in 1. At a mean follow-up of 2.1 years (range, 3 months to 4 years), two lesions had developed signs of further growth, yielding a local recurrence rate of 4.6%. Four of the 15 patients treated with curative intent remained disease-free under follow- up.

Key point 11

- RFA alone or in combination with surgery appears to be a useful 'cytoreductive' tool which can improve neuroendocrine symptomatology from metastatic neuroendocrine tumours.

RFA IN THE TREATMENT OF RENAL TUMOURS

Renal tumours represent some 2% of all human tumours. Despite considerable research into immunotherapy and other agents, little advance has been achied in the treatment of metastatic renal cell carcinoma and only 5–10% of patients will be alive at 5 years.[51] The incidence of renal cell carcinoma has also continued to rise by 38% between 1974 and 1990.[52] Against this background, the 5-year survival rate from renal cell carcinoma has steadily improved from 37% in the 1960s to 58% between 1983 and 1989.[52] This is at least partly attributable to the improved radiological detection of early stage disease.

An increasing body of opinion has acknowledged the morbidity and mortality of radical surgery for often small and probably low-grade tumours.[53] This has paved the way for nephron-sparing surgery or partial nephrectomy.[54] However, compared with standard nephrectomy, partial nephrectomy can be a technically demanding procedure and carries its own morbidity.[55] RFA is a minimally invasive technique and may represent a useful therapeutic option (Fig. 5). In 1999, McGovern *et al.*[56] reported the first use of RFA to treat renal cell carcinoma in a patient with 3.5 cm renal lesion who refused surgery. Three months following ablation, a CT follow-up confirmed non-enhancement of the treated lesion.

To date, most reported studies of RFA for renal cell carcinoma have been in terms of safety and local efficacy although patient outcomes, with moderate cohorts, out to the mid-term are now accruing. Gervais *et al.*[57] have reported

A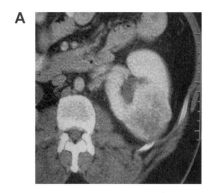

B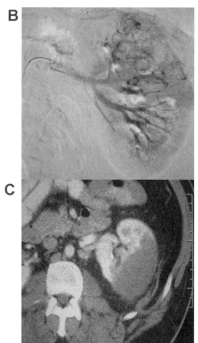

C

Fig. 5 (A) 6.5-cm interpolar renal cell carcinoma in a patient with spina bifida and stone disease and scarring of contralateral kidney. (B) Angiogram demonstrating neovascularity of the tumour prior to particulate embolisation. (C) Portal venous phase contrast enhanced CT following RFA. The tumour appears completely devascularised but, at this tumour size, careful follow-up imaging is indicated.

their experience with RFA in the treatment of 85 patients with 100 renal tumours showing that direct contiguity of tumour or zone of ablation to the collecting system did not increase the complication rate, although the obscuration of calyces by a central tumour was found to be a significant predictor of collecting system haemorrhage necessitating treatment ($P < 0.001$). In only one patient was a clinically significant urine leak reported and this was related to downstream obstruction. In addition, no bowel complications were reported despite 27 of the tumours being within 1 cm of bowel. The study showed that any residual disease was evident at 1–3 months (22/23 tumours) confirming the need for early and 6-month imaging after ablation, followed by longer intervals between imaging studies. Matsumoto *et al.*[58] reported their short-term follow-up results (1–3 years) using RFA to treat 109 small tumours (mean tumour size, 2.4 cm; range, 0.8–4.7 cm) in 91 patients. The initial ablation was successful in 107/109 tumours (98%) and two tumours were successfully retreated. Only one patient had a local recurrence during a mean follow-up of 19.4 months (range, 12–33 months) and this was successfully re-ablated so all 109 cases had no clinical or radiographic evidence of disease at last follow-up. (It is important to point out that this local recurrence occurred in a patient who had initially undergone laparoscopic cryoablation and, therefore, the RFA was a salvage attempt.)

Our own experience includes 97 tumours in 90 patients with a mean diameter of 34 mm (range, 15–68 mm) over a 6-year period, (mean follow-up, 30 months; range, 1–72 months). In 81 of 97 tumours, complete necrosis was obtained at a single sitting. Fourteen patients were retreated for viable tumour 'crescents' and, in two elderly patients with minor residual disease, a clinical decision was made not to re-treat.

Nine patients have died during follow-up. Only two patients have demonstrated metastatic renal disease. In one patient, a contralateral nephrectomy had been performed for a 7-cm tumour, 18 months earlier. A lung metastasis was noted 3 months post-RFA but may well have been related to the previous tumour. In a second case, a 67-year-old patient with Von Hippel Lindau disease had previously undergone nephrectomy and presented with four tumour foci in the remnant kidney. RFA was performed and the patient appeared disease-free for 18 months prior to the appearance of lung metastases. The metastatic disease was subsequently managed medically. In all these cases, no late local recurrence has been observed. All subtotal treatments were appreciated on the initial post-procedural study. There have been two major complications – a profuse, self-limiting haematuria and a thermal, perforating duodenal injury, which was repaired.

Key point 12

- Uro-oncological practice suggests there is a place for a minimally invasive therapy for the treatment of small volume (< 4 cm), T1a disease renal malignancy. Radiofrequency ablation under imaging guidance appears well suited to this task.

RFA IN LUNG CANCERS

Primary lung cancer is among the most commonly occurring malignancies in the world and the lungs are the second most frequent site of metastatic disease from extrathoracic cancers.[59]

Surgery is considered the treatment of choice in both lung cancer (NSCLC), which is the most frequent primary malignancy, and colorectal metastases. However, surgical treatment is not always possible due to patient co-morbidity, number and site of lesions; the mortality following lobectomy for stage Ia disease may reach 4%.[60]

Experimental studies have demonstrated the safety and effectiveness of RFA in induced malignancies of rabbit lungs.[61] Many studies have gone on to investigate its effectiveness in unresectable primary and secondary malignancies[62,63] showing excellent results in terms of lesion devascularisation. Possible complications of the procedure include pneumothorax, pleurisy/pleural effusion, haemorrhage and infection.

In 2003, Lencioni et al.[64] reported preliminary results of an on-going multicentre study including 71 patients with 117 lung primary and metastatic lesions, considered unfit for surgery and treated with RFA. The procedure was technically feasible in 70 patients (98%); major complications were pneumothorax requiring treatment ($n = 15$) and pneumonia ($n = 1$). Typically, a well-demarcated area of 'ground glass' change surrounded by a penumbral rind of injured haemorrhagic lung was seen around the ablated lesions on CT follow-up at 1 month. Forty-one patients were followed up for 6 months in whom 60 of 66 lesions (91%) showed no tumour progression. In 20 patients followed up for 1 year, CT confirmed no signs of recurrence. No difference of tumour response to ablation was observed between patients with NSCLC and those with metastases. In an international multicentre study including 493 percutaneous procedures in lung tumours, Steinke et al.[65] reported similar results.

The efficacy in this setting may be explained by the fact that solid lung tumours are surrounded by aerated lung, which provides an insulating effect, thus facilitating current flux and, thereby, thermal deposition within the tumour.

Moreover, due to the fact that central tumoural cells are normally hypoxic with reduced blood flow, they can be resistant to chemotherapy and radiotherapy. RFA may be a useful complementary treatment considering the increased sensitivity of cells to heat in the hypoxic state and the decreased heat loss due to reduced blood flow.

Key point 13

- RFA has shown to be feasible, effective and safe in the treatment of poorly resectable primary and secondary lung malignancies.

SUMMARY

Tumours in many organs are becoming smaller in size at the time of detection and characterisation. A minimally-invasive technique reducing the morbidity of resection is an increasingly attractive proposition. Ablative techniques such as radiofrequency ablation and cryotherapy are continuing to evolve and, with improved imaging guidance and radiological follow-up, look set to have a increasing role in the management of small volume tumours.

Key points for clinical practice

- Radiofrequency ablation works by converting electromagnetic energy into heat but its effectiveness is influenced by thermal conductivity and perfusion of the target tissue.

- Radiofrequency thermal ablation can be performed via a percutaneous approach, laparoscopically or during open laparotomy. The percutaneous approach offers lower mortality, morbidity and costs and should be used whenever possible.

- For liver and renal tumours, radiofrequency ablation is usually performed under ultrasound guidance. For lung tumours, the procedure is necessarily performed under computed tomography guidance.

- The ideal lesion for radiofrequency ablation using current technology is around 3 cm in diameter, not superficial and distant from large bowel and large vascular structures.

- Radiofrequency ablation in the liver is a safe technique with low mortality and morbidity rates, However, it should be only performed following adequate training.

- Caution should be taken when treating lesions near the proximal bile ducts, large vessels, diaphragm and gut to avoid possible complications such as bleeding, infection, bilomas, biliary strictures, haemothorax and colonic perforation due to heat transmission.

(continued on next page)

Key points for clinical practice *(continued)*

- Radical surgical resection remains the best treatment for discrete, non-transplantable hepatocellular carcinomas in favourable patients. RFA plays an important role as an alternative treatment of primary liver lesions when surgery is not possible and has been shown to be more effective than other local therapies such as percutaneous ethanol injection and cryotherapy.

- The nature of hepatocellular carcinoma lesions, often soft and encap-sulated, surrounded by firm, cirrhotic parenchyma, helps to maintain heat within the lesion and increases the efficiency of the thermal ablation 'oven effect', thereby reducing the risk of local recurrence.

- RFA plays an important role in the treatment of non-resectable liver colorectal metastases and as a complement to surgical resection.

- The fibrotic nature of the colorectal liver metastases, surrounded by normal parenchyma may compromise the efficacy of RFA. Lesions > 3 cm in diameter are considered at significantly higher risk of local recurrence.

- RFA alone or in combination with surgery appears to be useful 'cytoreductive' tool which can improve neuroendocrine symptomatology from metastatic neuroendocrine tumours.

- Uro-oncological practice suggests there is a place for a minimally invasive therapy for the treatment of small volume (< 4 cm), T1a disease renal malignancy. Radiofrequency ablation under imaging guidance appears well suited to this task.

- RFA has shown to be feasible, effective and safe in the treatment of poorly resectable primary and secondary lung malignancies.

References

1. D'Arsonval A. Action physiologique des courants alternatifs. *C R Soc Biol* (Paris) 1891; **43**: 283.
2. McGahan JP, Browning PD, Brock JM, Tesluk H. Hepatic ablation using radiofrequency electrocautery. *Invest Radiol* 1990; **25**: 267–270.
3. Rossi S, Fornari F, Pathies C *et al.* Thermal lesions induced by 480 kHz localized current field in guinea pig and pig liver. *Tumori* 1990; **76**: 54.
4. McGahan J, Gu WZ, Brock JM *et al.* Hepatic ablation using bipolar radiofrequency electrocautery. *Acad Radiol* 1996; **3**: 418.
5. Godelberg SN, Gazell GS, Solbiati SG *et al.* Radiofrequency tissue ablation: increased lesion diameter with a perfusion electrode. *Acad Radiol* 1996; **3**: 636.
6. Patterson EJ, Scudamore CH, Owen DA *et al.* Radiofrequency ablation of procrine liver *in vivo*: effects of blood flow and treatment time on lesion size. *Ann Surg* 1998; **227**: 559–565.
7. Siperstien AE, Gitomirski A. History and technological aspects of radiofrequency thermoablation. *Cancer J* 2000; **5**: 293–303.
8. Cosman ER, Nashold BS, Ovelman-Levitt J. Theoretical aspects of radiofrequency lesions in the dorsal root entry zone. *Neurosurgery* 1984; **15**: 945–950.
9. Organ LW. Electrophysiology principles of radiofrequency lesion making. *Appl Neurophysiol* 1996/1997; **39**: 69.
10. Corwin TS, Lindberg G, Traxer O *et al.* Laparoscopic radiofrequency thermal ablation of renal tissue with and without hilar occlusion. *J Urol* 2000; **166**: 281–284.

11. Shibata T, Yamamoto Y, Yamamoto N *et al*. Cholangitis and liver abscess after percutaneous ablation therapy for liver tumors: incidence and risk factors. *J Vasc Intervent Radiol* 2003; **14**: 1535–1542.

12. Lewin JS, Connell CF, Duerk JL *et al*. Interactive MRI-guided radiofrequency interstitial thermal ablation of abdominal tumors: clinical trial for evaluation of safety and feasibility. *J Magn Reson Imaging* 1998; **8**: 40–47.

13. Nour SG, Lewin JS. Radiofrequency thermal ablation: the role of MR imaging in guiding and monitoring therapy. *Magn Reson Imaging Clin North Am* 2005; **13**: 561–581.

14. Livraghi T, Solbiati L, Meloni MF, Gazelle GS, Halpern EF, Goldberg SN. Treatment of focal liver tumours with percutaneous radio-frequency ablation: complications encountered in a multicentre study. *Radiology* 2003; **226**: 441–451.

15. Belghiti J, Regimbeau JM, Durand F *et al*. Resection of hepatocellular carcinoma: a European experience on 328 cases. *Hepatogastroenterology*. 2002; **49**: 41–46.

16. Nicoli N, Casaril A, Abu Hilal M *et al*. A case of rapid intrahepatic dissemination of hepatocellular carcinoma after radiofrequency thermal ablation. *Am J Surg* 2004; **188**: 165–167.

17. McGahan JP, Dodd III GD. Radiofrequency ablation of the liver: current status. *AJR Am J Roentgenol* 2001; **176**: 3–16.

18. Solbiati L, Livraghi T, Goldberg SN *et al*. Percutaneous radio-frequency ablation of hepatic metastases from colorectal cancer: long-term results in 117 patients. *Radiology* 2001; **221**: 159–166.

19. Colombo M, De Franchis R, Del Ninno E *et al*. Hepatocellular carcinoma in Italian patients with cirrhosis. *N Engl J Med* 1991; **325**: 675–680.

20. Yoschizawa H. Hepatocellular carcinoma associated with hepatitis C virus infection in Japan: projection to other countries in the foreseeable future. *Oncology* 2002; **62 (Suppl 1)**: 8–17.

21. Utsunomiya T, Shimada M, Taguchi KI *et al*. Clinicopathologic features and postoperative prognosis of multicentric small hepatocellular carcinoma. *J Am Coll Surg* 2000; **190**: 331–335.

22. Pulvirenti A, Garbagnati F, Regalia J *et al*. Experience with radiofrequency ablation of small hepatocellular carcinomas before liver transplantation. *Transplant Proc* 2001; **33**: 1516–1517.

23. Mazzaferro V, Regalia E, Doci R *et al*. Liver transplantation for the treatment of small hepatocellular carcinomas in patients with cirrhosis. *N Engl J Med* 1996; **334**: 693–699.

24. Maeda T, Takenaka K, Tagichi K *et al*. Small hepatocellular carcinoma with minute satellite nodules. *Hepatogastroenterology* 2000; **47**: 1063–1066.

25. Arii S, Yamaoda Y, Futagawa S *et al*. Results of surgical and nonsurgical treatment for small-sized hepatocellular carcinomas: a retrospective and nationwide survey in Japan. The Liver Cancer Study Group of Japan. *Hepatology* 2000; **32**: 1224–1229.

26. Livraghi T, Meloni F, Goldberg SN, Lazzaroni S, Solbiati L, Gazelle GS. Hepatocellular carcinoma: radio-frequency ablation of medium and large lesions. *Radiology* 2000; **214**: 761–768.

27. Buscarini L, Buscarini E, Di Stasi M, Vallisa D, Quaretti P, Rocca A. Percutaneous radiofrequency ablation of small hepatocellular carcinoma: long-term results. *Eur Radiol* 2001; **11**: 914–921.

28. Garcea G, Lloyd TD, Aylott C *et al*. The emergent role of focal liver ablation techniques in the treatment of primary and secondary liver tumours. *Eur J Cancer* 2003; **39**: 2150–2164.

29. Livraghi T, Goldberg SN, Lazzaroni S *et al*. Small hepatocellular carcinoma treatment with radio-frequency ablation versus ethanol injection. *Radiology* 1999; **210**: 655–661.

30. Lin SM, Lin CJ, Lin CC, Hsu CW, Chen YC. Randomised controlled trial comparing percutaneous radiofrequency thermal ablation, percutaneous ethanol injection, and percutaneous acetic acid injection to treat hepatocellular carcinoma of 3 cm or less. *Gut* 2005; **54**: 1151–1156.

31. Vivarelli M, Guglielmi A, Ruzzenente A *et al*. Surgical resection versus percutaneous radiofrequency ablation in the treatment of hepatocellular carcinoma on cirrhotic liver. *Ann Surg* 2004; **240**: 102–107.

32. Matsumata T, Taketomi A, Kawahara N *et al*. Morbidity and mortality after hepatic resection in the modern era. *Hepatogastroenterology* 1995; **42**: 456–460.

33. Doci R, Gennari L, Bignami P *et al*. Morbidity and mortality after hepatic resection of metastases from colorectal cancer. *Br J Surg* 1995; **82**: 377–381.

34. Scheele J, Stangl R, Altendorf-Hofmann A. Hepatic metastases from colorectal carcinoma: impact of surgical resection on the natural history. *Br J Surg* 1990; **77**: 1241–1246.

35. Bradley AL, Chapman WC, Wright JK *et al*. Surgical experience with hepatic colorectal metastases. *Am Surg* 1999; **65**: 560–566.

36. Rees M, Plant G, Bygrave S. Late results justify resection for multiple hepatic metastases from colorectal cancer. *Br J Surg* 1997; **84**: 1136–1140.

37. Solbiati L, Livraghi T, Goldberg SN *et al*. Percutaneous radio-frequency ablation of hepatic metastases from colorectal cancer: long-term results in 117 patients. *Radiology* 2001; **221**: 159–166

38. de Baere T, Elias D, Dromain C *et al*. Radiofrequency ablation of 100 hepatic metastases with a mean follow-up of more than 1 year. *AJR Am J Roentgenol* 2000; **175**: 1619–1625.

39. Oshowo A, Gillams A, Harrison E, Lees WR, Taylor I. Comparison of resection and radiofrequency ablation for treatment of solitary colorectal liver metastases. *J Surg* 2003; **90**: 1240–1243.

40. Abdalla EK, Vauthey JN, Ellis LM *et al*. Recurrence and outcomes following hepatic resection, radiofrequency ablation, and combined resection/ablation f or colorectal liver metastases. *Ann Surg* 2004; **239**: 818–825.

41. Sutcliffe R, Maguire D, Ramage J, Rela M, Heaton N. Management of neuroendocrine liver metastases. *Am J Surg* 2004; **187**: 39–46.

42. Chamberlain RS, Canes D, Brown KT *et al*. Hepatic neuroendocrine metastases: does intervention alter outcomes? *J Am Coll Surg* 2000; **190**: 432–445.

43. Que FG, Nagorney DM, Batts KP *et al*. Hepatic resection for metastatic neuroendocrine carcinomas. *Am J Surg* 1995; **169**: 36–43.

44. Oberg K. The use of chemotherapy in the management of neuroendocrine tumours. *Endocrinol Metab Clin North Am* 1993; **22**: 941–952.

45. Que FG, Sarmiento JM, Nagorney DM. Hepatic surgery for metastatic gastrointestinal neuroendocrine tumors. *Cancer Control* 2002; **9**: 67–79.

46. Scudamore CH, Lee SI, Patterson EJ *et al*. Radiofrequency ablation followed by resection of malignant liver tumors. *Am J Surg* 1999; **177**: 411–417.

47. Sperstein AE, Rogers SJ, Hansen PD, Gitomirsky A. Laparoscopic thermal ablation of hepatic neuroendocrine tumor metastases. *Surgery* 1997; **122**: 1147–1154.

48. Chung MH, Pisegna J, Spirt M *et al*. Hepatic cytoreduction followed by a novel long-acting somatostatin analog: a paradigm for intractable neuroendocrine tumors metastatic to the liver. *Surgery* 2001; **130**: 954–962.

49. Gillams A, Cassoni A, Conway G, Lees W. Radiofrequency ablation of neuroendocrine liver metastases: the Middlesex experience. *Abdom Imaging* 2005; **30**: 435–441.

50. Hellman P, Ladjevardi S, Skogseid B, Akerstrom G, Elvin A. Radiofrequency tissue ablation using cooled tip for liver metastases of endocrine tumors. *World J Surg* 2002; **26**: 1052–1056.

51. Kosary CL, Mclaughlin JK. Kidney and renal pelvis. In: Miller BA, Ries LAG, Hankey BF *et al*. (eds) *SEER Cancer Statistics Review, 1973–1990*. Bethesda, MD: National Cancer Institute, 1993.

52. Motzer RJ, Bander NH, Nanus DM. Renal cell carcinoma. *N Engl J Med* 1996; **335**: 865–875.

53. Belldegrun A, Tsui KH, de Kernien JB, Smith RB. Efficacy of nephron-sparing surgery for renal cell carcinoma: analysis based on the new 1997 tumour-node-metastasis staging system. *J Clin Oncol* 1999; **17**: 2868–2875.

54. Uzzo RC, Novick AC. Nephron sparing surgery for renal tumors: indications, techniques and outcomes. *J Urol* 2001; **166**: 6–18.

55. Belldegrun A, Tsui KH, de Kernien JB, Smith RB. Efficacy of nephron-sparing surgery for renal cell carcinoma: analysis based on the new 1997 tumour-node-metastasis staging system. *J Clin Oncol* 1999; **17**: 2868–2875.

56. McGovern FJ, Wood BJ, Goldberg SN, Mueller PR. Radio frequency ablation of renal cell carcinoma via image guided needle electrodes. *J Urol*. 1999; **161**: 599–600.

57. Gervais DA, Arellano RS, McGovern FJ, McDougal WS, Mueller PR. Radiofrequency ablation of renal cell carcinoma: part 2, Lessons learned with ablation of 100 tumors. *AJR Am J Roentgenol* 2005; **185**: 72–80.

58. Matsumoto ED, Johnson DB, Ogan K *et al*. Short-term efficacy of temperature-based radiofrequency ablation of small renal tumors. *Urology* 2005; **65**: 877–881

59. Rusch VW. Pulmonary metastasectomy. Current indications. *Chest* 1995; **107**: 322S–331S.

60. Dowie J, Wildman M, Choosing the surgical mortality threshold for high risk patients with stage Ia non small lung cancer: insights from decision analysis. *Thorax* 2002; **57**: 3–4.

61. Miao Y, Ni Y, Bosmans H *et al*. Radiofrequency ablation for eradication of pulmonary tumor in rabbits. *J Surg Res* 2001; **99**: 265–271.

62. Steinke K, Habicht JM, Thomsen S, Soler M, Jacob AL. CT-guided radiofrequency ablation of a pulmonary metastasis followed by surgical resection. *Cardiovasc Intervent Radiol* 2002; **25**: 543–546.

63. Herrera LJ, Fernando HC, Perry Y *et al*. Radiofrequency ablation of pulmonary malignant tumors in nonsurgical candidates. *J Thorac Cardiovasc Surg* 2003; **125**: 929–937.

64. Lencioni R, Crocetti L, Glenn DW *et al*. Percutaneous radiofrequency ablation of pulmonary malignancies: a prospective, multicenter clinical trail. *Radiology* 2003: **229**: 437.

65. Steinke K, Sewell PE, Dupuy D *et al*. Pulmonary radiofrequency ablation – an international study survey. *Anticancer Res* 2004; **24**: 339–343.

Jake E.J. Krige Stephen J. Beningfield
Philip C. Bornman

7

Management strategies
in pancreatic trauma

Injuries to the pancreas are uncommon but may result in considerable morbidity and mortality due to the consequences of associated trauma and delay in diagnosis.[1-4] Prognosis is influenced by the cause and complexity of the pancreatic injury, the amount of blood lost, duration of shock, speed of resuscitation and quality and nature of surgical intervention.[5-9] Early mortality usually results from uncontrolled or massive bleeding due to associated vascular and adjacent organ injuries.[10,11] Late mortality is generally a consequence of infection or multiple organ failure. Neglect of a main pancreatic duct injury may lead to major complications including pseudocysts, fistulae, pancreatitis, sepsis and secondary haemorrhage.[1,3,12,13] Major injuries to the pancreas are among the most complex challenges a surgeon is likely to encounter. Successful treatment of complex injuries of the pancreas depends largely on initial correct assessment and appropriate treatment. This review provides a comprehensive approach to the management of pancreatic injuries.

EPIDEMIOLOGY

Traumatic injury to the pancreas is uncommon, occurring in 2–3% of severe abdominal injuries.[1,5–7,13,14] Recent data, however, reveal an increasing

Jake E.J. Krige FACS FRCS(Edin) FCS(SA) (for correspondence)
Associate Professor and Head, HPB Surgical Unit, Department of Surgery, Groote Schuur Hospital and University of Cape Town Health Sciences Faculty, Anzio Road, Observatory, 7925 Cape Town, South Africa. E-mail: jake@curie.uct.ac.za

Stephen J. Beningfield FF Rad(D) (SA)
Professor and Head, Division of Radiology, Groote Schuur Hospital and University of Cape Town Health Sciences Faculty, Anzio Road, Observatory, 7925 Cape Town, South Africa

Philip C. Bornman MMed(Surg) FCRS(Edin) FRCS(Glasg) FCS(SA)
Professor and Head, Surgical Gastroenterology Unit, Department of Surgery, Groote Schuur Hospital and University of Cape Town Health Sciences Faculty, Anzio Road, Observatory, 7925 Cape Town, South Africa

incidence of pancreatic trauma due to both high-speed automobile accidents and escalation in civil violence involving increasingly dangerous weapons.[5,6] In North American cities and South Africa, penetrating abdominal injuries from gunshot wounds are the most common cause of pancreatic trauma, while in Western Europe, England and Australia, traffic accidents predominate.[4–7,15] This geographical variation in aetiology results in considerable disparity in the reported severity and spectrum of pancreatic injuries.[6,13]

MECHANISM OF INJURY

The unique anatomical features of the pancreas influence the site and type of injury, with proximity of major vascular structures and surrounding viscera adding complexity. Leakage of pancreatic exocrine secretions due to duct disruption exacerbates the mechanical effects of direct pancreatic injury, with resultant peri-pancreatic oedema, tissue and fat necrosis.[7,8]

The nature and consequence of penetrating injuries due to gunshots depend on the type of missile and the kinetic energy of the missile. Penetrating injuries with adjacent contusions occur in single-fragment missile wounds, while severe pancreatic fragmentation is seen with shotgun wounds. High-velocity missiles may produce devastating, and often lethal, abdominal injuries.[3]

Blunt trauma to the pancreas and duodenum is usually the result of a direct blow to the epigastrium during assaults, pedestrian road traffic accidents or deceleration of the torso against an unyielding surface or steering wheel, as occurs in unrestrained drivers or passengers without a seat belt.[1,5,6] The mechanism of injury in blunt trauma depends on the magnitude and direction of the impact force and the retroperitoneal position of the pancreas closely applied to the lumbar spine.[8] Blunt, mid-line upper-abdominal trauma results in posterior compression of the anterior abdominal wall against the spine with injury to the intervening pancreas, usually in the part overlying or to the left of the portal vein and superior mesenteric vessels.[6] Impact forces concentrated to the right of the midline produce crush injuries of the pancreatic head and duodenum against the spine,[9] while those further to the left may damage the pancreatic tail and spleen.

Associated injuries

Isolated injuries to the pancreas are uncommon.[16–20] Serious associated injuries include liver lacerations and avulsions of the common bile duct and gastroduodenal, right and middle colic vessels, all of which further compound the effects of the pancreatic trauma.[3] The incidence of associated injuries ranges from 50–90%, with a mean of 3.5 organs injured.[21,22] These associated injuries cause most of the morbidity and mortality in patients with pancreatic trauma. The organs most commonly injured in association are the liver (42%), stomach (40%), major vessels (35%), thoracic viscera (31%), colon and small bowel (29%), central nervous system and spinal cord, skeleton and extremities (25%) and duodenum (18%).[1,6,7,23] Colonic injuries are more common after penetrating than blunt trauma, and increase the risk of postoperative sepsis.[6,13] Penetrating injuries also result in damage to retroperitoneal vessels in a third of patients.[7,13,21]

> **Key point 1**
>
> - Isolated injuries of the pancreas are infrequent, and the associated injuries which occur in 50–90% of patients are responsible for most of the morbidity and mortality in pancreatic trauma.

CLASSIFICATION OF INJURIES

Comparisons between various forms of treatment are often difficult to analyse as pancreatic injuries are infrequent. Experience in most centres is, therefore, limited, and there is no universally accepted classification system. Several have been proposed,[5,7] with the system initially devised by Lucas[24] the most widely used (Table 1).

Table 1 Modified Lucas classification of pancreatic injury[4,24]

Class 1	Simple superficial contusion or peripheral laceration with minimal parenchymal damage. Any portion of the pancreas can be affected, but the main pancreatic duct is intact
Class 2	Deep laceration, perforation or transection of the neck, body or tail of the pancreas, with or without pancreatic duct injury
Class 3	Severe crush, perforation or transection of the head of the pancreas, with or without ductal injury
Class 4	Combined pancreaticoduodenal injuries, subdivided into: (i) minor pancreatic injury (ii) severe pancreatic injury and duct disruption

MANAGEMENT

The principles of optimal management of pancreatic trauma include the need for early diagnosis and accurate definition of the site and extent of injury.[1,6,7,21] Serious sequelae follow if the injury is underestimated or inappropriately treated.[1,2,7] The treatment of combined injuries to the pancreas and duodenum is complex, especially where devitalised tissue and associated damage to contiguous vital structures including the bile duct, portal vein, vena cava, aorta or colon are present.[1,6,13,25] Major complications including pancreatic fistulae, pseudocysts, abscesses or haemorrhage occur in one-third of surviving patients.[1,6,8,21,26,27] Factors influencing overall mortality rates include the degree and duration of pre-operative shock, the number and magnitude of associated injuries and the location and complexity of the pancreatic injury.[7,13,16] The gravity of major pancreatic injuries and the resultant potentially serious complications necessitate a clear surgical strategy with a comprehensive and multidisciplinary approach to the management of complications.[1]

DIAGNOSIS

Delay in the diagnosis and appropriate intervention is the most important cause of increased morbidity and mortality.[1,3,4]. The retroperitoneal position of the pancreas contributes to the delay in diagnosis as clinical signs may be masked and late in onset, especially in patients with isolated injuries. Blunt trauma to the pancreas may be clinically occult, and parenchymal and duct injury may go unrecognised both during initial evaluation and subsequent surgery.[5] Awareness of this risk and recognition of the mechanism of injury should, therefore, lead to a high index of suspicion for pancreatic injury.[1,4]

Key point 2

- Delay in diagnosis and intervention causes increased morbidity and mortality in pancreatic trauma. The retroperitoneal location of the pancreas contributes to the delay in diagnosis as clinical signs may be masked and late in onset, especially with isolated injuries.

Serum amylase levels correlate poorly with the presence or absence of pancreatic trauma.[9] Amylase levels may be normal in patients with major pancreatic damage, or may be elevated when no demonstrable injury to the gland has occurred. The incidence of hyperamylasaemia in patients with proven blunt pancreatic trauma ranges from 3–75%.[28,29] Conversely, in patients with hyperamylasaemia after blunt abdominal trauma, the pancreas is found to be injured in 10–90% of patients.[28] Measuring serum amylase levels more than 3 h after blunt trauma may avoid false-negative results in pancreatic injuries, and a serially rising serum amylase level in a patient with abdominal tenderness and pain may be a better indicator of pancreatic injury.[29] Other causes for a raised serum amylase level after blunt trauma include prior alcohol intake, bowel infarction or direct injury to duodenum, stomach or small bowel.[1]

IMAGING

Plain abdominal radiographs

A plain radiograph of the abdomen may raise the suspicion of pancreatic trauma, especially when an associated duodenal injury is present. Gas bubbles in the retroperitoneum adjacent to the right psoas muscle, around the kidney or anterior to the upper lumbar vertebrae seen on frontal or cross-table radiographs, may indicate a duodenal injury.[13,21] Free intraperitoneal gas may occasionally be present. Fractures of the transverse processes of the lumbar vertebrae are collateral evidence of significant retroperitoneal trauma. Other indirect signs of pancreatic injury are displacement of the stomach or transverse colon, and a generalised 'ground-glass' appearance, due to intraperitoneal fluid.[21,24] Oral iodinated contrast may demonstrate a duodenal leak, with or without distortion of the duodenal C-loop.

Ultrasonography

Ultrasound imaging, as part of the initial assessment of trauma patients, is an effective and reliable technique for assessing the presence of free abdominal fluid, usually blood.[30–33] Focused abdominal ultrasound in trauma (FAST) has been widely used as the initial imaging modality to assess trauma patients. However, directed ultrasound evaluation to exclude pancreatic trauma is often difficult and unreliable due to associated abdominal injuries, overlying bowel gas, obesity or subcutaneous emphysema.[30,33]

Computerised tomography

Computerised tomography (CT) is well suited to the evaluation of pancreatic trauma as it is more sensitive and specific than ultrasonography.[34] The major role of CT is in haemodynamically stable patients with abdominal pain or tenderness following trauma who have a suspected pancreatic injury, and in the assessment of late complications of pancreatic trauma. An intravenous iodinated contrast bolus provides the optimal enhancement of the pancreas necessary to identify subtle fractures. The features of injury or post-traumatic pancreatitis include focal or diffuse pancreatic enlargement, oedema and infiltration of the peripancreatic soft tissues, thickening of the anterior pararenal fascia, with or without acute fluid collections in or around the pancreas.[34] Other, non-specific CT findings of pancreatic trauma include blood or fluid tracking along the mesenteric vessels, fluid in the lesser sac, fluid between the pancreas and splenic vein, or thickening of the anterior pararenal fascia.[1]

Key point 3

- Computerised tomography (CT) is the imaging investigation of choice as it is more sensitive and specific than ultrasonography in the evaluation of pancreatic trauma. The major role of CT is in haemo-dynamically stable patients with abdominal pain or tenderness following trauma who have a suspected pancreatic injury, and in the assessment of late complications of pancreatic trauma.

The features of pancreatic trauma may, however, be subtle, particularly in the immediate post-injury period and in adults with minimal retroperitoneal fat. Pancreatic contusions may appear as low-attenuations or heterogeneous focal or diffuse enlargements of the pancreas. Pancreatic lacerations may be seen as linear, irregular, low-attenuation areas within the normal parenchyma. Unless the two edges of a fracture or transected pancreas are separated by low-attenuation fluid or haematoma, the diagnosis of pancreatic transection may be difficult to recognise on CT (Fig. 1). The location of the pancreatic laceration or fracture, whether it is to the left or right of the superior mesenteric artery, and the depth of the laceration may help predict pancreatic duct disruption.[1]

Common CT pitfalls in diagnosing pancreatic injury include fluid in the lesser sac or unpacified bowel mimicking focal pancreatic enlargement or contusion, and streak artefacts or focal fatty replacement of pancreatic parenchyma simulating a pancreatic laceration.[1] Other CT findings that mimic pancreatic injury include blood or fluid tracking around the pancreas from injuries to the adjacent duodenum, spleen or left kidney, pelvic haematoma tracking superiorly in the retroperitoneum and retroperitoneal oedema from overvigorous intravenous fluid resuscitation.[1]

The ability of CT to demonstrate pancreatic injury accurately depends on the quality of the CT scanner, the technique used, including the volume and

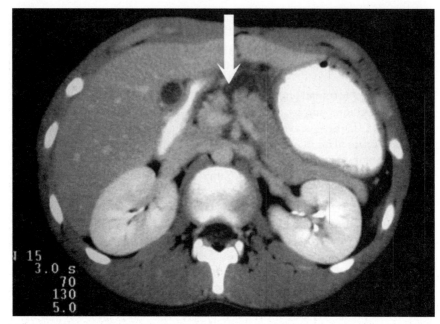

Fig. 1. CT scan showing low density fracture (arrow) at the pancreatic neck.

concentration of intravenous contrast administration, the experience of the observer and the timing of the examination in relation to the injury. The CT findings of post-traumatic pancreatitis are time-dependent and may, therefore, not be evident on scans performed soon after injury. CT is reported to have an 85% sensitivity within the first 24 h after the acute pancreatic injury, and a 90% sensitivity overall.[35] Within 12 h of a pancreatic injury, CT scans may be normal in a substantial proportion of patients due to obscured fracture planes, overlying or intervening blood or close apposition of the edges of the pancreatic injury. Repeat scanning 12–24 h after the injury may reveal an obvious injury which was initially subtle.

While the overall sensitivity of CT in detecting all grades of pancreatic injury has been estimated at 80%, major ductal injury detection is as low as 43%, even with modern imaging techniques.[33] Analysis of missed injuries suggests that CT is inaccurate in grading pancreatic injury, and often a lower grade of injury is adjudged on the CT than is found at laparotomy.[31–34].

Endoscopic retrograde cholangiopancreatography (ERCP)

Until recently, ERCP was the most accurate method of detecting pancreatic duct disruption by demonstrating extravastion of contrast from the duct (Fig. 2).[36–39] Pre-operative ERCP is seldom feasible in acute pancreatic trauma, as most patients require urgent laparotomy for bleeding or associated injuries.[5,40] ERCP in stable patients after blunt trauma to the pancreatic head or neck may also be technically difficult due to distortion of recognisable mucosal landmarks, including the papilla, caused by intramural haematoma or adjacent peripancreatic oedema.[40] The concept of intra-operative ERCP to define pancreatic duct anatomy is appealing as it avoids opening the duodenum and performing a potentially difficult operative cannulation of the

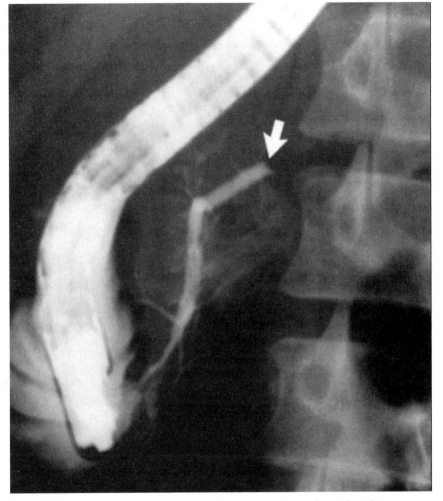

Fig. 2 ERCP showing pancreatic duct occlusion at site of injury (arrow) at the pancreatic neck.

papilla during laparotomy when a pancreatic duct injury is suspected.[41] However, even in centres with the necessary expertise, the logistical difficulties involved in performing an emergency intra-operative ERCP often outweigh the potential benefits. In addition, the patient's supine position, the need for high-quality X-ray facilities and the necessity for complete visualisation of the pancreatic duct add to the technical difficulties.

ERCP is also an invasive procedure associated with complications, including post-cannulation pancreatitis in 3% of patients. Successful completion pancreatography is operator-dependent, and failure to cannulate the ampulla or completely fill the pancreatic duct may occur in up to 10% of patients.[42] Patients with minor duct injury without leakage from the pancreatic parenchyma can be treated non-surgically.[43–46] Confirmation of major ductal injury with extravasation requires operative intervention in most patients, unless main duct continuity is present and facilities exist to place an endoscopic pancreatic stent.[43,47] ERCP has the added subsequent advantage of

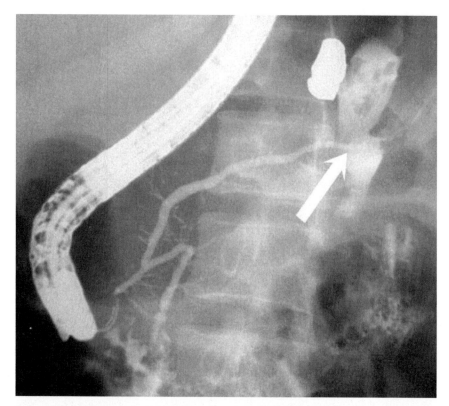

Fig. 3 ERCP via Santorini's duct demonstrating distal pancreatic fistula (arrow) after an abdominal gunshot injury.

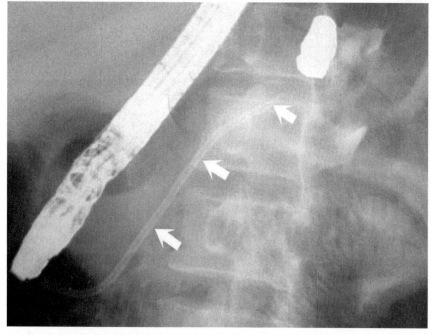

Fig. 4 Endoscopically placed pancreatic stent (arrows) to treat the fistula shown in Figure 3.

allowing endoscopic intervention with transpapillary stenting for persistent pancreatic fistulae (Figs 3 and 4)[48] or transgastric or transduodenal drainage of traumatic pancreatic pseudocysts.[12,36,49,50]

Magnetic resonance cholangiopancreatography (MRCP)

MRCP is a valuable additional imaging modality which provides a non-invasive, accurate and rapid assessment of the pancreatic duct. MRCP sequences depict the fluid-filled pancreatic and bile ducts as high-signal structures without the need for contrast material, thus avoiding the risks of ERCP-related complications.[51] MRCP findings indicating injury to the pancreatic duct include focal disruption or interruption of the duct, focal or diffuse dilation of the upstream duct (with a diameter 3 mm or greater), and communication between the duct and intrapancreatic or peripancreatic fluid collections. Unlike retrograde pancreatography, MRCP is able to provide additional useful information regarding the pancreatic duct anatomy upstream of the injury, even without ductal continuity.

The development of rapid MR imaging techniques and MR-compatible physiological monitoring and ventilation devices allows imaging to be performed on patients with acute injuries, although it may still be logistically difficult. Even though several images are required to show the pancreatic duct in various planes, scans can be completed in less than 10 min, which is an important advantage for the acutely and severely traumatised patient. Special sequences may also suppresses artefact formation from metallic objects such as surgical clips and bullet fragments.[51] Complementing MRCP with conventional MRI extends evaluation to the pancreatic parenchyma.[51]

OPERATIVE MANAGEMENT

The initial management of the patient with pancreatic trauma is similar to that of any patient with severe abdominal injury.[1,6,7] The priorities of primary management include establishing and maintaining a clear airway, urgent resuscitation, and ventilatory and circulatory support.[1–4,6,52] Venous access, blood grouping and cross-matching, volume replacement, haemoglobin concentration, white cell count, packed cell volume, urea, creatinine, electrolytes and blood gases are rapidly obtained.[6,7] The mechanism and type of injury are established while physical examination and resuscitation are in progress. In patients with blunt abdominal trauma, information should be sought regarding the mechanism of injury (*e.g.* steering wheel, bicycle or motorcycle handlebar, sports injury or assault) and the vector of force. The injury may seem trivial or innocuous and the initial clinical assessment may be misleading with scant physical signs because of the retroperitoneal location of the pancreas. A nasogastric tube and urinary catheter are essential.[10] Urgent laparotomy is required in all patients with evidence of major intraperitoneal bleeding, associated major visceral trauma or peritonitis.[1]

A long midline incision provides optimal exposure.[1,2,8] In the presence of shock and haemoperitoneum, the first priority is to identify the source of bleeding. Immediate survival is dependent upon successful control and repair of major vascular injuries.[1,2] The inaccessible retropancreatic positions of the superior mesenteric, splenic and portal veins make proximal and distal clamping or circumferential control of individual vessels impractical during massive bleeding. Rapid initial control is, therefore, best obtained by surgical packing or digital pressure.[2] Early duodenal mobilisation and bimanual compression of the bleeding site is helpful if there is suspicion of a major portal or superior mesenteric vein injury.[2] Resuscitation with red cells and blood components should continue until bleeding has been staunched and normovolaemia achieved. Attention is then directed to other priority visceral injuries before dealing with the pancreatic injury.[2]

Intra-operative evaluation of the pancreas

In most patients, the diagnosis of pancreatic injury is made at laparotomy.[1,2,17,18] Minor contusions or lacerations of the pancreatic substance do not usually require further definitive treatment, but this decision can only be made after careful local exploration to exclude a major duct injury. Determining the presence and extent of a pancreatic injury intra-operatively requires recognition of the features indicating a potential pancreatic injury, adequate exposure of the pancreas, definition of the integrity of the pancreatic parenchyma and determination of the status of the major pancreatic duct.[1,2] This may be complicated by the extent and severity of associated injuries. Gross inspection and palpation of the pancreas alone can be misleading, as retroperitoneal or subcapsular haematoma and peripancreatic oedema may mask major parenchymal and ductal injuries.[7] Clues suggesting the presence of a pancreatic injury include a lesser sac fluid collection, retroperitoneal bile-staining, and crepitus or haematoma overlying the pancreas at the base of the transverse mesocolon or visible through the gastrohepatic ligament.[14] Fat necrosis of the omentum or retroperitoneum may be present if there has been undue delay before laparotomy.[14] With these findings, complete visualisation of the gland and accurate determination of the integrity of the pancreatic duct is crucial, remembering that failure to recognise a major pancreatic duct injury is the principal cause of postoperative morbidity.

Key point 4

- Operative clues suggesting a major pancreatic injury include a lesser sac fluid collection, retroperitoneal bile staining, crepitus or haematoma overlying the pancreas at the base of the transverse mesocolon or fat necrosis of the omentum or retroperitoneum.

The lesser sac is entered through the gastrocolic omentum outside the gastroepiploic arcade[9,16] and, by retracting the transverse colon inferiorly and the stomach superiorly, exposure of the anterior surface and the superior and inferior borders of the body and tail of the pancreas is obtained.[8] Surrounding haematoma may complicate adequate assessment of the body and tail and further detailed evaluation may require division of the lateral peritoneal attachments. If necessary, the spleen, tail and body of the pancreas can be reflected forwards and medially by developing a plane between the kidney and the pancreas.[2,8] This manoeuvre allows full exposure and access for bimanual palpation of the tail and body of the pancreas. Findings which indicate an obvious main duct injury are a transected pancreas and a visible duct injury. In addition, other intra-operative features suggesting a major pancreatic duct injury include a laceration involving more than half of the width of the pancreas or a large central perforation.[7,53,54]

Intra-operative evaluation of the head of the pancreas includes assessment of the integrity of the main pancreatic duct, determining whether the pancreatic head or duodenum are devitalised, the presence and extent of duodenal injury, whether the ampulla is disrupted, if the bile duct is intact and whether a vascular injury has occurred. To provide the access for detailed inspection of the pancreatic head and uncinate process, both an extensive Kocher manoeuvre to mobilise the second part of the duodenum medially toward the superior mesenteric vessels and, if necessary, complete mobilisation at the ligament of Treitz are required.[1,55,56] Dissection and inferior reflection of the hepatic flexure of the colon and the right transverse mesocolon further improve exposure of the second portion of the duodenum and uncinate process.[4,11,55] All penetrating wounds should be traced through their entire intra-abdominal course to exclude an unsuspected pancreatic or other visceral injury.[9,11]

Key point 5

- Intra-operative evaluation of the head of the pancreas to determine the extent of injury and appropriate intervention includes assessment of the integrity of the main pancreatic duct, the presence and extent of duodenal injury, and whether the pancreatic head or duodenum is devitalised, the ampulla is disrupted, the bile duct is intact or whether a significant vascular injury has occurred.

Operative pancreatography

Several radiological methods of intra-operative evaluation of the biliary and pancreatic ducts have been recommended.[9] The easiest and most convenient is to perform a conventional operative cholangiogram through the cystic duct after removing the gall bladder or, alternatively, by inserting a 25-gauge butterfly needle into the common bile duct and injecting 10-ml full-strength iodinated contrast under fluoroscopic control. The images obtained may be useful to assess the intrapancreatic portion of the bile duct, the integrity of the ampulla and continuity of the pancreatic duct if there is fortuitous contrast reflux into the pancreatic duct. In the presence of an associated open duodenal injury, the papilla may be conveniently accessible and should be located.[1] A firm squeeze of the gallbladder helps to identify the ampullary opening by producing bile at the ampulla. A fine lacrimal probe passed through the papilla into the pancreatic duct in the neck may provide sufficient information by demonstrating the position of an intact duct to be away from the site of the parenchymal injury. A soft 5-Fr paediatric feeding tube can be used for operative pancreatography by cannulating the ampulla of Vater. Previously advised distal pancreatic resection to obtain a prograde pancreatogram is no longer acceptable because of subsequent complications. A skilled endoscopist may be of assistance in performing an intra-operative ERCP, if logistics permit.[40]

TREATMENT

CLASS 1: CONTUSIONS AND LACERATIONS WITHOUT DUCT INJURY

Of pancreatic injuries, 70% are minor and include contusions, haematomas and superficial capsular lacerations without underlying major ductal injury. Control of bleeding and simple external drainage without repair of capsular lacerations are sufficient treatment. Either a Penrose drain or a soft closed suction or sump drain can be used. A closed silastic suction drain is preferred as pancreatic secretions are then more effectively controlled, skin excoriation at the drain exit site is reduced, and bacterial colonisation is diminished.[21,54]

CLASS 2: DISTAL INJURY WITH DUCT DISRUPTION

Injury to the neck, body or tail of the pancreas with major lacerations or transections and associated pancreatic duct injury is best treated by distal pancreatectomy and splenectomy.[9,54] Optimal management of the divided pancreatic duct and the resection margin after distal pancreatectomy remain controversial. Some surgeons have advocated the use of a Roux-en-Y pancreatojejunostomy to incorporate and drain the resection margin to prevent the development of a pancreatic fistula.[6,7] Even in patients without multiple injuries, the added risk of an anastomotic leak is not warranted and this procedure, therefore, is not recommended.[9,25,53] A visible pancreatic duct at the resection margin should rather be ligated with a transfixing suture.[9] Oversewing or stapling the transected end of the pancreas and using simple methods to buttress or seal the cut margin are sufficient, and have not led to increased fistula formation.[9]

CLASS 3: PROXIMAL INJURY WITH PROBABLE DUCT DISRUPTION

Injuries to the head of the pancreas are best managed by simple external drainage. Even if there is a suspected isolated pancreatic duct injury (as may occur with a localised penetrating injury), provided there is no devitalisation and the ampulla is intact, external drainage of the injured area is often the safest option.[27,54,57–59] A controlled fistula thus created either settles spontaneously or may later require elective internal drainage after definition of the exact site of duct leakage. Techniques describing onlay Roux-en-Y loop anastomoses to incorporate an injured area in the head of the pancreas are not advisable because of the difficulty in assuring the integrity of the anastomosis in the acute situation.[6,7,9]

CLASS 4: COMBINED MAJOR PANCREATICODUODENAL INJURIES

Severe combined pancreatic head and duodenal injuries are uncommon, and usually result from gunshot wounds or blunt trauma, often with other associated intra-abdominal injuries. In determining the best option for patients with combined injuries, it is crucial to define the integrity of the common bile duct, pancreatic duct and ampulla and the viability of the duodenum. If the existing injury is in the second part of the duodenum, careful retraction of the edges of the wound or extension of the laceration in the direction of the papilla may provide adequate exposure of the papilla. As previously indicated, gentle passage of a fine lacrimal probe through the ampulla provides a convenient guide to the position of the pancreatic duct in relation to the injury.[1,2] Alternatively, a cholangiogram performed through the gallbladder, cystic or bile duct may provide the same information.[9] If there is unobstructed flow of contrast into the duodenum without extravasation, it can be assumed that the common bile duct and ampulla are intact. The presence of bile staining in the retroperitoneum or around the lower bile duct in the hepatoduodenal ligament is confirmation of bile duct injury or ampullary avulsion.[9]

If the common bile duct and ampulla are shown to be intact, the duodenal laceration is repaired and the pancreatic injury treated according to the site of the injury. As with Class 3 injuries, division or damage to the main pancreatic duct and parenchyma near the junction of head and neck are optimally managed by resection of the neck, body and tail. Penetrating injury in the pancreatic head without devitalisation is best treated by careful drainage of the area. Localised ischaemia at the site of the duodenal injury should be debrided before primary duodenal closure. If there is concern about the integrity of the duodenum, decompression using a carefully placed nasogastric tube in the duodenal loop is useful.[1,2]

With a severe injury to the duodenum in association with a lesser pancreatic head injury, some authors advise diversion of gastric and biliary contents away from the duodenal repair. Several complex and innovative techniques have been described to deal with this situation, including diversion by a duodenal 'diverticulisation' procedure with primary closure of the duodenal wound, a vagotomy, an antrectomy with an end-to-side gastrojejunostomy, a T-tube common bile duct drainage, and a tube duodenostomy.[59] The aim is to convert a potentially uncontrolled lateral duodenal fistula into a controlled end-fistula by diversion of gastric and biliary contents away from the duodenal injury, while making provision for early enteral nutrition via a gastrojejunostomy. An alternative option avoiding a vagotomy and antrectomy is the 'pyloric exclusion' procedure.[60] The pylorus is closed with an absorbable suture performed through a gastrotomy, and a side-to-side gastrojejunostomy provides temporary diversion of gastric flow away from the duodenum while the duodenal and pancreatic injuries heal. The pylorus opens when the sutures dissolve 3 or 4 weeks later, or the sutures can be removed endoscopically after an intact duodenum has been confirmed. In a small number of selected patients, pyloric exclusion has proved useful in managing severe duodenal injuries combined with pancreatic head injuries in which a Whipple procedure is not justified.[57] We believe, however, that the same objectives can be achieved by less complex procedures and, in this situation, we use primary duodenal closure, external catheter drainage near the site of the repair, a diverting gastrojejunostomy without closure of the pylorus and a fine-bore silastic nasojejunal feeding tube.[1-3]

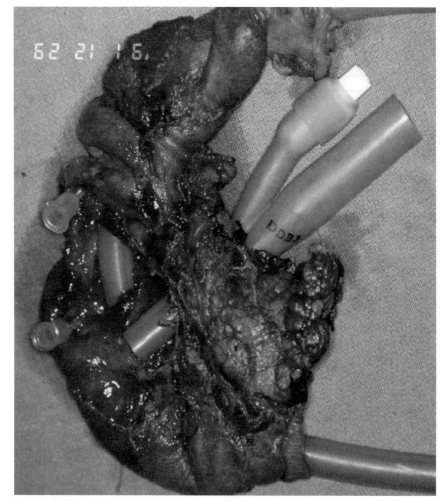

Fig. 5 Pancreaticoduodenectomy specimen showing disruption of the ampulla and duodenum.

Pancreaticoduodenectomy

Reconstruction may not be possible in some combined injuries of the proximal duodenum and head of the pancreas with extensive tissue devitalisation, with complete disruption of the ampulla involving the proximal pancreatic duct and distal common bile duct, or avulsion of the duodenum from the pancreas.[2,56,61,62] In these situations, the only rational option is resection (Fig. 5). Pancreaticoduodenectomy has the advantage of removing all injured tissue and allows reconstruction of the digestive tract and preservation of pancreatic function. The decision to resort to pancreaticoduodenectomy is based upon the extent of the pancreatic injury, the size and vascular status of any duodenal injury, the integrity of the distal common duct and ampulla of Vater, the status of the major peripancreatic vascular structures and the experience of the surgeon. Specific indications that have been proposed for pancreatico-duodenectomy for trauma are: (i) extensive devitalisation of the head of the pancreas and duodenum so that reconstruction is not possible; (ii) ductal disruption of the pancreatic head in association with injuries to the duodenum and distal common bile duct; (iii) injury to the ampulla of Vater, with disruption of the main pancreatic duct from the duodenum; (iv) uncontrollable bleeding from vessels in the head of the pancreas; and (v) inaccessible exsanguinating retropancreatic portal or superior mesenteric vein injury.[61,63,64]

Key point 6

- Pancreaticoduodenectomy may be required in a small group of patients with maximal combined injuries of the duodenum and head of the pancreas with extensive tissue devitalisation, or in those with complete disruption of the ampulla involving the proximal pancreatic duct and distal common bile duct, or avulsion of the duodenum from the pancreas.

Emergency pancreaticoduodenectomy for trauma is similar to the elective operation, but with appropriate modifications if the patient is hypotensive with active bleeding from the pancreas. In situations where there is exsanguinating bleeding due to an injury to the retropancreatic portal mesenteric venous system, the steps of the procedure change and are directed to accelerated exposure and control of the site of bleeding.[65] The duodenum and head of the pancreas are rapidly mobilised medially by the Kocher manoeuvre and the portal mesenteric venous system is compressed manually between the thumb on the anterior aspect of the pancreas and the second and third fingers inserted behind the head of the pancreas.[2] While the first assistant controls the bleeding by compression in this manner, the lesser sac is opened, the stomach is retracted superiorly, the hepatic flexure of the colon mobilised inferiorly, the superior mesenteric vein identified inferior to the neck of the pancreas and the portal vein identified superiorly.[2] The neck of the pancreas is divided to gain direct access to the region of the injury. Once exposure of the portal-mesenteric-splenic venous confluence has been achieved, the vascular injuries are identified and repaired.[65]

Associated inferior vena caval lacerations are best repaired by direct suture techniques. It may be possible to repair the vena cava both anteriorly and posteriorly without mobilising and clamping the cava above or below the injury. Digital or stick-sponge pressure applied superior and inferior to the rent usually controls bleeding while the defects are closed. A small posterior caval defect often can be sutured through a larger anterior rent, without rotating the vessel. This is especially helpful when the wound in the vena cava is at the level of the renal veins. If a posterior rent cannot be visualised in this area, the right kidney is mobilised, elevated and rotated medially, exposing the junction of right renal vein and vena cava.[66]

Pancreaticoduodenectomy may be necessary in 1–2% of isolated pancreatic injuries and in up to 10% of combined pancreaticoduodenal injuries.[65–72] The need for resection is usually obvious at first sight when there is massive destruction with gross devitalisation of the duodenum, or pancreatobiliary, duodenal and ampullary disruption is present. Blunt trauma may result in a

Table 2 Pancreaticoduodenectomy for trauma

		Patients (n)	Deaths	Mortality
Yellin[65]	1975	10	6	60%
Oreskovich[68]	1984	10	0	0%
Jones[16]	1985	12	7	58%
Feliciano[23]	1987	13	6	46%
Asensio[56]	2003	18	6	33%
Krige[72]	2005	17	3	17%
Overall		80	28	35%

near-complete *de facto* pancreaticoduodenectomy. Technical problems in the reconstruction of pancreatic and biliary anastomoses may arise due to the small size of the undilated ducts and jejunal oedema. The parenchyma of the pancreatic remnant is also frequently swollen if there has been a delay between the injury and the operation, and the pancreatic duct may be small or obscured if posteriorly located in the gland. Invagination of the end of the pancreas into a Roux-en-Y jejunal loop has been the most widely used pancreatic-enteric anastomosis. Pancreatogastrostomy has also been used in this situation, with minimal morbidity.[72] Biliary-enteric continuity is commonly restored by means of a side-to-side hepaticojejunostomy, using the high bile duct reconstruction technique with preplaced sutures. In desperate situations with a minute common bile duct, the gall bladder can be used for the anastomosis, after ligating the bile duct below the cystic duct insertion. Since major vascular injuries are frequent, massive blood loss, coagulopathy and hypothermia are often present at the time the pancreatic repair is undertaken. In the six largest series, overall mortality was 35% (Table 2).

In unstable patients with serious associated injuries, simple controlled drainage and delayed reconstruction may be the most judicious procedure.[73–75] Damage control surgery is advised in patients with haemodynamic instability despite full resuscitation, clinical or proven coagulopathy, hypothermia, associated complex and other major multiple visceral injuries, severe metabolic acidosis and intra-operative blood transfusion exceeding 10 units of packed red blood cells.[76–79]

POSTOPERATIVE CARE

The principles of postoperative care in patients undergoing resection for complex pancreatic injuries are similar to those in patients with other major abdominal injuries.[1] Attention is paid to ventilatory status, fluid balance, renal function, intestinal ileus and nasogastric tube losses. Meticulous charting of drain content and volume are important. Prolonged ileus and pancreatic complications may preclude normal oral intake in severely injured patients. The standard composition of regular tube feeds increases pancreatic secretions. The low-fat and higher pH (4.5) formulation of an elemental diet is less stimulating to the pancreas, and should be attempted before instituting parenteral nutrition. A catheter jejunostomy placed using a submucosal needle technique or a fine bore silastic nasogastric tube with a weighted tip placed at the initial operation in complex pancreatic injuries allows the option of early postoperative enteral feeding, rather than total parenteral nutrition. The enteral route is more efficient for nitrogen utilisation and may better restore immune competence, as well as being cheaper with less morbidity.[1]

COMPLICATIONS

The most common specific complication following pancreatic injury is a pancreatic fistula.[4,80–83] This occurs in 10–20% of major injuries to the pancreas. Most fistulae are minor and resolve spontaneously within 1 or 2 weeks of injury, provided adequate external drainage has been established. High-output fistulae (> 700 ml/day) usually indicate major pancreatic duct disruption and can be confirmed by measuring amylase levels. A sinogram is then useful to define the site of the fistula, as well as aid in the planning of further treatment if a high-output fistula fails to progressively decrease in volume or persists for longer than 10 days. Supplementary nutritional support is standard management, but the role of somatostatin and octreotide is unproven. Persistent fistulae require endoscopic pancreatography and transpapillary stent insertion, or, if this fails, operative intervention with distal pancreatic resection for leaks in the pancreatic tail or a Roux-en-Y cystjejunostomy for proximal leaks.[1]

Key point 7

- A pancreatic fistula is the most common complication after pancreatic injury and occurs in 10–20% of major injuries. Most fistulas are minor and resolve spontaneously within 1 or 2 weeks of injury, provided adequate external drainage has been established.

Peripancreatic, subhepatic and subphrenic fluid collections are commonly seen on ultrasonography or CT after pancreatic trauma.[84–86] An infected collection should be suspected in any patient who develops an elevated temperature, raised white cell count, prolonged ileus or unexplained upper abdominal tenderness postoperatively (Fig. 6). Ultrasonography or CT scan are necessary to confirm the diagnosis. Clinical evidence of intra-abdominal sepsis mandates guided needle aspiration to obtain fluid for bacteriology and amylase content. Empirical broad spectrum parenteral antibiotic therapy should be instituted to cover the full bacterial spectrum until definitive culture results become available. Percutaneous aspiration or catheter drainage is usually effective in patients with accessible unilocular collections and no evidence of pancreatic necrosis.

The presence of necrotic pancreatic tissue generally mandates surgery with debridement of non-viable tissue and generous external catheter drainage, although percutaneous insertion of large-bore drainage catheters may be beneficial in selected cases. Secondary haemorrhage from the pancreatic bed or surrounding vessels as a consequence of infected devitalised tissue and retroperitoneal autodigestion from uncontrolled pancreatic drainage is an uncommon, but formidable, complication after pancreatic trauma. If control cannot be obtained by angiographic embolisation, operative exposure, careful suture-ligation of vessels and packing with abdominal swabs may be life-saving.[1,2]

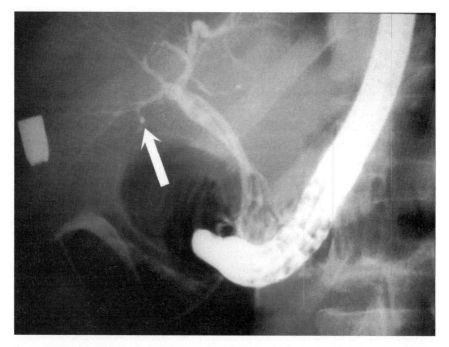

Fig. 6 ERCP after Whipple's resection showing small residual intrahepatic bile leak (arrow) due to bullet injury.

Pseudocysts after abdominal trauma may occur as a result of undetected pancreatic duct disruption with continued leakage of pancreatic enzymes and may present weeks or months after the original pancreatic injury (Fig. 7).[12,80,81,87] Surgical strategy in the management of traumatic pseudocysts will depend on the site and nature of the duct injury, the maturity and thickness of the cyst wall, proximity to stomach or duodenum and the clinical urgency.[87] If the pseudocyst is symptomatic or enlarging in size, MRCP or ERCP provide accurate anatomical delineation of the duct injury. If there is minimal communication with a side-duct or if the leak involves the distal duct, percutaneous ultrasound-guided aspiration should be attempted initially.[26] Pseudocysts with proximal major duct injury should be drained endoscopically[24] if there is adequate juxtaposition with stomach or duodenum and if there is a visible intraluminal bulge endoscopically and a thin interposing wall (< 10 mm) on imaging.[49,50] If endoscopic drainage is not feasible, internal surgical drainage as a cystgastrostomy, cystduodenostomy or cystjejunostomy is required.[12]

CONCLUSIONS

Most pancreatic injuries are minor and can be treated by external drainage.[5] The commonest major injury is a prevertebral laceration of the proximal body or neck of the pancreas which requires a distal pancreatectomy.[5,21] Major fractures to the right of the portal vein with an intact bile duct are similarly best treated by distal resection. Pancreaticoduodenectomy is reserved for severe injuries to the head of pancreas and duodenum in which salvage or reconstruction is not feasible.[2] All procedures should include effective

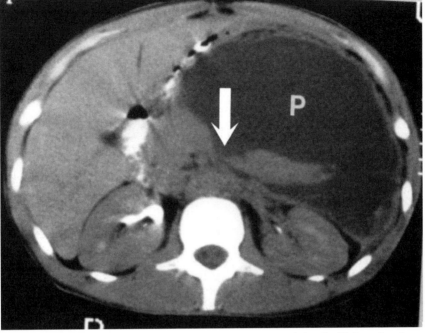

Fig. 7 CT scan of pancreatic pseudocyst (P) following blunt abdominal injury showing pancreatic fracture (arrow) over vertebral column.

drainage of the pancreatic injury. The trend to increasingly conservative surgery for most pancreatic injuries without elaborate enteric anastomoses or obligatory intra-operative pancreatography represents a simplification of past methods and allows preservation of pancreatic tissue without increasing morbidity.[5] With careful assessment of the injury by inspection, pancreatic complications can be reduced without the need for complex resections, enteric diversions and pancreaticoenteric anastomoses.[4,82,86]

Key points for clinical practice

- Isolated injuries of the pancreas are infrequent, and the associated injuries which occur in 50–90% of patients are responsible for most of the morbidity and mortality in pancreatic trauma.

- Delay in diagnosis and intervention causes increased morbidity and mortality in pancreatic trauma. The retroperitoneal location of the pancreas contributes to the delay in diagnosis as clinical signs may be masked and late in onset, especially with isolated injuries.

- Computerised tomography (CT) is the imaging investigation of choice as it is more sensitive and specific than ultrasonography in the evaluation of pancreatic trauma. The major role of CT is in haemodynamically stable patients with abdominal pain or tenderness following trauma who have a suspected pancreatic injury, and in the assessment of late complications of pancreatic trauma.

(continued on next page)

Key points for clinical practice *(continued)*

- Operative clues suggesting a major pancreatic injury include a lesser sac fluid collection, retroperitoneal bile staining, crepitus or haematoma overlying the pancreas at the base of the transverse mesocolon or fat necrosis of the omentum or retroperitoneum.

- Intra-operative evaluation of the head of the pancreas to determine the extent of injury and appropriate intervention includes assessment of the integrity of the main pancreatic duct, the presence and extent of duodenal injury, and whether the pancreatic head or duodenum is devitalised, the ampulla is disrupted, the bile duct is intact or whether a significant vascular injury has occurred.

- Pancreaticoduodenectomy may be required in a small group of patients with maximal combined injuries of the duodenum and head of the pancreas with extensive tissue devitalisation, or in those with complete disruption of the ampulla involving the proximal pancreatic duct and distal common

- A pancreatic fistula is the most common complication after pancreatic injury and occurs in 10–20% of major injuries. Most fistulas are minor and resolve spontaneously within 1 or 2 weeks of injury, provided adequate external drainage has been established.

References

1. Krige JEJ, Bornman PC, Beningfield SJ, Funnell IC. Pancreatic trauma. In: Pitt H, Carr-Locke D, Ferrucci J. (eds) *Hepatobiliary and pancreatic disease*. Philadelphia, PA: Little Brown, 1995; 421–435.
2. Krige JEJ, Bornman PC, Terblanche J. The role of pancreatoduodenectomy in the management of complex pancreatic trauma. In: Hanyu F, Takasaki K. (eds) *Pancreatoduodenectomy*. Tokyo: Springer, 1997; 49–62.
3. Krige JEJ. Pancreatic trauma. In: Nicol AJ, Steyn E. (eds). *Handbook of Trauma*. Cape Town: Oxford University Press, 2004; 258–265.
4. Farrell RJ, Krige JEJ, Bornman PC, Knottenbelt JD, Terblanche J. Operative strategies in pancreatic trauma. *Br J Surg* 1996; **83**: 934–937.
5. Chrysos E, Athanasakis E, Xynos E. Pancreatic trauma in the adult: current knowledge in diagnosis and management. *Pancreatology* 2002; **2**: 365–378.
6. Wilson RH, Moorehead RJ. Current management of trauma to the pancreas. *Br J Surg* 1991; **78**: 1196–1202.
7. Frey CF, Wardell JW. Injuries to the pancreas. In: Trede M, Carter DC. (eds) *Surgery of the pancreas*. Edinburgh: Churchill Livingstone, 1993; 565–589.
8. Smego DR, Richardson JD, Flint LM. Determinants of outcome in pancreatic trauma. *J Trauma* 1985; **25**: 771–776.
9. Patton Jr JH, Fabian TC. Complex pancreatic injuries. *Surg Clin North Am* 1996; **76**: 783–795.
10. Bradley 3rd EL, Young Jr PR, Chang MC *et al*. Diagnosis and initial management of blunt pancreatic trauma: guidelines from a multiinstitutional review. *Ann Surg* 1998; **227**: 861–869.
11. Jurkovich GJ, Carrico CJ. Pancreatic trauma. *Surg Clin North Am* 1990; **70**: 575–593.

12. Lewis G, Krige JEJ, Bornman PC, Terblanche J. Traumatic pancreatic pseudocysts. *Br J Surg* 1993; **80**: 89–93.

13. Glancy KE. Review of pancreatic trauma. *Western J Med* 1989; **151**: 45–51.

14. Olah A, Isselkutz A, Haulik L, Makay R. Pancreatic transection from blunt abdominal trauma: early versus delayed diagnosis and surgical management. *Dig Surg* 2003; **20**: 408–414.

15. Fleming WR, Collier NA, Banting SW. Pancreatic trauma: Universities of Melbourne HPB Group. *Aust NZ J Surg* 1999; **69**: 357–362.

16. Jones RC. Management of pancreatic trauma. *Am J Surg* 1985; **150**: 698–704.

17. Young Jr PR, Meredith JW, Baker CC, Thomason MH, Chang MC. Pancreatic injuries resulting from penetrating trauma: a multi-institution review. *Am Surg* 1998; **64**: 838–843, discussion 843–844.

18. Timberlake GA. Blunt pancreatic trauma: experience at a rural referral center. *Am Surg* 1997; **63**: 282–286.

19. Akhrass R, Yaffe MB, Brandt CP, Reigle M, Fallon Jr WF, Malangoni MA. Pancreatic trauma: a ten-year multi-institutional experience. *Am Surg* 1997; **63**: 598–604.

20. Vasquez JC, Coimbra R, Hoyt DB, Fortlage D. Management of penetrating pancreatic trauma: an 11-year experience of a level-1 trauma center. *Injury* 2001; **32**: 753–759.

21. Jurkovich GJ, Carrico CJ. Pancreatic trauma. *Surg Clin North Am* 1990; **70**: 575–593.

22. Stone HH, Fabian TC, Satiani B, Turkleson ML. Experiences in the management of pancreatic trauma. *J Trauma* 1981; **21**: 257–262.

23. Feliciano DV, Martin TD, Cruse PA *et al.* Management of combined pancreatoduodenal injuries. *Ann Surg* 1987; **205**: 673–680.

24. Lucas CE. Diagnosis and treatment of pancreatic and duodenal injury. *Surg Clin North Am* 1977; **57**: 49–65.

25. Cogbill TH, Moore EE, Kashuk JL. Changing trends in the management of pancreatic trauma. *Arch Surg* 1982; **117**: 722–728.

26. Funnell IC, Bornman PC, Krige JEJ, Beningfield SJ, Terblanche J. Endoscopic drainage of traumatic pancreatic pseudocysts. *Br J Surg* 1994; **81**: 879–881.

27. Wisner DH, Wold RL, Frey CF. Diagnosis and treatment of pancreatic injuries. An analysis of management principles. *Arch Surg* 1990; **125**: 1109–1113.

28. Bouwman DL, Weaver DW, Walt AJ. Serum amylase and its isoenzymes: a clarification of their implications in trauma. *J Trauma* 1984; **24**: 573–578.

29. Takishima T, Sugimoto K, Hirata M, Asari Y, Ohwada T, Kakita A. Serum amylase level on admission in the diagnosis of blunt injury to the pancreas: its significance and limitations. *Ann Surg* 1997; **226**: 70–76.

30. McKenney KL. Ultrasound of blunt abdominal trauma. *Radiol Clin North Am* 1999; **37**: 879–893.

31. Weishaupt D, Grozaj AM, Willmann JK, Roos JE, Hilfiker PR, Marincek B. Traumatic injuries: imaging of abdominal and pelvic injuries. *Eur Radiol* 2002; **12**: 1295–1311.

32. Gupta A, Stuhlfaut JW, Fleming KW, Lucey BC, Soto JA. Blunt trauma of the pancreas and biliary tract: a multimodality imaging approach to diagnosis. *Radiographics* 2004; **24**: 1381–1395.

33. Cirillo Jr RL, Koniaris LG. Detecting blunt pancreatic injuries. *J Gastrointest Surg* 2002; **6**: 587–598.

34. Mullinix AJ, Foley WD. Multidetector computed tomography and blunt thoracoabdominal trauma. *J Comput Assist Tomogr* 2004; **28**: 20–27.

35. Patel SV, Spencer JA, el-Hasani S, Sheridan MB. Imaging of pancreatic trauma. *Br J Radiol* 1998; **71**: 985–990.

36. Funnell IC, Bornman PC, Krige JEJ, Beningfield SJ, Terblanche J. Endoscopic drainage of traumatic pancreatic pseudocyst. *Br J Surg* 1994; **81**: 879–881.

37. Wind P, Tiret E, Cunningham C, Frileux P, Cugnenc PH, Parc R. Contribution of endoscopic retrograde pancreatography in management of complications following distal pancreatic trauma. *Am Surg* 1999; **65**: 777–783.

38. Harrell DJ, Vitale GC, Larson GM. Selective role for endoscopic retrograde cholangiopancreatography in abdominal trauma. *Surg Endosc* 1998; **12**: 400–404.

39. Chandler C, Waxman K. Demonstration of pancreatic ductal integrity by endoscopic retrograde pancreatography allows conservative surgical management. *J Trauma* 1996; **40**: 466–468.

40. Sugawa C, Lucas CE. The case for preoperative and intraoperative ERCP in pancreatic trauma. *Gastrointest Endosc* 1988; **34**: 145–147.

41. Blind PJ, Mellbring G, Hjertkvist M, Sandzen B. Diagnosis of traumatic pancreatic duct rupture by on-table endoscopic retrograde pancreatography. *Pancreas* 1994; **9**: 387–389.

42. Whittwell AE, Gomez GA, Byers P, Kreis Jr DJ, Manten H, Casillas VJ. Blunt pancreatic trauma: prospective evaluation of early endoscopic retrograde pancreatography. *South Med J* 1989; **82**: 586–591.

43. Takishima T, Hirata M, Kataoka Y *et al.* Pancreatographic classification of pancreatic ductal injuries caused by blunt injury to the pancreas. *J Trauma* 2000; **48**: 745–751, discussion 751–752.

44. Kim HS, Lee DK, Kim IW *et al.* The role of endoscopic retrograde pancreatography in the treatment of traumatic pancreatic duct injury. *Gastrointest Endosc* 2001; **54**: 49–55.

45. Hayward SR, Lucas CE, Sugawa C, Ledgerwood AM. Emergent endoscopic retrograde cholangiopancreatography. A highly specific test for acute pancreatic trauma. *Arch Surg* 1989; **124**: 745–746.

46. Clements RH, Reisser JR. Urgent endoscopic retrograde pancreatography the stable trauma patient. *Am Surg* 1996; **62**: 446–448.

47. Takishima T, Horiike S, Sugimoto K *et al.* Role of repeat computed tomography after emergency endoscopic retrograde pancreatography in the diagnosis of traumatic injury to pancreatic ducts. *J Trauma* 1996; **40**: 253–257.

48. Kim HS, Lee DK, Kim IW *et al.* The role of endoscopic retrograde pancreatography in the treatment of traumatic pancreatic duct injury. *Gastrointest Endosc* 2001; **54**: 49–55.

49. Beckingham IJ, Krige JEJ, Bornman PC, Terblanche J. Endoscopic management of pancreatic pseudocysts. *Br J Surg* 1997; **84**: 1638–1645.

50. Beckingham IJ, Krige JEJ, Bornman PC, Terblanche J. Long-term outcome of endoscopic drainage of pancreatic pseudocysts. *Am J Gastroenterol* 1999; **94**: 71–74.

51. Fulcher AS, Turner MA, Yelon JA *et al.* Magnetic resonance cholangiopancreatography (MRCP) in the assessment of pancreatic duct trauma and its sequelae: preliminary findings. *J Trauma* 2000; **48**: 1001–1007.

52. Sawyers JL, Carlisle BB, Sawyers JE. Management of pancreatic injuries. *South Med J* 1967; **60**: 382–386.

53. Heitsch RC, Knutson CO, Fulton RL, Jones CE. Delineation of critical factors in the treatment of pancreatic trauma surgery. *Surgery* 1976; **80**: 523–529.

54. Patton Jr JH, Lyden SP, Croce MA *et al.* Pancreatic trauma: a simplified management guideline. *J Trauma* 1997; **43**: 234–239.

55. Asensio JA, Demetriades D, Berne JD *et al.* A unified approach to the surgical exposure of pancreatic and duodenal injuries. *Am J Surg* 1997; **174**: 54–60.

56. Asensio JA, Petrone P, Roldan G, Kuncir E, Demetriades D. Pancreaticoduodenectomy: a rare procedure for the management of complex pancreaticoduodenal injuries. *J Am Coll Surg* 2003; **197**: 937–942.

57. Degiannis E, Levy RD, Velmahos GC, Potokar T, Florizoone MG, Saadia R. Gunshot injuries of the head of the pancreas: conservative approach. *World J Surg* 1996; **20**: 68–71.

58. Johnson CD. Pancreatic trauma. In: Taylor I, Johnson CD. (eds) *Recent Advances in Surgery*. Edinburgh: Churchill Livingstone, 1997; 57–68.

59. Berne CJ, Donovan AJ, White EJ, Yellin AE. Duodenal 'diverticulization' for duodenal and pancreatic injury. *Am J Surg* 1974; **127**: 503–507.

60. Vaughan GD, Frazier OH, Graham DY, Mattox KL, Petmecky FF, Jordan Jr GL. The use of pyloric exclusion in the management of severe duodenal injuries. *Am J Surg* 1977; **134**: 785–790.

61. Feliciano DV, Martin TD, Cruse PA *et al.* Management of combined pancreatoduodenal injuries. *Ann Surg* 1987; **205**: 673–680.

62. Koniaris LG. Role of pancreatectomy after severe pancreaticoduodenal trauma. *J Am Coll Surg* 2004; **198**: 677–678.

63. Bach RD, Frey CF. Diagnosis and treatment of pancreatic trauma. *Am J Surg* 1971; **121**: 20–29.

64. Lowe RJ, Saletta JD, Moss GS. Pancreaticoduodenectomy for penetrating pancreatic trauma. *J Trauma* 1977; **17**: 732–741.

65. Yellin AE, Rosoff L. Pancreatoduodenectomy for combined pancreatoduodenal injuries. *Arch Surg* 1975; **110**: 1117–1183.

66. Chambers RT, Norton L, Hinchey EJ. Massive right upper quadrant intra-abdominal injury requiring pancreaticoduodenectomy and partial hepatectomy. *J Trauma* 1975; **15**: 714–719.

67. Moore JB, Moore EE. Changing trends in the management of combined pancreatoduodenal injuries. *World J Surg* 1984; **8**: 791–797.

68. Oreskovich MR, Carrico CJ. Pancreaticoduodenectomy for trauma: a viable option? *Am J Surg* 1984; **147**: 618–623.

69. Heimansohn DA, Canal DF, McCarthy MC, Yaw PB, Madura JA, Broadie TA. The role of pancreaticoduodenectomy in the management of traumatic injuries to the pancreas and duodenum. *Am Surg* 1990; **56**: 511–514.

70. Gentillo LM, Cortes V, Buechter KJ, Gomez GA, Castro M, Zeppa R. Whipple procedure for trauma: is duct ligation a safe alternative to pancreaticojejunostomy? *J Trauma* 1991; **31**: 661–668.

71. Asensio JA, Demetriades D, Hanpeter DE, Gambaro E, Chahwan S. Management of pancreatic injuries. *Curr Probl Surg* 1999; **36**: 325–419.

72. Krige JEJ, Nico AJ, Navsaria PH, Jones O, Bornman PC. Emergency pancreatoduodenectomy for complex pancreatic trauma. *HPB* 2005; **7 (Suppl 1)**: 104.

73. Boffard KD, Brooks AJ. Pancreatic trauma – injuries to the pancreas and pancreatic duct. *Eur J Surg* 2000; **166**: 4–12.

74. Holcomb JB, Champion HR. Military damage control. *Arch Surg* 2001; **136**: 965–967.

75. Carrillo C, Fogler RJ, Shaftan GW. Delayed gastrointestinal reconstruction following massive abdominal trauma. *J Trauma* 1993; **34**: 233–235.

76. Eastlick L, Fogler RJ, Shaftan GW. Pancreaticoduodenectomy for trauma: delayed reconstruction: a case report. *J Trauma* 1990; **30**: 503–505.

77. Rotondo MF, Schwab CW, McGonigal MD *et al.* 'Damage control': an approach for improved survival in exsanguinating penetrating abdominal injury. *J Trauma* 1993; **35**: 375–382.

78. Hirshberg A, Mattox KL. 'Damage control' in trauma surgery. *Br J Surg* 1993; **80**: 1501–1502.

79. Koniaris LG, Mandal AK, Genuit T, Cameron JL. Two-stage trauma pancreaticoduodenectomy: delay facilitates anastomotic reconstruction. *J Gastrointest Surg* 2000; **4**: 366–369.

80. Beckingham IJ, Krige JEJ. Liver and pancreatic trauma. In: *ABC of Liver, Pancreas and Gallbladder*. London: British Medical Journal Publishing,. 2001; 44–46.

81. Beckingham IJ, Krige JEJ. Liver and pancreatic trauma. *BMJ* 2001; **322**: 783–785.

82. Lewis G, Knottenbelt J, Krige JEJ. Conservative surgery for trauma to the pancreatic head: is it safe? *Injury* 1991; **22**: 372–374.

83. Phelan HA, Minei JP. Pancreatic trauma: diagnostic and therapeutic strategies. *Curr Treat Options Gastroenterol* 2005; **8**: 355–363.

84. Lin BC, Chen RJ, Fang JF, Hsu YP, Kao YC, Kao JL. Management of blunt major pancreatic injury. *J Trauma* 2004; **56**: 774–778.

85. Kao LS, Bulger EM, Parks DL, Byrd GF, Jurkovich GJ. Predictors of morbidity after traumatic pancreatic injury. *J Trauma* 2003; **55**: 898–905.

86. Ivatury RR, Nallathambi M, Rao P, Stahl WM. Penetrating pancreatic injuries. Analysis of 103 consecutive cases. *Am Surg* 1990; **56**: 90–95.

87. Bornman PC, Krige JEJ, Beckingham IJ. Non-operative management of pancreatic pseudocysts. In: Schein M, Wise L. (eds) *Crucial Controversies in Surgery*, Vol 3. Baltimore, MD: Lippincott Williams & Wilkins, 1999; 170–181.

Brendan C. Visser Rowan W. Parks

8

Liver and splenic trauma

The liver and spleen are the two most commonly injured abdominal organs, accounting together for three-quarters of injuries in blunt abdominal trauma.[1] Though the injured spleen is easily removed, the surgical management of liver injuries remains a challenging problem. Paediatric surgeons first introduced the concept of non-operative management of splenic trauma. This approach was subsequently extended to adults with splenic injuries, and later to the management of blunt liver injuries. While a growing number of reports support non-operative management in haemodynamically stable adults, there still exists uncertainty about efficacy, patient selection and details of management. Interventional radiology has further increased the number of patients that can be treated without surgery. The progressive utilisation of non-operative management has, therefore, created its own set of complications and controversies.

This chapter will review the assessment and management (operative and non-operative) of liver and splenic trauma, and provide evidence-based practice guidelines.

EVALUATION OF THE TRAUMA PATIENT

The initial assessment of an injured patient should proceed according to the Advanced Trauma Life Support (ATLS) guidelines published by the American College of Surgeons. A detailed re-iteration of the ATLS algorithm is beyond the scope of this chapter. However, following the initial resuscitation, management may differ based on the mechanism of injury and the haemodynamic status of the patient.

Brendan C. Visser MD
Clinical Fellow, Edinburgh Royal Infirmary, Edinburgh EH16 4SA, UK

Rowan W. Parks (for correspondence)
Senior Lecturer in Surgery and Honorary Consultant Surgeon, Edinburgh Royal Infirmary, Edinburgh
EH16 4SA, UK. E-mail: r.w.parks@ed.ac.uk

119

Road traffic accidents and assault account for the vast majority of liver and splenic injuries, though the relative frequency varies according to geography. For example, in the UK and Europe, the majority of injuries are due to road traffic accidents,[2,3] while in South Africa and the US there is a somewhat higher proportion of penetrating trauma.[4,5] Due to its size and relatively protected anatomical position, splenic injuries are more frequently associated with blunt trauma than penetrating trauma.[6]

Following blunt trauma, a conscious patient who is haemodynamically unstable and has generalised peritonitis should undergo immediate laparotomy. Patients with neurological impairment or with equivocal physical signs traditionally underwent diagnostic peritoneal lavage. However, diagnostic peritoneal lavage is invasive and time consuming. Moreover, it is non-specific and oversensitive for the presence of blood, factors that contribute to a high rate of non-therapeutic laparotomies.[7] Diagnostic peritoneal lavage has, therefore, largely been replaced by ultrasonography. The Focused Abdominal Sonography in Trauma (FAST) examination is non-invasive, repeatable, and easily taught to clinicians.[8] The FAST examination can be performed in the resuscitation area while other assessments are being carried out, and in less time than required for diagnostic peritoneal lavage. The principal drawback of ultrasonography is that it remains operator dependent. While easily adopted in high-volume trauma centres in North America, the utility of FAST is yet to be proven in lower volume centres where individual surgeons and emergency physicians may not easily get sufficient experience to master the learning curve.[9] In such centres, examinations performed by radiologists may have a role.

Key point 1

- Ultrasonography (using the FAST examination) is an important tool for triaging unstable patients after blunt abdominal trauma.

If the patient is haemodynamically stable following blunt injury, time permits more thorough radiological assessment. CT scanning has become the gold standard for the diagnosis of solid organ injury. Importantly, CT allows assessment for other visceral injuries that may require operative management. Early reports based on conventional CT suggested that radiological findings following solid organ injury did not correlate exactly with findings at laparotomy.[10] However, with the advent of multidetector CT, scanning times have decreased and resolution has continued to improve. Furthermore, CT findings in both liver and splenic trauma have been demonstrated to be occasionally helpful in predicting the success of non-operative management and the utility of angiographic embolisation.[11,12]

Key point 2

- CT remains the gold standard for evaluating solid organ injuries due to blunt abdominal trauma.

Table 1 Liver injury scale (grade and description)[13]

I	Subcapsular haematoma < 10% surface area, laceration < 1 cm deep
II	Subcapsular haematoma 10–50% surface area, laceration 1–3 cm deep; < 10 cm in length
III	Subcapsular haematoma > 50% surface area or expanding, laceration > 3 cm deep
IV	Parenchymal disruption involving 25–75% of hepatic lobe or 1–3 Couinaud's segments in a single lobe
V	Parenchymal disruption > 75% of lobe or > 3 Couinaud's segments; juxtahepatic venous injuries (retrohepatic vena cava/hepatic veins)
VI	Hepatic avulsion

Penetrating trauma to the abdomen more frequently demands operative exploration. However, recent reports have documented successful non-operative management in selected patients with stab wounds and even low velocity gunshot wounds to the abdomen (see below).

LIVER TRAUMA

GRADING SYSTEM FOR LIVER INJURIES

The grading system proposed by the American Association for the Surgery of Trauma (AAST), initially drafted in 1989 and modified in 1994,[13] has been adopted internationally (Table 1). Grade I or II injuries are considered minor, represent 80–90% of cases, and rarely require operative intervention. Grades III–V are severe and more often require angiographic or surgical intervention. Grade VI injuries are incompatible with life.

NON-OPERATIVE MANAGEMENT OF BLUNT HEPATIC TRAUMA

Paediatric surgeons were the first to realise that the injured liver could be managed without surgery. In 1990, Knudson and colleagues[14] published the first retrospective series of selected adult patients (*n* = 52) managed successfully without laparotomy. Since that time, there have been a significant number of case series, largely retrospective, confirming the success of non-operative management in selected patients, and this has become the strategy of choice for haemodynamically stable patients following blunt liver trauma.[15] These findings have also been confirmed by several more recent prospective studies.[16,17] These reports have broadened the selection criteria to include patients with other intra-abdominal injuries not requiring operation, higher grades of hepatic injury, and older patients. The results have shown that non-operative management is associated with fewer liver-related and intra-abdominal complications than operative management, and that non-operative management does not result in a greater need for blood transfusion. In addition, although much of the benefit of non-operative management is attributed to avoidance of an operation, the mortality of liver injuries appears to have decreased.[18]

Key elements have slowly emerged: neither grade of injury nor degree of haemoperitoneum on CT reliably predicts the outcome of non-operative management.[17] The haemodynamic status of the patient is, therefore, the most reliable criterion for non-operative management. Between half and two-thirds of patients suffering blunt hepatic injury meet criteria for non-operative management, and the overall success of non-operative treatment in appropriately selected patients exceeds 95%.[19,20]

If a non-operative strategy is selected, it should be borne in mind that the risk of hollow organ injury increases in proportion to the number of solid organs injured[21] and that there is a small, but significant, risk of delayed haemorrhage.[22] However, it appears that the natural course of liver injuries is more analogous to that of lung or kidney injuries, rather than splenic injuries, in that any deterioration is usually gradual, with a fall in haemoglobin level or an increase in fluid requirement, rather than acute haemodynamic decompensation.[23] Therefore, with close supervision, patients who fail with an initial non-operative approach can be detected early and treated appropriately. Though in the past some authors recommended follow-up CT scans following non-operative management of liver injury, the evidence supporting this practice in asymptomatic patients is poor and these scans seldom alter management.[24]

Key point 3

- Selection of patients for non-operative management of liver injuries should be dictated primarily by haemodynamic stability.

NON-OPERATIVE MANAGEMENT OF PENETRATING HEPATIC INJURIES

Mandatory surgical exploration for penetrating wounds to the abdomen has been surgical dictum for the greater part of the last century. Initially motivated by the sheer volume of patients and limited resources, several centres in South America and South Africa began to practice selected non-operative management of abdominal stab wounds. Though not universally accepted, the success of this strategy has subsequently been demonstrated in larger prospective series.[25,26] Selective non-operative management of stab wounds specifically to the liver has been reported. If haemodynamically stable, a patient with a stab wound that is either directly over the liver or apparently tangential (without likely entrance into the peritoneal cavity) may be evaluated by CT. If the CT suggests an isolated liver injury and a knife tract unlikely to have caused other visceral injury, non-operative management may be pursued. Close serial abdominal examination is essential, and any evidence of generalised peritonitis mandates laparotomy.

Until recently, there has been a broad consensus that a gunshot wound to the abdomen is an indication for laparotomy.[27] However, this strategy has been challenged in selected patients with isolated gunshot wounds of the liver. Demetriades and colleagues[28] reported 52 patients with isolated liver injuries due to abdominal gunshot wounds, of whom 16 were initially managed non-operatively. Five patients subsequently required laparotomy for peritonitis (4) or an abdominal compartment syndrome (1). Eleven patients were, therefore, successfully managed without laparotomy. Given that this represented just 7% of all liver gunshot injuries and 21% of isolated liver injuries in the series, the non-operative approach applies in only very selected cases. A more recent prospective series from South Africa attempted non-operative management in 33 of 124 (27%) patients with liver gunshot injuries, avoiding laparotomy in 31 (94%).[29] These included 14 AAST grade III, 8 grade IV, and 3 grade V injuries, demonstrating success with selective non-operative management in even higher grade injuries. Though experience is mounting with this strategy, at present there is insufficient evidence to justify wide-spread adoption of a non-operative management in gunshot wounds of the liver.

OPERATIVE MANAGEMENT OF LIVER TRAUMA

The trauma laparotomy

Primary operative intervention is indicated for liver injury if the patient is haemodynamically unstable despite adequate initial resuscitation. A long mid-line incision is employed for an emergency laparotomy, although access to the liver can be improved by converting the incision into a 'T' by adding a right transverse component. In situations where surgery is undertaken after initial conservative management, a subcostal incision affords excellent access.

The trauma laparotomy is conducted in a routine fashion – four quadrant packing, control of gross enteric spillage, systematic inspection for injuries, and finally definitive management of injuries. Liver haemorrhage can usually be initially controlled by direct pressure using packs. Additional techniques include the Pringle manoeuvre (digital compression of the portal triad), bimanual compression of the liver, or manual compression of the aorta above the coeliac trunk. At this point, further evaluation of the extent of liver injury should be delayed until the anaesthetist has adequately replenished the intravascular volume. A key element of the resuscitation is the availability of adequate blood products: packed red blood cells, platelets, fresh frozen plasma, and cryoprecipitate. Recently, recombinant Factor VIIa has been used as an adjunctive agent in trauma patients with severe coagulopathic bleeding.[30]

After intra-operative resuscitation, the liver must be mobilised adequately to allow a thorough examination of the injury. If necessary, the Pringle manoeuvre may be maintained with a vascular clamp to allow further assessment and operative remedy. A normal liver can tolerate inflow occlusion for up to 1 h; however, the ability of a damaged liver to tolerate ischaemia may be impaired. Depending on the injury and the experience of the surgeon, a variety of surgical techniques are then available.

Key point 4

- The principles of operative management of hepatic injuries are:
  (i) Arrest haemorrhage and enteric contamination, **Before** (ii) Careful systematic inspection for injuries, and (iii) **D**efinitive management by an appropriately trained surgeon.

Techniques for haemostasis

Perihepatic packing: In situations where it is thought that definitive control of haemorrhage cannot be obtained, the liver injury should be packed, the incision closed and the patient transferred to a specialist centre for definitive treatment. Packing can also be employed as a damage control strategy in patients who are critically unstable, coagulopathic or acidotic and, therefore, would not tolerate a prolonged operative procedure. In this setting, packing must be employed before the patient has deteriorated to a point that survival is unlikely under any circumstances. Finally, packing can occasionally also be used in conjunction with interventional techniques.

Packing is remarkably effective at controlling major haemorrhage from liver injuries, even in patients with caval or hepatic venous injuries.[31] The technique of packing involves manual closure or approximation of the parenchyma, followed by sequential placing of dry abdominal packs or a single rolled gauze around the liver and directly over the injury in an attempt to provide tamponade to a bleeding wound. Most surgeons employ skin closure only, leaving the fascia for primary closure at the subsequent procedure for pack removal.

Hepatorrhaphy: Absorbable sutures on a curved blunt-tipped needle can be used to approximate a fissured parenchymal injury and thus control haemorrhage as an alternative to exploration of the depths of the injury. These sutures are placed as large horizontal mattress stitches, often in conjunction with a bolster of haemostatic material. Though occasionally useful in minor injuries, the disadvantages of this technique are that parenchymal vessels may continue to bleed resulting in a cavitating haematoma, bile duct injuries may not be detected and the suture itself may cause further bleeding, ischaemia or intrahepatic bile duct injury.

Hepatotomy with direct suture ligation: This technique involves extending the liver laceration using the finger fracture technique or the ultrasonic dissector to expose injured vessels. The bleeding vessels can be suture ligated or clipped to achieve haemostasis. Diathermy coagulation can also be used; in this context, the argon beam coagulator (which 'sprays' the diathermy current on an argon beam) is invaluable. This strategy has proved particularly effective in penetrating liver trauma.[32]

Omental packing: Stone and Lamb[33] reported in 1975 that the greater omentum could be employed as a pedicled flap to fill a defect in the liver parenchyma. This omental pedicle helps stop oozing from the low-pressure venous system of the liver parenchyma and may fill dead space that might later be predisposed to form an abscess. This technique is used infrequently today.

Mesh wrapping: The use of an absorbable polyglactin mesh to wrap major parenchymal disruptions has also been described.[34] This technique is not indicated where juxtacaval or hepatic vein injury is suspected. Advocates claim that it provides the benefits of packing without the disadvantages (a second laparotomy is not required for removal, abdominal closure is much easier, and respiratory or renal function are less compromised).[35] However, there is some concern about the amount of time needed to apply the mesh wrap in a haemodynamically unstable patient who might be best treated with rapid insertion of perihepatic packs.

Resectional debridement: This technique involves removal of devitalised liver tissue using the lines of the injury, rather than anatomical planes, as the boundaries of the resection. The optimum timing may be to combine debridement with pack removal, as necrotic tissue will be well demarcated 48-h after injury.

Anatomical liver resection: The practical difficulties of undertaking formal anatomical resection in a patient with a significant liver injury (frequently associated with shock, coagulopathy, and concomitant injury) are substantial. Though anatomical resections should be reserved for situations in which no other procedure adequately achieves haemostasis, excellent results have been reported from experienced centres.[36]

Selective ligation of the hepatic artery: This strategy is rarely required. Hepatic arterial ligation to control haemorrhage should only be performed when other manoeuvres have failed, when selective ligation has been unsuccessful and when pedicle clamping has been demonstrated to arrest haemorrhage. Acute gangrenous cholecystitis is a well-recognised complication of hepatic artery ligation, and thus, cholecystectomy must be performed.

Management of hepatic venous and retrohepatic caval injury: Suspicion that one of these serious injuries is present should be raised if the Pringle manoeuvre fails to arrest haemorrhage. There is no consensus on an optimal management strategy. Total vascular exclusion (clamping of the inferior vena cava and suprahepatic cava in addition to the Pringle manoeuvre) may be used. However clamping the vena cava seriously compromises venous return in a patient with major trauma. Veno-venous bypass (shunt from common femoral vein to left internal jugular or axillary vein) has the advantage of preserving venous return but has been infrequently used in the trauma setting. Atriocaval shunting via a chest tube through the right atrial appendage into the inferior vena cava, introduced by Schrock in 1968,[37] allows total vascular isolation of the liver whilst preserving venous return, but this technique undoubtedly has produced more manuscripts than survivors. Packing can effectively control bleeding from retrohepic caval injuries,[38] and this is the authors' preference, only using vascular exclusion as a last resort.

Liver transplantation: Several reports have been published of severe liver trauma treated by total hepatectomy followed by liver transplantation.[39,40] Though experience of this sort of surgery is extremely infrequent, awareness of the therapeutic potential is useful.

ROLE OF INTERVENTIONAL RADIOLOGY

Interventional radiological techniques have become important adjuncts to both non-operative, and occasionally operative, management of liver trauma. Angiography and embolisation have been successfully employed as an extension of resuscitation in the non-operative management of patients with

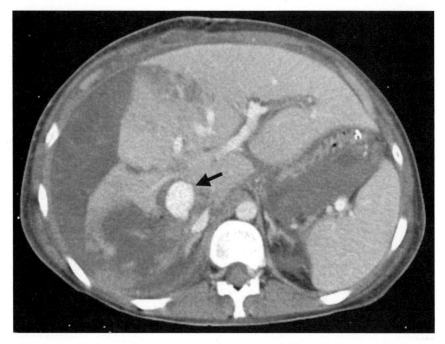

Fig. 1 Grade IV injury with 'blush' of pseudo-aneurysm from right hepatic artery (arrow).

blunt hepatic injuries. Most authors recommend angiography in haemodynamically stable patients with a 'blush' (suggesting active arterial extravastion of contrast) on the initial CT scan. Pooling of contrast may occur within the liver parenchyma or in the peritoneal cavity. While the former is appropriately, and often successfully, managed by embolisation, patients with extravasation of contrast into the peritoneal cavity often quickly become unstable and hence require laparotomy. Transcatheter embolisation is reported to be technically successful in about 80% of cases,[41,42] and has been described in non-operative management of penetrating injuries.[43] A small percentage of patients may re-bleed despite a technically successful initial embolisation. These patients may require a second angiogram and embolisation, or laparotomy if unstable.

Angiography may also be helpful in conjunction with 'damage control laparotomy'.[44] In the case illustrated in Figures 1–3, the patient sustained a Grade IV injury due to a road traffic accident. At the initial laparotomy, profound haemorrhage was controlled by packing. A subsequent CT demonstrated a pseudo-aneurysm of the right hepatic artery (Fig. 1). This was successfully coiled (Fig. 2), with complete resolution of the pseudo-aneurysm on a follow-up CT (Fig. 3). Complications of embolisation include hepatic necrosis and gallbladder infarction.

Key point 5

- Angiography and embolisation are important adjuncts to both non-operative, and occasionally operative, management of liver trauma.

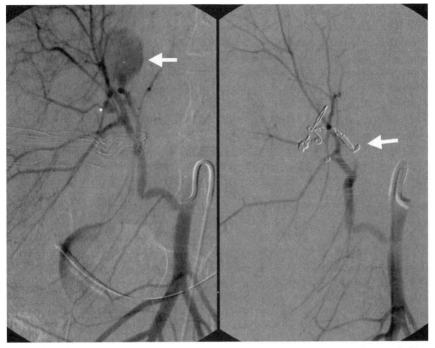

Fig. 2 Pseudo-aneurysm from right hepatic artery (right). Successful coil embolisation (left).

COMPLICATIONS OF NON-OPERATIVE AND OPERATIVE MANAGEMENT

Non-operative management of liver trauma can result in two important categories of complications. First, co-existing intra-abdominal injuries may not

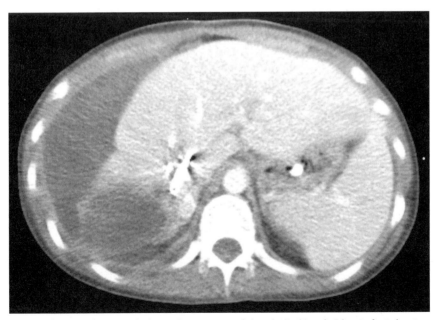

Fig. 3 Follow-up CT 2 weeks later shows successful embolisation (with artefact due to coils) and significant healing of hepatic parenchyma.

be recognised at the time of initial presentation or may only become apparent after initial delay. A small portion of patients that 'fail' non-operative management do so only because they require laparotomy for other intra-abdominal injuries.[16,19] The second type of complication is that related to the liver injury itself. Septic complications such as intra-abdominal abscess and bile leak are recognised late complications and may require radiological, endoscopic or surgical intervention.

The complications after liver surgery for trauma are largely similar to those encountered after any form of hepatic surgery. Haemorrhage due to coagulopathy requires correction with fresh frozen plasma and platelets. If haemorrhage occurs despite normal coagulation, angiography may provide diagnostic information and may permit therapeutic embolisation. Other complications include haemobilia, arterioportal fistulas, and sepsis due to infected collections of bile, blood or related to devitalised liver parenchyma.

OUTCOME/VOLUME RELATIONSHIP

Mounting evidence suggests that victims of significant trauma are best served at specialised, high-volume trauma centres.[45,46] However, patients with liver trauma often present initially to surgeons without specialist hepatobiliary experience. The surgeon operating on a patient in this situation should, therefore, attempt to control bleeding by packing, and then transfer the patient to the care of a specialist hepatobiliary surgeon.

Key point 6

- Centres without specialist hepatobiliary experience should transfer patients with complex liver injuries as soon as stability permits.

SPLENIC TRAUMA

The spleen is the second most frequently injured organ in abdominal trauma, and a missed splenic injury is the most common cause of preventable death in trauma patients.[47] Published series of splenectomies following trauma from the first half of the 20th century cited mortality rates of 50% or more.[6] In the absence of diagnostic imaging, these patients presented with peritonitis and shock necessitating laparotomy. Splenic injuries presenting in this fashion were, not surprisingly, significant, and the standard treatment was, therefore, splenectomy. This practice was further supported by scattered reports of 'delayed splenic rupture' as a complication of blunt trauma. The published results following trauma splenectomy improved significantly as a result of the experience of the Second World War. However, enthusiasm was soon blunted as case reports and small studies began appearing in the 1950s describing a fulminant, rapidly progressive and frequently lethal systemic infection following splenectomy.[48] The development of diagnostic peritoneal lavage in the 1960s and later CT scanning resulted in many laparotomies for more minor splenic injuries. Splenorrhaphy became the management of choice. Following the lead of paediatric surgeons, non-operative management of splenic trauma has gained increasing momentum since the 1980s. Non-operative management is now the preferred treatment for the majority of patients with blunt splenic trauma. Immediate laparotomy and splenectomy is reserved for patients presenting with peritonitis and shock. The management of splenic injuries thus appears to have come full circle.

> **Key point 7**
> • Selection of patients for non-operative management of splenic injuries depends primarily on haemodynamic stability.

GRADING SYSTEM FOR SPLENIC INJURIES

The standard grading system proposed by the American Association for the Surgery of Trauma (AAST) is shown in Table 2.[13]

NON-OPERATIVE MANAGEMENT

In recent large series, about two-thirds of adults with blunt splenic injuries are initially managed non-operatively, with success in more than 85% of cases.[49–51] An even higher percentage of paediatric patients may be managed non-operatively, exceeding 80% at trauma centres, especially if cared for by paediatric surgeons.[52] A variety of factors have been hypothesised to account for the observed difference between paediatric and adult patients: the presence of a more elastic rib cage in children, differences in the splenic capsule, and the differences in mechanism of injury. The most likely explanation is the latter – the higher percentage of road traffic accidents in adults (with more sports injuries, bicycle accidents, and falls in children) results in higher injury severity scores, lower Glasgow Coma Scale scores, and higher mortality.[53] A greater number of associated extra-abdominal and intra-abdominal injuries precludes a non-operative approach in a higher percentage of adults.

As with non-operative management of liver trauma, non-operative management of splenic injuries does not carry with it a greater need for transfusion than operative management. In fact, several studies suggest that the need for transfusion is less with non-operative management than it is with operative management for injuries of similar grades.[54]

Table 2 Splenic injury scale (grade and description)[13]

I	Subcapsular haematoma < 10% of surface area, laceration < 1 cm deep
II	Subcapsular haematoma 10–50% of surface area, laceration 1–3 cm deep
III	Subcapsular haematoma > 50% surface area or expanding, intraparenchymal haematoma > 5 cm or expanding
IV	Laceration involving segmental or hilar vessels with major devascularisation
V	Completely shattered spleen, hilar vascular injury with devascularised spleen.

OPERATIVE MANAGEMENT

Splenectomy

Splenectomy is indicated under the following circumstances: (i) the patient is haemodynamically unstable; (ii) other intra- or extra-abdominal injuries require prompt attention; (iii) the spleen is extensively injured with ongoing bleeding; and (iv) bleeding is associated with hilar injury.

Splenorrhaphy

Though utilised frequently in the 1970s and 1980s, the use of this technique has gradually decreased as non-operative management has become more widely adopted. However, a significant, and perhaps under-reported cause of splenic trauma for which splenorrhaphy is appropriate, is iatrognic injury during intra-abdominal or retro-peritoneal surgery.[55]

There are four basic techniques of splenorrhaphy: (i) superficial haemostatic strategies; (ii) suture repair; (iii) absorbable mesh wrap; and (iv) resectional debridement. Temporary clamping of the splenic artery may aid in all of these techniques. Superficial haemostatic approaches (diathermy or argon beam coagulation, cellulose, absorbable gelatin sponge, topical thrombin) are typically only useful in low-grade (AAST I and II) injuries. Suture repair, especially if bolstered by pledgets to avoid tearing the splenic parenchyma, may be useful in somewhat higher-grade injuries. The use of rolled oxidised cellulose in conjunction with suture splenorrhaphy has proven particularly effective.[56] Perhaps the most effective technique for significant splenic injuries is wrapping the spleen with absorbable polyglactin mesh.[57] The basic strategy is similar to that in liver injuries. A keyhole is cut into the mesh to accommodate the hilar vessels, and the mesh is secured around the spleen to compress the parenchyma and tamponade bleeding. Mesh wrapping has also more recently been used in cases of intra-operative iatrogenic splenic injury.[58] Finally, resectional debridement is occasionally useful for upper or lower pole fractures. Topical techniques or sutures are then used to control bleeding from the cut margin. Subtotal splenectomy does appear experimentally to preserve the immune function of the spleen.[59]

ROLE OF INTERVENTIONAL RADIOLOGY

As is the case with liver trauma, interventional radiological techniques are playing a growing role in the management of splenic trauma. The presence of extravasation of contrast on the arterial phase of the abdominal CT, also termed 'blush', portends failure of non-operative management.[12,60] This finding represents a pseudo-aneurysm within the spleen or on-going bleeding (*e.g.* extravasation from a laceration into the peritoneal cavity adjacent to the spleen). In addition to a standard arterial phase, delayed CT images may better demonstrate subtle pooling of intravenous contrast. Growing evidence suggests that angiography and transarterial embolisation for patients with a 'contrast blush' on CT improves the success of non-operative management.[61,62] The preferred technique is distal superselective embolisation of the involved splenic artery branch using a microcatheter, though more proximal embolisation may be required if superselective embolisation is not technically possible or for multiple pseudo-aneurysms.

> **Key point 8**
>
> - Angiography and embolisation are important adjuncts to management of splenic injuries.

POST-SPLENECTOMY INFECTION

Though initially documented some 50 years ago, the true risk and appropriate prevention measures of post-splenectomy infections are still poorly documented. These life-threatening infections have been termed 'overwhelming post-splenectomy infection' (OPSI). Reasonable estimates of the annual incidence of OPSI derived from cohort studies are 0.2–0.4% per year[63] with a life-time risk of about 5%.[64] The risk is higher in children, in those who undergo splenectomy for haematological conditions or malignancy, and in those who have another cause for immunosuppression (*e.g.* corticosteroids). Adult patients who undergo splenectomy following trauma appear to be at the lowest risk. OPSI carries a mortality of about 50%.[64]

Recommendations following splenectomy for trauma vary. Almost universally, meningococcal, *Haemophilus influenzae* type b, pneumococcal, and influenza vaccinations are recommended. Life-long prophylactic antibiotics (oral phenoxymethylpenicillin or erythromycin) are advised in the UK,[65] though this is not widely prescribed elsewhere. There is concern that this practice will contribute to emerging resistance. An alternative is that antibiotics should be available at home and used whenever travelling and immediately should infective symptoms develop. All patients should be advised to seek immediate medical help if infective symptoms arise.

> **Key point 9**
>
> - Following successful non-operative management of blunt splenic trauma, repeat imaging should be considered in those patients with subcapsular haematomas and more severe injuries (Grade III or higher).

REPEAT IMAGING

The risk of delayed splenic haemorrhage following blunt splenic injury has been well documented and appears to occur in about 1–2% of patients.[6] Given that the majority of patients suffer low grade (I–II) injuries with little risk of delayed rupture, the utility of routine follow-up imaging is debated. However, a subset of patients may benefit from a repeat CT scan before discharge (Table 3).

SUMMARY

The management of liver and splenic injuries is summarised in Figure 4. Following blunt trauma, haemodynamically unstable patients require laparotomy. Stable patients may be evaluated with CT. Approximately two-

Table 3 Recommended indications for repeat imaging after non-operative management in patients with splenic trauma[15]

- Active extravasation on initial scan
- Subcapsular haematoma on initial scan
- Underlying splenic pathology
- Coagulopathy
- Grade III or higher injuries
- Athletes
- Unreliable patients

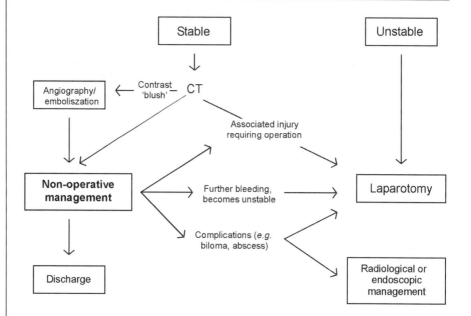

Fig. 4 Management algorithm for patients with blunt trauma to liver or spleen.

thirds of patients are suitable for non-operative management in a closely monitored setting, which is successful in more than 80% of cases. Angiography and embolisation improve the success of this strategy further. Subsequent deterioration, associated injuries, or complications of non-operative management may ultimately require surgical intervention.

As a general rule, most patients who suffer penetrating trauma with injury to the liver or spleen will require a laparotomy. However, a small subset with isolated liver injuries may be managed non-operatively. Current data are insufficient to recommend wide-spread adoption of this strategy.

Key points for clinical practice

- Ultrasonography (using the FAST examination) is an important tool for triaging unstable patients after blunt abdominal trauma.

- CT remains the gold standard for evaluating solid organ injuries due to blunt abdominal trauma.

> **Key points for clinical practice** *(continued)*
>
> - Selection of patients for non-operative management of liver injuries should be dictated primarily by haemodynamic stability.
>
> - The principles of operative management of hepatic injuries are: (i) **A**rrest haemorrhage and enteric contamination, **B**efore (ii) **C**areful systematic inspection for injuries, and (iii) **D**efinitive management by an appropriately trained surgeon.
>
> - Angiography and embolisation are important adjuncts to both non-operative, and occasionally operative, management of liver trauma.
>
> - Centres without specialist hepatobiliary experience should transfer patients with complex liver injuries as soon as stability permits.
>
> - Selection of patients for non-operative management of splenic injuries depends primarily on haemodynamic stability.
>
> - Angiography and embolisation are important adjuncts to management of splenic injuries.
>
> - Following successful non-operative management of blunt splenic trauma, repeat imaging should be considered in those patients with subcapsular haematomas and more severe injuries (Grade III or higher).

References

1. Cox EF. Blunt abdominal trauma. A 5-year analysis of 870 patients requiring celiotomy. *Ann Surg* 1984; **199**: 467–474.
2. Scollay JM, Beard D, Smith R *et al*. Eleven years of liver trauma: the Scottish experience. *World J Surg* 2005; **29**: 744–749.
3. Bergqvist D, Hedelin H, Karlsson G *et al*. Abdominal trauma during thirty years: analysis of a large case series. *Injury* 1981; **13**: 93–99.
4. Krige JE, Bornman PC, Terblanche J. Liver trauma in 446 patients. *S Afr J Surg* 1997; **35**: 10–15.
5. Feliciano DV, Mattox KL, Jordan Jr GL *et al*. Management of 1000 consecutive cases of hepatic trauma (1979–1984). *Ann Surg* 1986; **204**: 438–445.
6. Richardson JD. Changes in the management of injuries to the liver and spleen. *J Am Coll Surg* 2005; **200**: 648–669.
7. Jansen JO, Logie JR. Diagnostic peritoneal lavage – an obituary. *Br J Surg* 2005; **92**: 517–518.
8. Boulanger BR, McLellan BA, Brenneman FD *et al*. Prospective evidence of the superiority of a sonography-based algorithm in the assessment of blunt abdominal injury. *J Trauma* 1999; **47**: 632–637.
9. Gracias VH, Frankel HL, Gupta R *et al*. Defining the learning curve for the Focused Abdominal Sonogram for Trauma (FAST) examination: implications for credentialing. *Am Surg* 2001; **67**: 364–368.
10. Croce MA, Fabian TC, Kudsk KA *et al*. AAST organ injury scale: correlation of CT-graded liver injuries and operative findings. *J Trauma* 1991; **31**: 806–812.
11. Poletti PA, Mirvis SE, Shanmuganathan K *et al*. CT criteria for management of blunt liver trauma: correlation with angiographic and surgical findings. *Radiology* 2000; **216**: 418–427.
12. Shanmuganathan K, Mirvis SE, Boyd-Kranis R *et al*. Nonsurgical management of blunt splenic injury: use of CT criteria to select patients for splenic arteriography and potential endovascular therapy. *Radiology* 2000; **217**: 75–82.

13. Moore EE, Cogbill TH, Jurkovich GJ *et al*. Organ injury scaling: spleen and liver (1994 revision). *J Trauma* 1995; **38**: 323–324.

14. Knudson MM, Lim Jr RC, Oakes DD, Jeffrey Jr RB. Nonoperative management of blunt liver injuries in adults: the need for continued surveillance. *J Trauma* 1990; **30**: 1494–1500.

15. Knudson MM, Maull KI. Nonoperative management of solid organ injuries. Past, present, and future. *Surg Clin North Am* 1999; **79**: 1357–1371.

16. Velmahos GC, Toutouzas KG, Radin R *et al*. Nonoperative treatment of blunt injury to solid abdominal organs: a prospective study. *Arch Surg* 2003; **138**: 844–851.

17. Croce MA, Fabian TC, Menke PG *et al*. Nonoperative management of blunt hepatic trauma is the treatment of choice for hemodynamically stable patients. Results of a prospective trial. *Ann Surg* 1995; **221**: 744–753, discussion 753–755.

18. David Richardson J, Franklin GA, Lukan JK *et al*. Evolution in the management of hepatic trauma: a 25-year perspective. *Ann Surg* 2000; **232**: 324–330.

19. Pachter HL, Knudson MM, Esrig B *et al*. Status of nonoperative management of blunt hepatic injuries in 1995: a multicenter experience with 404 patients. *J Trauma* 1996; **40**: 31–38.

20. Christmas AB, Wilson AK, Manning B *et al*. Selective management of blunt hepatic injuries including nonoperative management is a safe and effective strategy. *Surgery* 2005; **138**: 606–611.

21. Nance ML, Peden GW, Shapiro MB *et al*. Solid viscus injury predicts major hollow viscus injury in blunt abdominal trauma. *J Trauma* 1997; **43**: 618–622, discussion 622–623.

22. Shilyansky J, Navarro O, Superina RA *et al*. Delayed hemorrhage after nonoperative management of blunt hepatic trauma in children: a rare but significant event. *J Pediatr Surg* 1999; **34**: 60–64.

23. Meredith JW, Young JS, Bowling J, Roboussin D. Nonoperative management of blunt hepatic trauma: the exception or the rule? *J Trauma* 1994; **36**: 529–534, discussion 534–535.

24. Ciraulo DL, Nikkanen HE, Palter M *et al*. Clinical analysis of the utility of repeat computed tomographic scan before discharge in blunt hepatic injury. *J Trauma* 1996; **41**: 821–824.

25. Demetriades D, Rabinowitz B. Selective conservative management of penetrating abdominal wounds: a prospective study. *Br J Surg* 1984; **71**: 92–94.

26. Demetriades D, Rabinowitz B, Sofianos C. Non-operative management of penetrating liver injuries: a prospective study. *Br J Surg* 1986; **73**: 736–737.

27. Marr JD, Krige JE, Terblanche J. Analysis of 153 gunshot wounds of the liver. *Br J Surg* 2000; **87**: 1030–1034.

28. Demetriades D, Gomez H, Chahwan S *et al*. Gunshot injuries to the liver: the role of selective nonoperative management. *J Am Coll Surg* 1999; **188**: 343–348.

29. Omoshoro-Jones JA, Nicol AJ, Navsaria PH *et al*. Selective non-operative management of liver gunshot injuries. *Br J Surg* 2005; **92**: 890–895.

30. Dutton RP, McCunn M, Hyder M *et al*. Factor VIIa for correction of traumatic coagulopathy. *J Trauma* 2004; **57**: 709–718, discussion 718–719.

31. Krige JE, Bornman PC, Terblanche J. Therapeutic perihepatic packing in complex liver trauma. *Br J Surg* 1992; **79**: 43–46.

32. Moore FA, Moore EE, Seagraves A. Nonresectional management of major hepatic trauma. An evolving concept. *Am J Surg* 1985; **150**: 725–729.

33. Stone HH, Lamb JM. Use of pedicled omentum as an autogenous pack for control of hemorrhage in major injuries of the liver. *Surg Gynecol Obstet* 1975; **141**: 92–94.

34. Brunet C, Sielezneff I, Thomas P *et al*. Treatment of hepatic trauma with perihepatic mesh: 35 cases. *J Trauma* 1994; **37**: 200–204.

35. Reed 2nd RL, Merrell RC, Meyers WC, Fischer RP. Continuing evolution in the approach to severe liver trauma. *Ann Surg* 1992; **216**: 524–538.

36. Strong RW, Lynch SV, Wall DR, Liu CL. Anatomic resection for severe liver trauma. *Surgery* 1998; **123**: 251–257.

37. Schrock T, Blaisdell FW, Mathewson Jr C. Management of blunt trauma to the liver and hepatic veins. *Arch Surg* 1968; **96**: 698–704.

38. Beal SL. Fatal hepatic hemorrhage: an unresolved problem in the management of complex liver injuries. *J Trauma* 1990; **30**: 163–169.

39. Ringe B, Pichlmayr R. Total hepatectomy and liver transplantation: a life-saving procedure in patients with severe hepatic trauma. *Br J Surg* 1995; **82**: 837–839.

40. Ginzburg E, Shatz D, Lynn M *et al*. The role of liver transplantation in the subacute trauma

patients. *Am Surg* 1998; **64**: 363–364.

41. Ciraulo DL, Luk S, Palter M *et al*. Selective hepatic arterial embolization of grade IV and V blunt hepatic injuries: an extension of resuscitation in the nonoperative management of traumatic hepatic injuries. *J Trauma* 1998; **45**: 353–358, discussion 358–359.

42. Wahl WL, Ahrns KS, Brandt MM *et al*. The need for early angiographic embolization in blunt liver injuries. *J Trauma* 2002; **52**: 1097–1101.

43. Velmahos GC, Demetriades D, Chahwan S *et al*. Angiographic embolization for arrest of bleeding after penetrating trauma to the abdomen. *Am J Surg* 1999; **178**: 367–373.

44. Johnson JW, Gracias VH, Gupta R *et al*. Hepatic angiography in patients undergoing damage control laparotomy. *J Trauma* 2002; **52**: 1102–1106.

45. Demetriades D, Martin M, Salim A *et al*. The effect of trauma center designation and trauma volume on outcome in specific severe injuries. *Ann Surg* 2005; **242**: 512–517, discussion 517–519.

46. Nathens AB, Jurkovich GJ, Maier RV *et al*. Relationship between trauma center volume and outcomes. *JAMA* 2001; **285**: 1164–1171.

47. Cales RH, Trunkey DD. Preventable trauma deaths. A review of trauma care systems development. *JAMA* 1985; **254**: 1059–1063.

48. King H, Shumacker Jr HB. Splenic studies. I. Susceptibility to infection after splenectomy performed in infancy. *Ann Surg* 1952; **136**: 239–242.

49. Bee TK, Croce MA, Miller PR *et al*. Failures of splenic nonoperative management: is the glass half empty or half full? *J Trauma* 2001; **50**: 230–236.

50. Myers JG, Dent DL, Stewart RM *et al*. Blunt splenic injuries: dedicated trauma surgeons can achieve a high rate of nonoperative success in patients of all ages. *J Trauma* 2000; **48**: 801–805, discussion 805–806.

51. Cocanour CS, Moore FA, Ware DN *et al*. Age should not be a consideration for nonoperative management of blunt splenic injury. *J Trauma* 2000; **48**: 606–610, discussion 610–612.

52. Mooney DP, Forbes PW. Variation in the management of pediatric splenic injuries in New England. *J Trauma* 2004; **56**: 328–333.

53. Powell M, Courcoulas A, Gardner M *et al*. Management of blunt splenic trauma: significant differences between adults and children. *Surgery* 1997; **122**: 654–660.

54. Schwartz MZ, Kangah R. Splenic injury in children after blunt trauma: blood transfusion requirements and length of hospitalization for laparotomy versus observation. *J Pediatr Surg* 1994; **29**: 596–598.

55. Cassar K, Munro A. Iatrogenic splenic injury. *J R Coll Surg Edinb* 2002; **47**: 731–741.

56. Aidonopoulos AP, Papavramidis ST, Goutzamanis GD *et al*. Splenorrhaphy for splenic damage in patients with multiple injuries. *Eur J Surg* 1995; **161**: 247–251.

57. Fingerhut A, Oberlin P, Cotte JL *et al*. Splenic salvage using an absorbable mesh: feasibility, reliability and safety. *Br J Surg* 1992; **79**: 325–327.

58. Berry MF, Rosato EF, Williams NN. Dexon mesh splenorrhaphy for intraoperative splenic injuries. *Am Surg* 2003; **69**: 176–180.

59. Traub A, Giebink GS, Smith C *et al*. Splenic reticuloendothelial function after splenectomy, spleen repair, and spleen autotransplantation. *N Engl J Med* 1987; **317**: 1559–1564.

60. Gavant ML, Schurr M, Flick PA *et al*. Predicting clinical outcome of nonsurgical management of blunt splenic injury: using CT to reveal abnormalities of splenic vasculature. *AJR Am J Roentgenol* 1997; **168**: 207–212.

61. Davis KA, Fabian TC, Croce MA *et al*. Improved success in nonoperative management of blunt splenic injuries: embolization of splenic artery pseudoaneurysms. *J Trauma* 1998; **44**: 1008–1013, discussion 1013–1015.

62. Haan JM, Bochicchio GV, Kramer N, Scalea TM. Nonoperative management of blunt splenic injury: a 5-year experience. *J Trauma* 2005; **58**: 492–498.

63. Ejstrud P, Kristensen B, Hansen JB *et al*. Risk and patterns of bacteraemia after splenectomy: a population-based study. *Scand J Infect Dis* 2000; **32**: 521–525.

64. Davidson RN, Wall RA. Prevention and management of infections in patients without a spleen. *Clin Microbiol Infect* 2001; **7**: 657–660.

65. Davies JM, Barnes R, Milligan D. Update of guidelines for the prevention and treatment of infection in patients with an absent or dysfunctional spleen. *Clin Med* 2002; **2**: 440–443.

Kellee Slater Jonathan Fawcett

9

Live donor liver transplantation

The most effective treatment for end-stage liver disease is transplantation. The increasing demand for transplant and a relatively low rate of cadaveric organ donation has resulted in long waiting lists. Waiting list mortality in some centres has reached 10%.[1]

The shortage of donors has driven the search for alternate organ sources. Split liver transplantation, marginal and non-heart beating donors make optimal use of cadaveric grafts but living donors offer another way to expand the donor organ pool.

The first successful living-donor liver transplant (LDLT) was performed in 1989 in a child, using a left lateral segment resected from his parent.[2] Since then, LDLT has gained acceptance as an excellent treatment for end-stage liver disease in children.[3]

In the 1990s, living-donor liver transplantation was developed extensively in Asia for both adults and children, where cultural beliefs discourage cadaveric organ donation. Currently, almost all liver transplantations performed in Asia involve a living donor.[4]

In the US and Europe, the technique of LDLT using a left lateral segment has met with far less success in adult recipients. The smaller left lobe provides insufficient hepatic mass for most Western adults who are physically larger than Asian patients. Clinicians have looked to the larger volume right lobe and the first adult-to-adult transplantation of a right hepatic lobe was reported in 1994 in Japan[5] and in the US in 1997.[6]

Kellee Slater FRACS (for correspondence)
Fellow in HPB Surgery, Queensland Liver Transplant Service, Princess Alexandra Hospital, Ipswich Road, Woolloongabba, Brisbane, QLD 4102, Australia
E-mail: j.fawcett@uq.edu.au

Jonathan Fawcett DPhil FRCS FRACS
Professor of Surgery, Consultant General and HPB Surgeon, and Deputy Director of Queensland Liver Transplant Service, Princess Alexandra Hospital, Ipswich Road, Woolloongabba, Brisbane, QLD 4102, Australia

Right lobe LDLT remains controversial in many respects. Significant complications and deaths after donor surgery have lead many centres not to introduce LDLT into their programmes. Despite this, the technique has rapidly expanded around the world. In the US between 1997 and 2003, LDLT increased from 2.1% to 5.6% of all liver transplants being performed.[7] Currently, the numbers being performed have decreased somewhat because of the concerns mentioned above, regarding complications.[8] In particular, two highly publicised donor deaths[9,10] signalled the need for caution. Furthermore, there has been uncertainty regarding the possible accelerated recurrence of hepatitis C virus (HCV) infection after LDLT.

RATIONALE

The driving force for the implementation of LDLT is the lack of donor cadaveric organs as illustrated in Figure 1.

The precedent for LDLT of solid organs was set half a century ago, with a successful renal transplant between mono-zygotic twin brothers.[11] Since then, reduced size and split liver transplantation has proven that segmental liver anatomy can be applied to liver transplantation. With advances in the safety of elective liver resection, it was appreciated that procurement of a hemiliver from a living donor was feasible. The first LDLTs were performed with left-sided resections for transplanting children. Subsequently, the more major right-sided resections for donation to adults were undertaken with the driving force being a shortage of cadaveric organs for transplant.

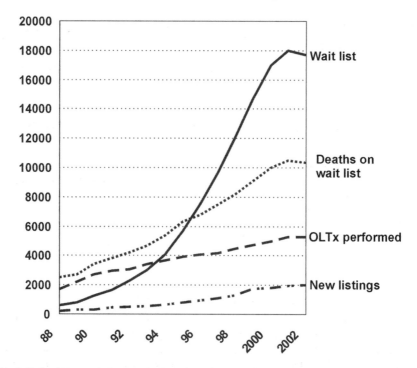

Fig. 1 United Network Organ Sharing data showing the increase in the deaths on the waiting list for cadaveric liver transplant in the US.[7]

A second stimulus for instituting LDLT has been access to transplant organs. Currently, most LDLTs are done within accepted indications for cadaveric transplantation. Eligibility criteria, though, exclude many patients with malignancy, as they have poorer outcomes than those with end-stage liver disease. Whilst these patients' chances of survival are less, they may still have a better outcome than with no treatment at all. Surgery and other therapies are routinely offered to patients with oesophageal and pancreatic cancer, with low survival rates. The only limitation to offering a cure to patients with non-resectable hepatocellular carcinoma is the scarcity of cadaveric organs and not the efficacy of the treatment itself. LDLT is, therefore, a viable option as long as the donor offers informed consent and understands possible outcomes.[12] Since LDLT falls outside organ allocation protocols, in the future one may expect to see reports of patients transplanted who do not meet cadaveric eligibility criteria.

Key point 1

- In the future, we may see LDLT applied to recipients who fall outside of current transplant eligibility criteria.

BENEFITS

These can briefly be listed as:

1. Shorter time on waiting list for the recipient.

2. Performed as elective surgery allowing the stabilisation of the recipient and increasing the likelihood of success.

3. An organ from a healthy donor is of better quality than a liver from a deceased person with a fatal illness, who may have been maintained on mechanical ventilation and vasopressor therapy.

4. The donor liver experiences minimal cold ischaemic time because implant occurs immediately after procurement.

5. The use of a living donor adds another liver to the donor pool, allowing a cadaveric liver to go to another recipient. This could potentially shorten the waiting time and improve survival for cadaveric recipients.[13,14]

All of these benefits are to the recipient; there is no benefit to the donor except the satisfaction of an altruistic act.

RISKS TO THE DONOR

The most divisive issue in adult right-lobe LDLT remains the safety of the donor. It should be remembered, though, that the donor is given the opportunity to aid in the cure of a dying family member.[15]

Nonetheless, for many clinicians, the prospect of performing unnecessary surgery on a healthy donor violates the fundamental principle of 'first do no harm'.

To date, there have been three reported donor deaths in the US, four in

Table 1 Issues to discuss during the donor consent procedure[18,19]

General risks of donation
- A 0.3% risk of procedure-related death
- Acute liver failure or chronic hepatic dysfunction requiring urgent liver transplant
- Anaesthesia-related complications
- Blood-borne infection and other transfusion-related morbidity
- Risks associated with intensive care and hospital admission (methicillin-resistant *Staphylococcus aureus*, vancomycin-resistant *Enterococcus* spp.)
- Infections and other complications related to intubation, mechanical ventilation and invasive monitoring

Pre-operative risks
- Risk of diagnosis of previously undiscovered disease
- Bleeding and complications of liver biopsy
- Allergic reaction of contrast media

Postoperative risks
- A 10–67% incidence of postoperative complications
- Potential complications of any abdominal surgery
- Complications specific to major liver resection (biliary leaks/strictures, bilomas, hepatic artery/portal vein thrombosis, hepatic failure)
- Incisional pain and hernia
- Impairment of quality of life
- Compromised success of future abdominal surgery in the donor
- Potential for short-term or long-term disability that might affect employment status, interpersonal relationships
- Financial hardship
- Deterioration in relationship between donor and recipient[19,20]

Europe, and one each in Japan, India, Egypt and South America. Three other donors have required liver transplantation and one donor is in a persistent vegetative state due to complications from donation.[10,16,17] These data are difficult to translate into an accurate overall operative mortality because the exact number of living donor operations performed world-wide has not been recorded in all countries.[18]

Fundamental to donation is the concept that voluntary and informed consent is obtained. In obtaining consent, the clinician needs to present a risk/benefit analysis to the family (Table 1).

EVALUATION OF THE DONOR

When a recipient's relative or friend volunteers as a potential donor, basic medical information is obtained. In this interview, co-morbidities may come to light that preclude further evaluation. The donor should have no medical problems, nor significant family history of genetic problems. The body-mass index (BMI) of the donor may be an important exclusion criterion; 76% of donors with a BMI greater than 28 have substantial hepatic steatosis.[21] Fatty livers function poorly after transplantation and thus most programmes exclude a patient with a BMI greater than 28. A close physical size match between donor and recipient is also important.[22]

If initial screening is suitable, the donor is checked for ABO blood type compatibility with the recipient.

The donor is then required to undergo a 'cooling-off' period, where time is taken to consider their choice. The donor is also offered a 'get-out' option, so they can decline to donate confidentially and be 'given' a medical reason for exclusion.

If the donor still wishes to proceed, a detailed medical, physical, psychological and social work analysis is undertaken.

Routine blood examination is performed to detect abnormalities. The donor then proceeds to more invasive testing. A computed tomography (CT) scan with volumetric studies of the liver ensures there is adequate liver volume in the right and left lobes to sustain both patients. It also identifies incidental pathology. CT angiography defines the hepatic artery, portal and hepatic vein anatomy. Magnetic resonance cholangiopancreatography (MRCP) images the biliary tree. Pre-operative percutaneous liver biopsy is performed if there is a clinical or radiological suspicion of fatty infiltration of the liver. Most centres now find they need to biopsy only a minority of patients.

When all testing is complete, the patient gives informed consent and a date for an elective liver transplant is set.

SELECTION OF THE RECIPIENT

Patients considered for LDLT should fall into current acceptable criteria for transplantation (see above). These are:[15]

1. End-stage liver disease that has failed medical and surgical management with an estimated survival of less than 1 year. Patients with advanced decompensation may not do as well as patients with earlier stage disease.

2. Non-cirrhotic metabolic liver disease, *e.g.* familial amyloid polyneuropathy.

3. Certain types of malignancy, *e.g.* hepatocellular carcinoma, within 'Milan' or other locally accepted criteria.[23]

4. Fulminant liver failure.

Not all patients benefit from LDLT and an evaluation of relative risk to donor and recipient must be made in each case.

There are two types of patients who are typically suited for LDLT. The first, are patients with hepatocellular carcinoma (HCC). These patients are usually given priority on waiting lists, but still may wait a substantial period during which the malignancy may advance rendering them untransplantable. The other group are patients whose severity of disease is not accurately reflected by their laboratory tests; examples include patients with primary sclerosing cholangitis or those with ascites, uncontrolled encephalopathy or severe cachexia.[24]

Outcomes for fulminant liver failure are not as good as for elective LDLT. In this situation there is an overwhelming desire for a relative to save a loved one's life. The urgency removes the time for reflection and reconsideration, which are basic steps in the living donor process. Serious consideration as to the positive outcome for the recipient must be made and the transplant team must act as gatekeepers in not allowing heroic relatives to participate in an unworthy enterprise when the chance of survival of the recipient is poor.[25]

RISKS TO THE RECIPIENT

Generally, the risk to the recipient is the same as receiving a partial graft from a split procedure performed on a cadaver liver which is a generally accepted procedure. Some specific points are worth highlighting.

GRAFT VOLUME

Extremes of size mismatch in LDLT may be detrimental. A 'small-for-size' syndrome is recognised in adult recipients and appears more likely in patients with advanced states of decompensation; therefore, the transplant team should endeavour to transplant grafts whose weight is at least 1% of the recipient's body weight.[26] Consideration must be given to the extent of right lobectomy in the donor. A graft made from an extended right lobe resection including the main trunk of the middle hepatic vein could guarantee optimal outcomes even in recipients with severe decompensation. This might compromise donor safety, though, and the majority of transplant centres currently advocate a standard right hemihepatectomy (Couinaud's segments 5–8), preserving the main trunk of the MHV in the donor.

Excluding the middle hepatic vein from the graft has caused concerns about venous congestion of the anterior segment of the liver (V and VIII) and subsequent non-function of the graft.[27] Many surgeons advocate the reconstruction of the right tributary of the middle hepatic vein to provide improved outflow. Opponents to this technique suggest there are sufficient collateral veins to render this unnecessary.

BILIARY COMPLICATIONS IN THE RECIPIENT

There is good evidence to suggest that biliary complications in the recipient are much higher after LDLT than after cadaveric transplant. These include leakage (anastomosis, cut-surface), stricture, sludge, choledocholithiasis and biliary sepsis. These biliary complications in recipients who are critically ill may have fatal consequences.[28]

The reported incidence of complications differs considerably among centres and ranges from 1–60%.[29] The increased risk of biliary complications is attributable to a reduced sized graft often having two or more biliary anastomoses and a smaller duct size.

Key point 2

- LDLT has a higher rate of biliary complications in the recipient than cadaveric transplants.

RECURRENCE OF HEPATITIS C

The most common indication for liver transplantation is HCV. Virtually all grafts are re-infected with the virus and in some this results in graft loss. One of the most highly debated issues in LDLT is the possibility of increased severity of recurrent HCV in recipients.[30]

Relevant factors may be:[20]

1. HLA matching between donor and recipient is higher in LDLT than in cadaveric transplantation (which are matched on ABO group alone) and this closer concordance may contribute to recurrence.

2. The smaller hepatic mass transplanted during LDLT results in the reduced metabolism of immunosuppressant drugs and can lead to over-immuno-suppression, a factor known to facilitate hepatitis C recurrence.

3. Regeneration of living donor livers following transplantation may promote the uptake of HCV particles into hepatocytes and enhance viral translation and replication.

Two large studies have shown that the incidence and severity of HCV recurrence does not differ between cadaveric liver transplant and LDLT;[31,32] others, however, have found that the incidence of cholestatic hepatitis, a particularly virulent and rapidly destructive form of recurrent HCV, is significantly greater in LDLT recipients.[33]

On the other hand, flexibility in the timing of LDLT can allow an attempt at pre-transplant viral eradication in the recipient. If the recipient is negative for serum HCV RNA on therapy, there is a very low percentage (10%) of post-transplant viral recurrence after LDLT. This may make possible a cure for hepatitis C through transplantation, which is very rarely possible with cadaveric liver transplant.[8]

Key point 3

- Questions regarding an increased rate of recurrence of hepatitis C in the recipient remain unanswered at this time.

THE TECHNIQUE

DONOR SURGERY

The recipient operation consists of a thorough laparotomy and appraisal of the liver including vascular and biliary anatomy (with cholangiography) to confirm correct pre-operative assessment.

The hilar structures are isolated but not divided, with the exception of the right hepatic duct, which must be transected well away from the confluence to avoid donor biliary stricture. The liver is mobilised off the diaphragm and inferior vena cava, slinging the right hepatic vein and any short hepatic vein > 1 cm (for separate anastomosis). Transection of the liver is undertaken along the principal plane preserving the middle hepatic vein for the donor.

When both donor and recipient surgery teams are ready, the right-sided donor vessels are divided and the right hemiliver is flushed on the back-table with cold heparinised saline or preservation solution via the inflow vessels.

RECIPIENT SURGERY

The recipient surgery is commenced in an adjacent room, as soon as the donor team indicates they can proceed. A standard hepatectomy is undertaken preserving the recipient inferior vena cava. The right lobe can be implanted in the same fashion as a right split graft, in the following sequence: right hepatic vein-inferior vena cava anastomosis, portal vein anastomosis, reperfuse, hepatic artery anastomosis and finally biliary anastomosis, either duct-to-duct or choledochojejunostomy-en-Y. The transected surface of the graft usually requires very little work to achieve haemostasis and close any bile leaks.

IMPACT AND FUTURE DEVELOPMENTS

NOT ALL PATIENTS ARE SUITABLE RECIPIENTS AND DONORS

Proponents of LDLT initially thought that the majority of patients listed for transplantation could be suitable for LDLT, thus decreasing the cadaveric waiting list. The reality is that using the current donor and recipient selection criteria, only a fraction of patients are able to undergo the procedure.

Trotter[24] reported that, of the one in three patients on the waiting list with sufficient need for urgent transplant, half are eliminated for technical reasons in the recipient that would jeopardise the success of the surgery (*e.g.* vascular thrombosis). Of the remaining patients, half are unable to identify a suitable donor for evaluation. Of the remaining one in twelve who have a donor evaluated, two-thirds had suitable donors. Finally, therefore, only 5% of patient listed were able to undergo LDLT.

Key point 4

- LDLT initially promised to greatly increase the pool of donor organs, however this seems unlikely due to lack of suitable donors and recipients.

ETHICAL AND SOCIAL CONSIDERATIONS

Until recently, donors for LDLT have been family members or people with a strong emotional connection to recipients. In the US, two new, and highly controversial, categories of donation are emerging:

1. Directed donation to a stranger, whereby donors choose to give to a specific person with whom they have no prior emotional connection. These situations usually occur when a patient advertises for an organ publicly, or the recipient is chosen on the basis of race, religion or ethnic group. The ethics of donation in these situations must be on a case-by-case basis.

2. Non-directed donation, in which the donor gives an organ to the general pool to be transplanted into the recipient at the top of the waiting list. This is a particularly difficult situation for the transplant team. The radical altruism that compels a person to make a potentially life-threatening sacrifice for a stranger, calls for careful scrutiny.[34]

Advertising for an organ over the internet, on billboards or through other advertising also raises the concern over the potential for financial exploitation. Laws have been passed in many countries to prohibit this practice. Further controversy surrounds the internet site MatchingDonors.com. This organisation is a venue where patients and potential donors can meet and communicate. As of 1 July 2005, 12 transplantations have taken place as a result of this web site, all of them renal.[35] As yet, no centres have permitted this kind of donation for liver transplants.

Key point 5

- LDLT raises many ethical and social issues regarding the safety of the donor and the possibility of solicitation of organs.

OUTCOMES

United Network of Organ Sharing data indicate that in the US, the 3-year patient and graft survival rates following LDLT (73% and 66%) are similar to cadaveric donation (78% and 72%, respectively). Europe and Japan quote similar outcomes.[28,36,37] However, LDLT recipients are usually not as ill at the time of transplantation as cadaveric recipients. There is no doubt that patients with a higher Childs-Pugh or model for end-stage liver disease score (MELD) have poorer outcomes; this may be compounded by using reduced sized allografts.[38,39] Adjusting for these factors, the relative rates of patient and graft loss appear significantly higher compared to adult cadaveric donation.[24] Results for those with fulminant hepatic failure are not as good as elective transplantation with a 1-year survival of 66%,[1,40] but the yardstick by these results are measured is comparison with the likelihood of not getting a graft at all, when mortality may approach 100%.

Key point 6

- Results for LDLT are probably not as good as cadaveric transplantation.

Key points for clinical practice

- In the future, we may see LDLT applied to recipients who fall outside of current transplant eligibility criteria.

- LDLT has a higher rate of biliary complications in the recipient than cadaveric transplants.

- Questions regarding an increased rate of recurrence of hepatitis C in the recipient remain unanswered at this time.

- LDLT initially promised to greatly increase the pool of donor organs, however this seems unlikely due to lack of suitable donors and recipients.

- LDLT raises many ethical and social issues regarding the safety of the donor and the possibility of solicitation of organs.

- Results for LDLT are probably not as good as cadaveric transplantation.

References

1. White SA, Al-Mukhtar A, Lodge JP, Pollard SG. Progress in living donor liver transplantation. *Transplant Proc* 2004; **36**: 2720–2726.
2. Strong RW, Lynch SV, Ong TH, Matsunami H, Koido Y, Balderson GA. Successful liver transplantation from a living donor to her son. *N Engl J Med* 1990; **322**: 1505–1507.
3. Takada Y, Tanaka K. Living related liver transplantation. *Transplant Proc* 2004; **36 (2 Suppl)**: 271S–273S.
4. Trotter JF, Wachs M, Everson GT, Kam I. Adult-to-adult transplantation of the right hepatic lobe from a living donor. *N Engl J Med* 2002; **346**: 1074–1082.
5. Yamaoka Y, Washida M, Honda K *et al*. Liver transplantation using a right lobe graft from a living related donor. *Transplantation* 1994; **57**: 1127–1130.
6. Wachs ME, Bak TE, Karrer FM *et al*. Adult living donor liver transplantation using a right hepatic lobe. *Transplantation* 1998; **66**: 1313–1316.
7. United Network of Organ Sharing (UNOS)– Organ Procurement and Transplantation Network. National transplant data reports. Available at <http://www.ortn.org/latestData/step2.asp?>.
8. Brown RS. Hepatitis C and liver transplantation. *Nature* 2005; **436**: 973–978.
9. Russo MW, Brown Jr RS. Adult living donor liver transplantation. *Am J Transplant* 2004; **4**: 458–465.
10. Miller C, Florman S, Kim-Schluger L *et al*. Fulminant and fatal gas gangrene of the stomach in a healthy live liver donor. *Liver Transplant* 2004; **10**: 1315–1319.
11. Merrill JP, Murray JE, Harrison JH, Guild WR. Successful homotransplantation of the human kidney between identical twins. *JAMA* 1956; **160**: 277–282.
12. Broelsch CE, Testa G, Alexandrou A, Malago M. Living related liver transplantation: medical and social aspects of a controversial therapy. *Gut* 2002; **50**: 143–145.
13. Trotter JF, Wachs M, Trouillot T *et al*. Evaluation of 100 patients for living donor liver transplantation. *Liver Transplant* 2000; **6**: 290–295.
14. Trotter JF. Selection of donors and recipients for living donor liver transplantation. *Liver Transplant* 2000; **6 (Suppl 2)**: S52–S58.
15. Blumgart LH, Fong Y. (eds) *Surgery of the Liver and Biliary Tract*, 3rd edn. Edinburgh: W.B. Saunders, 2003.
16. Akabayashi A, Slingsby BT, Fujita M *et al*. The first donor death after living-related liver transplantation in Japan. *Transplantation* 2004; **77**: 634.
17. Surman OS. The ethics of partial-liver donation. *N Engl J Med* 2002; **346**: 1038.
18. Kadry Z, McCormack L, Clavien PA. Should living donor liver transplantation be part of every liver transplant program? *J Hepatol* 2005; **43**: 32–37.
19. Schiano TD, Kim-Schluger L, Gondolesi G, Miller CM. Adult living donor liver transplantation: the hepatologist's perspective. *Hepatology* (2001; **33**: 3–9.
20. Tuttle-Newhall JE, Collins BH, Desai DM, Kuo PC, Heneghan MA. The current status of living donor liver transplantation. *Curr Probl Surg* 2005; **42**: 144–183.
21. Rinella ME, Alonso E, Rao S *et al*. Body mass index as a predictor of hepatic steatosis in living liver donors. *Liver Transplant* 2001; **7**: 409–414.
22. Marsman WA, Wiesner RH, Rodriguez L *et al*. Use of fatty donor liver is associated with diminished early patient and graft survival. *Transplantation* 1996; **62**: 1246–1251.
23. Mazzaferr V, Regalia E, Doci R *et al*. Liver transplantation for the treatment of small hepatocellular carcinomas in patients with cirrhosis. *N Engl J Med* 1996; **334**: 693-699.
24. Trotter JF. Living donor liver transplantation: is the hype over? *J Hepatol* 2005; **42**: 20–25.
25. Strong RW, Lynch SV. Ethical issues in living related donor liver transplantation. *Transplant Proc* 1996; **28**: 2366–2369.
26. Ben-Haim M, Emre S, Fishbein TM *et al*. Critical graft size in adult-to-adult living donor liver transplantation: impact of the recipient's disease. *Liver Transplant Surg* 2001; **7**: 948.
27. de Villa VH, Chen CL, Chen YS *et al*. Right lobe living donor liver transplantation – addressing the middle hepatic vein controversy. *Ann Surg* 2003; **238**: 275–282.
28. Tanaka K, Yamada T. Living donor liver transplantation in Japan and Kyoto University: what can we learn? *J Hepatol* 2005; **42**: 25–28.
29. Todo S, Furukawa H, Kamiyama T. How to prevent and manage biliary complications in living donor liver transplantation? *J Hepatol* 2005; **43**: 22–27.

30. Sugawara Y, Makuuchi M. Should living donor liver transplantation be offered to patients with hepatitis C virus cirrhosis? *J Hepatol* 2005; **42**: 472–475.

31. Russo MW, Galanko J, Beavers K, Fried MW, Shrestha R. Patient and graft survival in hepatitis C recipients after adult living donor liver transplantation in the United States. *Liver Transplant* 2004; **10**: 340–346.

32. Shiffman ML, Stravitz RT, Contos MJ *et al*. Histologic recurrence of chronic hepatitis C virus in patients after living donor and deceased donor liver transplantation. *Liver Transplant* 2004; **10**: 1248–1255.

33. Gaglio PJ, Malireddy S, Levitt BS *et al*. Increased risk of cholestatic hepatitis C in recipients of grafts from living versus cadaveric liver donors. *Liver Transplant* 2003; **9**: 1028–1035.

34. Truog RD. The ethics of organ donation by living donors. *N Engl J Med* 2005; **353**: 444–446.

35. Steinbrook R. Public solicitation of organ donors. *N Engl J Med* 2005; **353**: 441–444.

36. Adam R, Lucidi V, Karam V. Liver transplantation in Europe: is there a room for improvement? *J Hepatol* 2005; **42**: 33–40.

37. Williams RS, Alisa AA, Karani JB, Muiesan P, Rela SM, Heaton ND. Adult-to-adult living donor liver transplant: UK experience. *Eur J Gastroenterol Hepatol* 2003; **15**: 7–14.

38. Brown Jr RS, Russo MW, Lai M *et al*. A survey of liver transplantation from living adult donors in the United States. *N Engl J Med* 2003; **348**: 818–825.

39. Todo S, Furukawa H, Jin MB, Shimamura T. Living donor liver transplantation in adults: outcome in Japan. *Liver Transplant* 2000; **6 (Suppl 2)**: S66–S72.

40. Heaton ND, Maguire D. Adult living donations: lessons learned. *Transplant Proc* 2002; **34**: 2450–2453.

Henry Hook Ross Carter

10

Management of severe acute pancreatitis

The majority of patients with acute pancreatitis will settle quickly with conservative management; in these patients, the only consideration is towards the prevention of further episodes. A detailed discussion of the anatomy, physiology, aetiology, investigation and management of mild acute pancreatitis is beyond the scope of this chapter, which will concentrate on the assessment and potential for intervention in patients with severe physiological disturbance secondary to pancreatic inflammation.

DEFINITION OF SEVERITY

There have been many attempts to stratify patients with acute pancreatitis according to biochemical or clinical parameters. The original concept that a severe attack could be predicted through biochemical scoring systems has changed as it was recognised that organ dysfunction had to be present before serological abnormalities became evident. The close relationship between secondary organ dysfunction and outcome has now been recognised.[1-3] The Atlanta definitions of mild and severe pancreatitis are illustrated in Table 1.

Strict application of the Atlanta definitions has proven of minimal clinical use as organ dysfunction is either present or absent, and the definitions are inflexible regarding the dynamic changes in organ function that occur with time,[3] or the clinical difference between a patient with mild respiratory compromise and one with multi-organ dysfunction syndrome(MODS; Table 2).

Henry Hook BSc MBBS FRACS
Lister Surgical Fellow, West of Scotland Pancreatic Unit, Lister Department of Surgery, Glasgow Royal Infirmary, Glasgow G31 2ER, UK

Ross Carter MBChB FRCS MD FRCS(Gen) (for correspondence)
Consultant Surgeon and Honorary Senior Lecturer, West of Scotland Pancreatic Unit, Lister Department of Surgery, Glasgow Royal Infirmary, Glasgow G31 2ER, UK
E-mail: r carter@clinmed.gla.ac.uk

Table 1 Atlanta definitions of severity

Mild acute pancreatitis

Mild acute pancreatitis is associated with minimal organ dysfunction and an uneventful recovery. The predominant feature is interstitial oedema of the gland

Severe acute pancreatitis

Severe acute pancreatitis is associated with organ failure and/or local complication such as necrosis (with infection) pseudocyst or abscess. Most often, this is an expression of the development of pancreatic necrosis although patients with oedematous pancreatitis may manifest clinical features of a severe attack.

Table 2 Definitions of SIRS and MODS[1]

Systemic inflammatory response syndrome (SIRS)
Response to a variety of severe clinical insults, manifested by two or more of the following conditions
    Temperature > 38°C or < 36°C
    Heart rate > 90 beats/min
    Respiratory rate > 20/min or $PaCO_2$ < 32 mmHg (< 4.3 kPa)
    WBC > 12,000 cells/mm^3, < 4000 cells/mm^3, or > 10% immature (band) forms

Multiple organ dysfunction syndrome (MODS)
Presence of altered organ function in an acutely ill patient such that homeostasis cannot be maintained without intervention

Resource limitations prevent the transfer of patients with potential rather than established problems. Therefore, outwith a study environment where stratification is important, the separation into mild and severe disease is largely academic, and the management algorithm is based more on a holistic assessment of the patient's clinical condition.

MANAGEMENT

Management issues of acute pancreatitis can be separated into: (i) early phase resuscitation and support; and (ii) management of complications. The UK guidelines[4] on the management of acute pancreatitis from 1998 suggested early referral to a specialist centre was indicated for patients with severe disease; however, adequate resourcing of centres to make this a feasible option has not been made available. Whilst there is value in the early discussion of patient management with a specialist centre, it is also inappropriate to transfer a sick patient when the receiving centre has no planned therapeutic intervention, other than continuing organ support. There are relatively few indications for early intervention even in the acutely unwell patient with multiple organ failure. An initial period of management within the intensive care unit of the admitting hospital may well be appropriate, transfer being made if intervention becomes necessary.

EARLY PHASE INVESTIGATION AND MANAGEMENT

Brevity limits a discussion of optimal early management of a patient with organ compromise; however, this differs little from that of any surgical patient with a significant fluid deficit. Inadequate resuscitation may convert potentially reversible organ compromise into established organ failure, and resuscitation within a high dependency or intensive care environment, with invasive monitoring and real-time reassessment should be the norm for a patient with suspected severe disease.

Other than organ support, there are two early potential decisions which may affect management: (i) should the patient receive prophylactic antibiotics; and (ii) is an ERCP/sphincterotomy indicated? Neither has any role in mild disease and their role in severe disease outwith specific circumstances remains controversial. The decision regarding each will also determine what early investigation is required in the patient with clinically severe pancreatitis.

Key point 1

- Resuscitation within a high dependency or intensive care environment, with invasive monitoring and real time re-assessment, should be the norm for a patient with suspected severe disease.

Role of prophylactic antibiotics

The rationale for antibiotic use is to decrease the incidence of septic complications so as to reduce the late mortality associated with sepsis-derived organ failure. There have been a number of trials of antibiotics[5–10] although, unfortunately, none has been sufficiently powered to address mortality. Study design has also allowed the use of antibiotics in the control arms and, until recently, the inclusion criteria tended to be 'predicted severe' acute pancreatitis rather than the presence of suspected necrosis on computed tomography (CT). Although septic complications in general have tended to be reduced, concern has also been raised regarding the development of bacterial resistance,[11,12] and there has been an inconsistent effect on mortality. Recent trials,[10,57] limited to patients with proven necrosis, have failed to confirm the initial promise of the Italian and Finnish studies.

As noted in a Cochrane review, the evidence for and against the use of antibiotics is currently inadequate to make firm recommendations. Misuse of antibiotics is unfortunately commonplace, where an initial prophylactic course extrapolates into a sequence of increasingly broad-spectrum antibiotics in the face of a continuing SIRS response but without bacteriological evidence of infection. Secondary infection, when it eventually supervenes, is usually with resistant or fungal organisms. If used, antibiotics should be given for a defined course and then discontinued.

At this time, it is our policy not to use antibiotics prophylactically; however, where patients have already started a course prior to referral, this is completed. Invasive procedures may be covered by a single intra-operative prophylactic dose. Line sepsis or clinically relevant infections (as opposed to

Key point 2

- The evidence supporting the use of antibiotics is equivocal and no firm recommendations can be made. In units where prophylaxis is the policy of choice, early CT may be useful in identifying those patients with necrosis with the highest risk of septic complications. If antibiotics are given, this should be for a defined period avoiding cyclical escalation in attempting to treat a non-infection driven SIRS response.

bacterial culture), are treated with a short, well-defined course of an appropriate agent in consultation with a microbiology team.

Contrast-enhanced CT

CT scanning is sensitive and quite specific in the diagnosis of pancreatitis and may be useful in the context of delayed presentation when serum markers (amylase) have reduced to non-specific levels. Non-specific elevation in amylase may occur with other acute abdominal conditions and a diagnosis of pancreatitis should not be accepted without a corroboratory CT in these circumstances. More than 90% of patients with acute pancreatitis will have a raised amylase on admission; although serum lipase or pancreatic-specific amylase may be more accurate, these are not universally available in clinical practice. The identification of pancreatic hypoperfusion/necrosis on CT (Fig.1) is common; however, apart from identifying those patients in whom the use of prophylactic antibiotics may be appropriate (see above), it has little role in influencing early management. The transfer of a critically ill patient to the CT

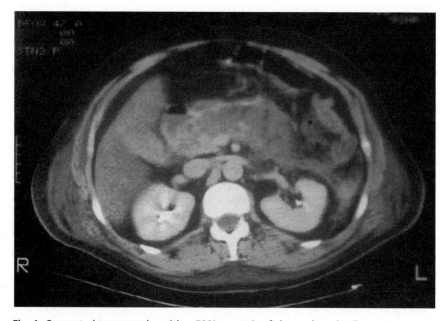

Fig. 1 Computed tomography with > 50% necrosis of the neck and tail.

suite is not without its dangers; consequently, although frequently done, unless there is a desire to identify necrosis to stimulate the prescription of prophylactic antibiotics, there is little logical role for CT in the first week. CT severity scoring systems[13] have also been advocated, but again do not effect early management, and are not used routinely in UK clinical practice.

Logistic difficulties with the availability of MRI-compatible intensive care equipment limit its usefulness, particularly in the early phase. Its role currently lies in the subsequent assessment of aetiology or follow-up during recovery from the acute episode.

Role of early ERCP

The role of early ERCP is equally controversial. Trans-abdominal ultrasound should be performed within the first 48 h following admission, especially in the jaundiced patient.[14] Patients with proven cholangitis occasionally present with associated hyperamylasaemia; in these patients, the organ dysfunction is driven by the cholangitis and not pancreatic inflammation. Urgent ERCP and duct drainage is indicated in this small proportion of patients.[15] Outwith this scenario, the role of early ERCP is much more debatable,[16] and the key question whether sphincter decompression in itself alters the course of the disease remains unanswered by any of the trials.

Of stones, 80% will have passed spontaneously by the time an ERCP is performed. There have been three randomised trials[17–19] investigating the role of early ERCP in acute pancreatitis, but the study design of these has failed to clarify optimal management. Jaundice (and, therefore, potentially cholangitis) was not an exclusion criterion in two of these studies. In others, sphincter decompression was only permitted when a stone was present, and was therefore performed in less than 50% of patients. In the absence of evidence supporting early ERCP in the non-jaundiced patient, due to the potential for procedure-associated morbidity, our current policy is to reserve early ERCP for those with suspected cholangitis.

Key point 3

- Early ERCP is indicated in those with suspected cholangitis and associated hyperamylasaemia; however, there is no proven role outwith this scenario.

SPECIFIC PHARMACOLOGICAL THERAPIES

Over the latter half of the 20th century, several pharmacological agents for acute pancreatitis were assessed for their efficacy in randomised, controlled trials. Acid suppression is commonly used in prevention of stress ulceration but does not alter the course of the disease. Pharmacological treatments include attempts to: (i) suppress pancreatic function with intravenous glucagon,[20,21] somatostatin or the somatostatin analogue, octreotide;[22–26] (ii) support the endogenous anti-protease defence mechanisms with aprotinin (Trasylol),[27] gabexate mesilate,[28] or FFP;[29,30] and (iii) interrupt the pro-inflammatory cytokine cascade with

Lexipafant. Although some of the initial pilot work showed promise there is currently no evidence that any pharmacological intervention alters the course of the disease.

Key point 4

- There is no pharmacological treatment of proven benefit in acute pancreatitis.

NUTRITIONAL SUPPORT IN ACUTE PANCREATITIS

In the majority of patients, the disease will run a benign course and normal diet is restored within a few days. Severe pancreatitis, especially when complicated by sepsis, places a huge metabolic burden on the patient. Profound catabolism with muscle wasting is a frequent accompaniment where nutritional intake may be compromised for months. There are two considerations in this regard:

1. Is there any evidence that the chosen method of nutritional support has any effect on the disease process and, therefore, potentially outcome?

2. If nutritional support is required, what is the best method of meeting the nutritional needs of the patient?

The first consideration is whether maintaining gut rest is beneficial. Traditional management typically involved a period of fasting until certain criteria (*e.g.* normal serum amylase) were met; however, the evidence to support gut rest is sparse. There has yet to be a randomised trial of enteric feeding versus no feeding, even in the first week of the illness. Early feeding, however, as evidenced from comparative studies of enteric and parenteral nutritional support,[31,32] does not appear to exacerbate the inflammatory response associated with the disease. Feeding distal to the ligament of Treitz (naso-jejunal) also seems to confer little benefit over the nasogastric route in our own randomised study,[33] and naso-jejunal tube insertion is not without morbidity; however, gastric stasis can limit the tolerance of nasogastric feeding.

Total parenteral feeding (TPN) and gut rest was standard management in the 1980s but the only trial of TPN versus no feeding showed no benefit.[34] If anything, randomised trials have shown a reduction in morbidity with naso-jejunal feeding compared to TPN in acute pancreatitis,[35–37] although this is largely due to catheter-related complications in the TPN groups rather than a beneficial effect of enteric feeding on the disease process. In addition, studies have suggested a possible benefit from maintaining the gut barrier function,[38] reducing translocation through improved mucosal nutrition, but these studies have been insufficiently powered to address clinically meaningful end-points.

Therefore, whilst there are theoretical advantages to distal enteric feeding, in practice providing nutritional support either proximally (nasogastric/oral) or by the parenteral route seems to have minimal bearing on the inflammatory response and overall disease progression. We have developed a pragmatic approach to nutritional support in severe acute pancreatitis. Where food is tolerated, it is encouraged; where supplementation is needed, we initially use the nasogastric approach; where gastric stasis limits intake, we feed nasally distal to the ligament of Treitz; and, where the gastrointestinal tract is non-functional or calorific targets cannot be met, we supplement this with parenteral nutrition.

SPECIFIC INTERVENTIONS

Blood glucose management

There are now strong data from prospective, randomised trials showing aggressive serum glucose management reduces mortality in critical illness.[39,40] Previous target levels of < 12 mmol/l are probably inadequate and a level of 6 mmol/l has been shown to confer survival advantage and a reduction in septic complications. Logistic nursing problems, and the possibility of severe hypoglycaemia necessitating close monitoring, means that this treatment is reserved for patients with severe pancreatitis admitted in an HDU/ICU setting. Whilst these trials have not specifically been performed in patients with severe pancreatitis, it would appear logical to extrapolate results especially as many have disturbed glucose control.

Role of cholecystectomy

The role of cholecystectomy in protecting patients from further episodes of pancreatitis is well established. A large number of units exercise a policy of cholecystectomy prior to discharge.[4] In the patients who have followed an uncomplicated course and do not have necrosis or fluid collections, this is feasible and not associated with a higher complication rate. There is some evidence to suggest that early cholecystectomy in patients with more severe pancreatitis, specifically those with persisting fluid collections, may lead to increased septic complications.[41] These patients may benefit from a period of observation and repeat imaging prior to cholecystectomy.

Regardless of timing, the cholecystectomy should be complimented by an operative cholangiogram to exclude persistent choledocholithiasis (Fig. 2). In the event of stones being found, several algorithms are possible. These range from trans-cystic exploration/formal choledochotomy to postoperative ERCP. The relative merits of each technique are beyond the scope of this chapter.

Role of surgery early in the disease (< 2 weeks)

A small number of patients with pancreatitis enter a spiral of progressive organ failure in the first week that fails to respond to supportive therapy, which leads to the early peak in mortality. The temptation to operate and remove devitalised tissue when all else has failed is understandable; however, incomplete separation of devitalised tissue leads to resective procedures if more than simple drainage is to be achieved and operative mortality is prohibitive. There is one randomised trial of early versus late surgery,[43] which was discontinued prematurely due to the mortality in the early surgery group. Uncommon, early-phase complications that may require intervention include colonic infarction or perforation. Active haemorrhage requiring intervention due to large vessel disruption (as opposed to haemorrhagic pancreatitis) is also very rare in the early phase; whilst angiographic embolisation is the treatment of choice, surgery may occasionally be required to obtain haemostasis.

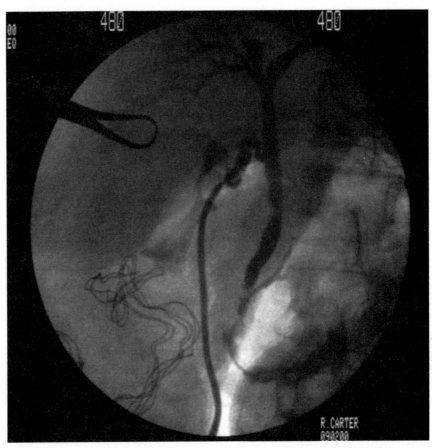

Fig. 2 Intra-operative cholangiogram showing a stone at the lower end of the common bile duct despite non-dilated ducts, a common ampullary channel,[42] and free reflux into the pancreatic duct.

Key point 5

- The role of surgery within the first 7–10 days is limited to the management of complications.

In summary, early deaths in pancreatitis are due to SIRS-induced multiple organ failure. In the absence of evidence indicating the presence of a surgically amenable condition, there is no evidence that outcome can be influenced by intervention, and an agonal laparotomy is to be discouraged.

LATE-PHASE MANAGEMENT

Pancreatic necrosis

Pancreatic necrosis arises in about 15% of patients with acute pancreatitis. Non-enhancement of at least 30% of the pancreatic parenchyma on contrast CT is the current gold standard for diagnosis.[44] The necrotic process is not limited to the pancreas and extensive necrosis of peripancreatic fat can be present despite apparently reasonable parenchymal perfusion. This peripancreatic necrosis is central to why obesity is an independent predictor of both morbidity and mortality.[45] There is little doubt that increasing amounts of necrosis has prognostic significance in acute pancreatitis.[13] Mortality is much less common in simple oedematous pancreatitis and the degree of organ dysfunction less. The risk of septic complications appears to increase proportionately to the degree of necrosis.

Traditional thinking has suggested that it is the necrosis, and particularly where infection supervenes, that drives the organ dysfunction, and resolution will not take place until this is removed. In the 1980s, it was, therefore, common-place to consider debridement for both sterile and infected necrosis. However, it has since been shown repeatedly that sterile necrosis can be managed conservatively with acceptable mortality.[46-48] Thus, while pancreatic necrosis remains a significant entity and a predictor of poor outcome, it is the sepsis-driven organ failure complicating it that determines outcome.

Key point 6

- The majority of patients with sterile necrosis may be managed conservatively. The role of surgery, in the patient who is failing to progress, to debride sterile necrosis is debatable and early elective intervention is, in general, to be discouraged, the ethos being aimed at late intervention when demarcation is complete.

SEPSIS AND INFECTED NECROSIS

Secondary infection in and around the pancreas is an ever-looming spectre and is the commonest life-threatening complication in severe acute pancreatitis. Of those with > 30% necrosis, about 40% will develop secondary infection and, if untreated, mortality approaches 100%.[49] Presence of infection in a tissue bed lacking perfusion has obvious ramifications for antibiotic therapy, which rarely results in resolution without intervention. Late infection of peripancreatic acute fluid collections (pancreatic abscess) are perhaps more frequent than true infected necrosis and require just as prompt treatment; however, the mortality and morbidity of the management of these is much less and they should be considered a separate entity.

The development of infection usually has a dramatic effect on organ function, and a biochemical or clinical deterioration in a patient who has either been stable or improving must raise the suspicion of sepsis and should be pursued aggressively. The source of infection is still debated but the high incidence of gut pathogens isolated suggests gut translocation may be a key player. Frank fistulisation from colon or small bowel may occur and should be suspected when copious gas is present in the collection. Another important contributor to sepsis is instrumentation, and ERCP can cause infection of sterile fluid collections, which dampens some of the enthusiasm for ERCP early in acute pancreatitis. Bacteraemia from central venous lines, feeding lines, arterial lines and urinary catheters may also contribute, and demands fastidious aseptic insertion.

We have recently recognised that the identification of bacteria within pancreatic necrosis is not always associated with clinical deterioration, although this is usually the case. Occasionally, sequential CT will identify gas within a collection, and bacterial contamination may be confirmed on culture; however, the patient remains clinically well. Drawing a parallel from the cholangitic patient, it has been recognised for many years that the presence of bacteria alone within the biliary tree is insufficient, as the combination of obstruction resulting in infection under pressure is required to cause a clinical illness. In this scenario, relieving the obstruction is more important than complete biliary clearance. This has led to a paradigm shift in surgical approach: the prior obsession with the urgent, complete removal of necrosis following the identification of bacterial contamination has moderated to simply ensuring adequate control of surgical sepsis, removal of necrosis being a secondary consideration.

Diagnosis

Acute pancreatitis results in an acute inflammatory process sufficient to cause cell death, and is associated with an acute SIRS response[1] with tachycardia, pyrexia, haematological (white cell count) and biochemical (CRP) indices of inflammation. Despite resolution of the initial initiating event, as a consequence of a large quantity of necrotic material remaining within the retroperitoneum, the SIRS response may persist for many weeks in the absence of any complications and, in particular, infection. The differentiation of sepsis from on-going SIRS is not always easy but there are some objective tools to help clinical judgement.

The development of sepsis will most often be manifest as a clinical deterioration, and any increase in requirement for organ support or deterioration in laboratory indices should raise suspicion. The combination of worsening clinical parameters (increasing tachycardia, worsening organ failure) and serum markers (rising CRP, white cell count) suggest possible sepsis and demand CT evaluation. Imaging with CT is a vital component in the diagnosis of sepsis related to the pancreas. The presence of gas in the pancreas or peripancreatic collections is strong evidence of infection. In the absence of gas, CT will still identify collections in the abdomen, pelvis and chest accurately.

Role of CT

Whilst early scanning is perhaps overdone, sequential CT is key to the identification and late management of the complications of severe acute pancreatitis. All scans should be performed with both oral and intravenous contrast and, where possible, on a high-quality multislice, spiral unit. It is the gold standard for assessment of pancreatic and peripancreatic necrosis and also identifies fluid collections with great anatomical accuracy. Indirect evidence of infection (gas), perforation, pseudo-aneurysm formation, portal/splenic thrombosis or extension of collections into the pelvis or chest may be identified.

The role of CT (or ultrasonography) guided fine needle aspirate (FNA) for culture is controversial. The detrimental influence of a laparotomy in the absence of infection led to the search for confirmatory evidence of infection before committing to necrosectomy. CT-guided aspiration of pancreatic or peri-ancreatic fluid for bacteriology was popularised as a pre-operative procedure in the 1990s; it is routinely employed in some large centres and certainly has reasonable sensitivity and good specificity. In recent years, the approach to infected necrosis has changed (see below); consequently, FNA no longer forms an integral part of the management algorithm.

Key point 7

- Indications for intervention are not absolute and judgement is required. Some patients with evidence of bacterial contamination may remain well and not require surgery. Clinical and biochemical signs of escalating sepsis in general require intervention.

Surgical intervention for infected necrosis

Until recently, the identification of bacteria within the pancreatic or peripancreatic necrosis was sufficient to demand urgent, aggressive, surgical intervention. Significant improvements in survival have followed general improvements in supportive care, and the adoption of debridement procedures in the 1970s rather than attempts at pancreatic resection, which were associated with mortality rates of at least 50%.[50] A 'necrosectomy' involves a wide exposure of the abdomen, usually through a bilateral subcostal/roof-top incision. Both colonic flexures are mobilised to expose the retroperitoneum, the paracolic gutters, and the lesser sac. The abscess is drained and the contained necrotic material removed using a blunt 'finger' dissection technique, leaving all viable tissue. The procedure also includes a cholecystectomy, operative cholangiogram and often a feeding jejunostomy. Whilst there has been debate regarding the optimal postoperative management of the necrotic cavity, blunt finger debridement has remained the most widely used approach for infected pancreatic necrosis.

With simple drainage, recurrent sepsis requiring repeated procedures is common and various approaches (including open laparostomy,[51] closed drainage[52] or packing,[53] and closed lesser sac lavage[54]) to the management of the debrided retroperitoneum have been described with, in some cases, truly remarkable results;[55] however, when each approach has been applied to our own population, mortality remained above 30%. This high operative risk tends to be deemed acceptable in view of the known outcome of untreated infected necrosis. Open debridement in its various forms still constitutes gold standard management of infected necrosis; indeed, a young fit patient, without organ failure and in whom the operative risk is relatively low, may be best served by a single definitive laparotomy with classical debridement and drainage.

Perhaps the biggest change in management has been the realisation, as mentioned above, that the key is adequate control of sepsis, the eventual removal of the necrosis being a secondary consideration. Following any intervention in a critically ill patient, organ dysfunction deteriorates to some degree prior to the hoped for recovery. Our experience of the massive surgical stimulus of necrosectomy was that the magnitude of this deterioration was

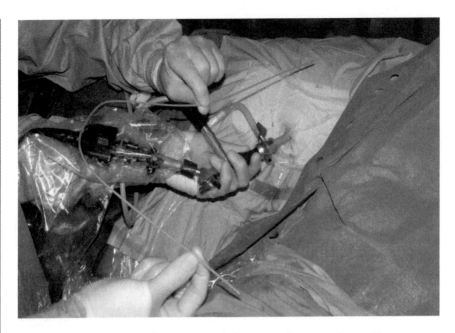

Fig. 3 Intra-operative percutaneous necrosectomy showing operating rod lens endoscope, Amplatz sheath and guiding catheter to maintain access whilst inserting lavage drain.

such that death within 48 h was common. This led to a search for a minimally invasive approach that would allow an adequate debridement coupled with a reduction in the surgical stimulus and we developed the technique of percutaneous necrosectomy (Fig. 3).[56] This involves dilating the tract of a radiologically-placed drain and introducing a modified nephroscope into the cavity. Necrosectomy is performed piecemeal with laparoscopic grasping forceps. Whilst initially our aim was to mirror the open approach by performing an adequate necrosectomy at one sitting, it became evident that a staged necrosectomy, whilst ensuring adequate sepsis control by continual postoperative cavity lavage, reduced complications; leaving significant amounts of necrosis for interval removal appeared to have no adverse effects. Radiological percutaneous drainage of peripancreatic collections fell into disrepute as the small bore catheters used, which often resulted in a temporary improvement, became blocked if the collection contained any solid component. We would now suggest the problem was not with the percutaneous approach, but rather that the drains were allowed to block resulting in further episodes of inadequately drained sepsis with an inevitable deterioration in organ failure.

Our current approach, when faced with a patient with suspected infection and a drainable peri-pancreatic collection, is to proceed with a CT-guided percutaneous drain for sepsis control, subsequent dilatation of the tract and percutaneous necrosectomy with a view to maintain adequate drainage; necrosectomy taking place over a number of weeks as a staged procedure. Critical assessment of the various operative and non-operative strategies for management of infected necrosis is made extremely difficult by the diversity of the cohorts. We believe that, as a result of this diversity, no one treatment should be regarded as gold standard for every patient. The various techniques, properly assessed, should be regarded as complimentary rather than mutually exclusive.

Key point 8

- There is no agreement as to the optimal approach, which is usually determined by local expertise and preference. There is a trend toward adopting a more minimally invasive approach (radiological, endoscopic, or percutaneous) where possible, particularly in the patient with multi-organ failure.

HAEMORRHAGE, DIAGNOSIS AND TREATMENT

Whilst infection of pancreatic necrosis is the commonest complication overall, secondary haemorrhage is the commonest complication in those patients that subsequently die from the disease. Haemorrhage in the early phase of the disease is very uncommon but tends to occur in the context of sepsis within the pancreatic bed and, as such, rarely occurs before the third week and often following surgical intervention.

Pseudo-aneurysm formation within the coeliac or superior mesenteric circulations may lead to rupture and massive haemorrhage. Bleeding presents most commonly as a fresh secondary haemorrhage into a surgical drain, but may also manifest as gastrointestinal haemorrhage or by sudden onset of abdominal pain and a fall in haemoglobin where the bleed is contained within an established pseudocyst. A contained bleed such as this is less likely to cause haemodynamic instability. Experience has shown us that fresh bleeding into a surgical drain must always be regarded as a 'herald' bleed and should be pursued aggressively, as exanguinating haemorrhage often follows. Obviously, upper gastrointestinal bleeds will occur in sick pancreatitis patients secondary to non-aneurysmal causes (e.g. stress ulceration) and endoscopy should be used freely to clarify this.

Haemorrhage into a surgical drain in a patient with severe acute pancreatitis mandates an urgent selective mesenteric angiogram with a view to embolisation of any bleeding point. A screening CT angiogram may be normal as bleeding may occur in the absence of a pseudo-aneurysm. Pseudo-aneurysms occur most frequently along the splenic or gastroduodenal arteries. Both of these may be embolised with acceptable risk of complication. Collateral circulation via the short gastrics tends to prevent splenic or duodenal infarction/perforation. Vigilance must be maintained post-embolisation to identify ischaemic complications.

Key point 9

- Twenty-four hour access to interventional radiology is a mandatory requirement for a unit wishing to manage patients with pancreatic necrosis.

MANAGEMENT OF LATE COLLECTIONS

In many hospitals, patients with true infected necrosis are considered in the same way as those who develop infection within an acute inflammatory collection/pseudocyst perhaps 8–12 weeks following onset of symptoms. A detailed discussion of the management of late collections/abscess is beyond the scope of this chapter; however, these patients are rarely in organ failure and mortality associated with treatment is low. In this diverse group, intervention is determined by the position of the collection relative to the gastrointestinal tract, and may involve open surgical, laparoscopic or endoscopic transmural drainage or, on occasion, percutaneous drainage. Once again, the principle of management is control of sepsis followed or accompanied by removal of any solid component; in most cases, the patient will recover regardless of the chosen approach.

Key points for clinical practice

- Resuscitation within a high dependency or intensive care environment, with invasive monitoring and real time re-assessment, should be the norm for a patient with suspected severe disease.

- The evidence supporting the use of antibiotics is equivocal and no firm recommendations can be made. In units where prophylaxis is the policy of choice, early CT may be useful in identifying those patients with necrosis with the highest risk of septic complications. If antibiotics are given, this should be for a defined period avoiding cyclical escalation in attempting to treat a non-infection driven SIRS response.

- Early ERCP is indicated in those with suspected cholangitis and associated hyperamylasaemia; however, there is no proven role outwith this scenario.

- There is no pharmacological treatment of proven benefit in acute pancreatitis.

- The role of surgery within the first 7–10 days is limited to the management of complications.

- The majority of patients with sterile necrosis may be managed conservatively. The role of surgery, in the patient who is failing to progress, to debride sterile necrosis is debatable and early elective intervention is, in general, to be discouraged, the ethos being aimed at late intervention when demarcation is complete.

- Indications for intervention are not absolute and judgement is required. Some patients with evidence of bacterial contamination may remain well and not require surgery. Clinical and biochemical signs of escalating sepsis in general require intervention.

- There is no agreement as to the optimal approach, which is usually determined by local expertise and preference. There is a trend toward adopting a more minimally invasive approach (radiological, endoscopic, or percutaneous) where possible, particularly in the patient with multi-organ failure.

- Twenty-four hour access to interventional radiology is a mandatory requirement for a unit wishing to manage patients with pancreatic necrosis.

References

1. Bone RC, Balk RA, Cerra FB *et al*. Definitions for sepsis and organ failure and guidelines for the use of innovative therapies in sepsis. The ACCP/SCCM Consensus Conference Committee. American College of Chest Physicians/Society of Critical Care Medicine. *Chest* 1992; **101**: 1644–1655.
2. Tenner S, Sica GA, Hughes M *et al*. Relationship of necrosis to organ failure in severe acute pancreatitis. *Gastroenterology* 1997; **113**: 899–903.
3. Buter A, Imrie CW, Carter CR, Evans S, McKay CJ. Dynamic nature of early organ dysfunction determines outcome in acute pancreatitis. *Br J Surg* 2002; **89**: 298–302.
4. Glazer G, Mann DV. United Kingdom guidelines in the management of acute pancreatitis. *Gut* 1998; **42 (Suppl 2)**: S1–S13.
5. Pederzoli P, Bassi C, Vesentini S, Campedelli A. A randomized multicenter clinical trial of antibiotic prophylaxis of septic complications in acute necrotizing pancreatitis with imipenem. *Surg Gynecol Obstet* 1993; **176**: 480–483.
6. Sainio V, Kemppainen E, Puolakkainen P *et al*. Early antibiotic treatment in acute necrotising pancreatitis. *Lancet* 1995; **346**: 663–667.
7. Schwarz M, Meyer H, Isenmann R, Beger HG. Antibiotic prophylaxis for reduction of complications in acute necrotizing pancreatitis. *Zentralbl Chir* 1998; **123**: 28–31.
8. Delcenserie R, Yzet T, Ducroix JP. Prophylactic antibiotics in treatment of severe acute alcoholic pancreatitis. *Pancreas* 1996; **13**: 198–201.
9. Delcenserie R, Delion-Lozinguez MP, Nord CHU *et al*. Prophylactic ciprofloxacin treatment in acute necrotising pancreatitis: a prospective randomised multicentre clinical trial. *Gastroenterology* 2003; **120 (Suppl 1)**: A25–A119.
10. Isenmann R, Runzi M, Kron M *et al*. Prophylactic antibiotic treatment in patients with predicted severe acute pancreatitis: a placebo-controlled, double-blind trial. *Gastroenterology* 2004; **126**: 997–1004.
11. Eatock FC, Brombacher GD, Hood J, Carter R, Imrie CW. Fungal infection of pancreatic necrosis is associated with increased mortality [abstract]. *Br J Surg* 1999; **86 (Suppl 1)**: 78.
12. Grewe M, Tsiotos GG, Luque-de Leon E, Sarr M. Fungal infection in acute necrotising pancreatitis. *J Am Coll Surg* 1999; **188**: 408–413.
13. Balthazar EJ, Robinson DL, Megibow AJ, Ranson JHC. Acute pancreatitis: value of CT in establishing prognosis. *Radiology* 1990; **174**: 331–336.
14. Johnson CD *et al*. Working Party of the British Society of Gastroenterology; Association of Surgeons of Great Britain and Ireland; Association of Upper GI Surgeons of Great Britain and Ireland. UK guidelines for the management of acute pancreatitis. *Gut* 2005; **54 (Suppl 3)**:iii1–9.
15. Neoptolemos JP, Carr-Locke DL, Leese T, James D. Acute cholangitis in association with acute pancreatitis: incidence, clinical features and outcome in relation to ERCP and endoscopic sphincterotomy. *Br J Surg* 1987; **74**: 1103–1106.
16. Ayub K, Imada R, Slavin J. Endoscopic retrograde cholangiopancreatography in gallstone-associated acute pancreatitis. *Cochrane Database Syst Rev* 2004; CD003630.
17. Fan S-T, Lai ECS, Mok FPT, Lo C-M, Zheng S-S, Wong J. Early treatment of acute biliary pancreatitis by endoscopic papillotomy. *N Engl J Med* 1993; **328**: 228–232.
18. Neoptolemos JP, London NJ, James D, Carr-Locke DL, Bailey IA, Fossard DP. Controlled trial of urgent endoscopic retrograde cholangiopancreatography and endoscopic sphincterotomy versus conservative treatment for acute pancreatitis due to gallstones. *Lancet* 1988; **2**: 979–983.
19. Folsch UR, Nitsche R, Ludtke R, Hilgers RA, Creutzfeldt. Early ERCP and papillotomy compared with conservative treatment for acute biliary pancreatitis. *N Engl J Med* 1997; **336**: 237–242.
20. Kronborg O, Bulow S, Joergensen PM, Svendsen LB. A randomized double-blind trial of glucagon in treatment of first attack of severe acute pancreatitis without associated biliary disease. *Am J Gastroenterol* 1980; **73**: 423–425.
21. Regan PT, Malagelada JR, Go VL, Wolf AM, DiMagno EP. A prospective study of the antisecretory and therapeutic effects of cimetidine and glucagon in human acute pancreatitis. *Mayo Clin Proc* 1981; **56**: 499–503.
22. Paran H, Neyfeld D, Mayo A *et al*. Preliminary report of a prospective randomized study of octreotide in the treatment of severe acute pancreatitis. *J Am Coll Surg* 1995; **181**: 121–124.

23. Beechey-Newman N. Controlled trial of high-dose octreotide in treatment of acute pancreatitis. Evidence of improvement in disease severity. *Dig Dis Sci* 1993; **38**: 644–647.
24. Karakoyunlar O, Sivrel E, Tanir N, Denecli AG. High dose octreotide in the management of acute pancreatitis. *Hepatogastroenterology* 1999; **46**: 1968–1972.
25. McKay C, Baxter J, Imrie C. A randomized, controlled trial of octreotide in the management of patients with acute pancreatitis. *Int J Pancreatol* 1997; **21**: 13–19.
26. Uhl W, Buchler MW, Malfertheiner P, Beger HG, Adler G, Gaus W and German Pancreatitis Study Group. A randomised double blind multicentre trial of octreotide in moderate to severe acute pancreatitis. *Gut* 1999; **45**: 97–104.
27. Trapnell JE, Rigby CC, Talbot CH. Controlled trial of Trasylol in the treatment of acute pancreatitis. *Br J Surg* 1974; **61**: 177–180.
28. Pederzoli P, Cavallini G, Falconi M, Bassi C. Gabexate mesilate vs aprotinin in human acute pancreatitis (GA.ME.P.A.): a prospective, randomized, double-blind multicenter study. *Int J Pancreatol* 1993; **14**: 117–124.
29. Leese T, Holliday M, Heath D, Hall AW, Bell PRF. Multicentre clinical trial of low volume fresh frozen plasma therapy in acute pancreatitis. *Br J Surg* 1987; **74**: 907–911.
30. Leese T, Holliday M, Watkins M *et al.* A multicentre controlled clinical trial of high-volume fresh frozen plasma therapy in prognostically severe acute pancreatitis. *Ann R Coll Surg Engl* 1991; **73**: 207–214.
31. Powell JJ, Murchison JT, Fearon KC, Ross JA, Siriwardena AK. Randomized controlled trial of the effect of early enteral nutrition on markers of the inflammatory response in predicted severe acute pancreatitis. *Br J Surg* 2000; **87**: 1375–1381.
32. Windsor ACJ, Kanwar S, Li AGK *et al.* Compared with parenteral nutrition, enteral feeding attenuates the acute phase response and improves disease severity in acute pancreatitis. *Gut* 1998; **42**: 431–435.
33. Eatock FC, Chocg P, Menezes N *et al.* A randomized study of early nasogastric versus nasojejunal feeding in severe acute pancreatitis. *Am J Gastroenterol* 2005; **100**: 432–439.
34. Sax HC, Warner BW, Talamini MA *et al.* Early total parenteral nutrition in acute pancreatitis: lack of beneficial effects. *Am J Surg* 1987; **153**: 117–124.
35. Kalfarentzos F, Kehagias J, Mead N, Kokkinis K, Gogos CA. Enteral nutrition is superior to parenteral nutrition in severe acute pancreatitis: results of a randomized prospective trial. *Br J Surg* 1997; **84**: 1665–1669.
36. McClave SA, Greene LM, Snider HL *et al.* Comparison of the safety of early enteral vs parenteral nutrition in mild acute pancreatitis. *J Parenter Enter Nutr* 1997; **21**: 14–20.
37. Abou-Assi S, Craig K, O'Keefe SJ. Hypocaloric jejunal feeding is better than total parenteral nutrition in acute pancreatitis: results of a randomized comparative study. *Am J Gastroenterol* 2002; **97**: 2255–2262.
38. Ammori BJ. Role of the gut in the course of severe acute pancreatitis. *Pancreas* 2003; **26**: 122–129.
39. Pittas AG, Siegel RD, Lau J. Insulin therapy for critically ill hospitalized patients: a meta-analysis of randomized controlled trials. *Arch Intern Med* 2004; **164**: 2005–2011.
40. Van den Berghe G, Wouters PJ, Bouillon R *et al.* Outcome benefit of intensive insulin therapy in the critically ill: insulin dose versus glycemic control. *Crit Care Med* 2003; **31**: 359–366.
41. Nealon WH, Bawduniak J, Walser EM. Appropriate timing of cholecystectomy in patients who present with moderate to severe gallstone-associated acute pancreatitis with peripancreatic fluid collections. *Ann Surg* 2004; **239**: 741–749.
42. Opie EL. The etiology of acute hemorrhagic pancreatitis. *Bull Johns Hopkins Hosp* 1901; **12**: 182–188.
43. Meir J, Luque-de Leon E, Castillo A, Robledo F, Blanco R. Early versus late necrosectomy in severe necrotising pancreatitis. *Am J Surg* 1997; **173**: 71–75.
44. Balthazar EJ, Ranson JHC, Naidich DP, Megibow AJ, Caccavale R, Cooper MM. Acute pancreatitis: prognostic value of CT. *Radiology* 1985; **156**: 767–772.
45. Johnson CD, Toh SK, Campbell MJ. Combination of APACHE-II score and an obesity score (APACHE-O) for the prediction of severe acute pancreatitis. *Pancreatology* 2004; **4**: 1–6.
46. Hartwig W, Werner J, Muller CA, Uhl W, Buchler MW. Surgical management of severe pancreatitis including sterile necrosis. *J Hepatobiliary Pancreat Surg* 2003; **9**: 429–435.

47. Rau B, Pralle U, Uhl W, Schoenberg MH, Beger HG, Bradley E III. Operative vs non-operative management in sterile necrotizing pancreatitis. *HPB Surg* 1997; **10**: 188–191.
48. Bradley III EL. A prospective longitudinal study of observation versus surgical intervention in the management of necrotizing pancreatitis. *Am J Surg* 1991; **161**: 19–25.
49. Rau B, Pralle U, Mayer JM, Beger HG. Role of ultrasonographically guided fine-needle aspiration cytology in the diagnosis of infected pancreatic necrosis. *Br J Surg* 1998; **85**: 179–184.
50. Watts CT. Total pancreatectomy for fulminant pancreatitis. *Lancet* 1963; **2**: 384–389.
51. Bradley III EL. Management of infected pancreatitis necrosis by open drainage. *Ann Surg* 1987; **206**: 542–550.
52. Warshaw AL, Jin G. Improved survival in 45 patients with pancreatic abscess. *Ann Surg* 1985; **202**: 408–415.
53. Fernandez-Del CC, Rattner DW, Makary MA, Mostafavi A, McGraft D, Warshaw AL. Debridement and closed packing for the treatment of necrotizing pancreatitis. *Ann Surg* 1998; **228**: 676–684.
54. Beger HG, Buchler M, Bittner R, Oettunger W, Block S, Nevalainen T. Necrosectomy and postoperative local lavage in patients with necrotizing pancreatitis: results of a prospective clinical trial. *World J Surg* 1988; **12**: 255–262.
55. Farkas G, Marton J, Mandi Y, Szederkenyi E. Surgical strategy and management of infected pancreatic necrosis. *Br J Surg* 1996; **83**: 930–933.
56. Carter CR, McKay CJ, Imrie CW. Percutaneous necrosectomy and sinus tract endoscopy in the management of infected pancreatic necrosis: an initial experience. *Ann Surg* 2000; **232**: 175–180.
57. Dellinger EP , Tellado JM, Soto N. Prophylactic antibiotic treatment in patients with severe acute necrotizing pancreatitis: a double-blind placebo-controlled study. ICAAC Meeting Abstract. 2005.

Sohail A. Choksy James Keir John R. Bottomley

11

Pseudoaneurysms: minimally invasive management

A pseudoaneurysm (false aneurysm) is an extravascular haematoma that communicates with the intravascular space as a result of disruption of the arterial wall. As a consequence, leakage of blood at arterial pressure results in a haematoma, which is confined by fascial planes in adjacent tissues. If an arterial wall thrombus plug fails to form, or is dislodged or breaksdown, the haematoma (prior to thrombosis) maintains communication with the vascular compartment and is known as a pseudoaneurysm. Delayed liquefaction of a haematoma and breakdown or dislodgement of the arterial defect thrombus plug may also leave a cavity into which blood will flow forming a pseudoaneurysm.

Pseudoaneurysms can occur in any vascular territory and arise due to a variety of aetiologies. The rapid expansion of endovascular interventions has seen a substantial rise in the incidence of iatrogenic femoral artery pseudoaneurysms which is reported to range between < 1% to 7%.[1,2] Although small, uncomplicated, asymptomatic pseudoaneurysms may be treated conservatively,[3] the remainder require treatment due to the potential for high morbidity and mortality.

Traditionally, most iatrogenic pseudoaneurysms were repaired surgically. Since the early 1990s, the treatment has evolved towards minimally invasive techniques. These include ultrasound-guided compression (USGC), ultrasound-guided thrombin injection (USTI), endovascular embolisation and pseudoaneurysm

Sohail A. Choksy BSc MBBS FRCS (for correspondence)
Senior Registrar in Vascular Surgery, Sheffield Vascular Institute, Herries Road, Northern General Hospital, Sheffield S5 7AU, UK
E-mail: sohail.choksy@sheffield.ac.uk

James Keir DOHNS MRCS
Specialist Registrar, Queens Medical Centre, Nottingham University Hospital NHS Trust, Derby Rd, Nottingham NG7 2UH, UK

John R. Bottomley MBChB FRANZCR
Consultant Vascular Radiologist, Sheffield Vascular Institute, Northern General Hospital, Herries Road, Sheffield S5 7AU, UK.

exclusion by endovascular placement of stent grafts. Surgical repair is now reserved for failure of less invasive methods, for infected pseudoaneurysms, rapid expansion, concomitant distal ischaemia, neurological deficit, or compromised soft tissue viability due to pressure effects from the pseudo-aneurysm.

The aim of this article is to outline the methods, results and pitfalls of various techniques and to discuss the role of each in the management of this potentially life-threatening condition.

Key point 1

- The majority of pseudoaneurysms occur following superficial femoral artery catheterisation. Most uncomplicated pseudo-aneurysms can be managed either conservatively or with minimally invasive techniques.

AETIOLOGY

Pseudoaneurysms may be caused by blunt or penetrating trauma, inflammation (*e.g.* pancreatitis) or infections; however, most are caused by a variety of iatrogenic arterial injuries. These include percutaneous biopsy or drain placement, orthopaedic, vascular and transplant surgery,[4] as well as following insertion of arterial lines for patient monitoring. The great majority of iatrogenic causes of pseudoaneurysms occur at the arterial access site following endovascular procedures. The Royal College of Radiologists' guidelines recommend an acceptable upper limit of pseudoaneurysm rate of 0.5% after endovascular procedures.[36]

Surgical causes of pseudoaneurysms include inadvertent, inadequately controlled and unrecognised arterial injury and the breakdown of the vascular anastomoses. This may be immediate (due to poor anastomotic technique, suture breakage, or mechanical distraction at the anastomosis), or delayed (due to graft infection, graft or suture material deterioration).

Although pseudoaneurysms are diagnosed more frequently, there has been a real increase in the incidence due to the increase in the number and complexity of endovascular procedures. The incidence depends upon the type of intervention used and ranges from 0.2–2%[1] for diagnostic angiography to 3.2–7.7% for interventions in which large bore sheaths are used.[2] Other risk factors include older age, obesity, anticoagulation, fibrinolytic therapy, calcified arteries, hypertension, obesity, and too brief or ineffective manual compression.[2,5] Failure to puncture the common femoral artery (CFA) over the femoral head, in particular low punctures into the superficial femoral (SFA) or profunda femoral artery, can also result in ineffective manual compression at the end of the procedure with consequent pseudoaneurysm formation.[5]

Arteriotomy closure devices (ACDs) have recently emerged as an alternative means of 'sealing off' arterial punctures following endovascular intervention. There are many devices available, all of which have moderate associated learning curves prior to their regular safe and effective deployment. Two recent meta-analyses assessed the safety of ACDs versus mechanical compression in patients undergoing percutaneous coronary interventions

(PCIs). The first concluded, based on the analysis of 30 randomised trials (many of poor methodological quality), that there is only marginal evidence that ACDs are effective and there is reason for concern that these devices may increase the risk of haematoma and pseudoaneurysm.[6] In the second, the risk of access-site related complications was similar for ACDs compared with mechanical compression after diagnostic angiography. In the setting of PCI, angioseal and perclose were similar to mechanical compression. The rate of complications after PCIs was higher with Vasoseal compared to mechanical compression.[7]

Despite these conclusions, the advantages of quicker time to haemostasis, ambulation and discharge, as well as patient satisfaction and cost effectiveness, particularly with newer generations of arterial closure devices remain to be evaluated.

Key point 2

- Arteriotomy closure devices are in wide-spread use but remain controversial in the prevention of access-site related complications. Newer generations of devices appear to be as safe and effective as manual compression.

CLINICAL FEATURES

It may be difficult to clinically differentiate a pseudoaneurysm from a haematoma. A palpable thrill, pulsatile mass or an audible bruit may be present. Pseudoaneurysms may be asymptomatic and may be diagnosed incidentally on imaging performed for another indication. Many of these smaller lesions may occlude spontaneously.[3,8,9]

Larger pseudoaneurysms may cause local pressure effects by compression of adjacent tissues and structures. In the groin, for example, the pseudoaneurysm may compress the femoral nerve causing neurological symptoms. Compression of the femoral vein may cause venous occlusion, oedema and may result in deep venous thrombosis. Communication with an adjacent vein may result in an arteriovenous fistula. This may result in steal syndrome and even cardiac failure.[10] Pressure on adjacent tissue may be painful, especially if complicated by infection, and may cause necrosis of overlying skin and subcutaneous tissue. Distal arterial thrombo-embolism may arise from the pseudoaneurysm itself or its treatment.

The risk of pseudoaneurysm rupture is unpredictable and is the most common cause of death in patients with a pseudoaneuysm. Blood loss may be obvious (*e.g.* haemorrhage and a rapidly expanding mass) or it may be occult (*e.g.* retroperitoneal bleeding following external iliac arterial puncture). The latter may be associated with a significant delay in diagnosis. Bleeding may be difficult to diagnose in rarer pseudoaneurysms in the gut, biliary system and pelvic spaces. Haemorrhage may also manifest as sentinel bleeds heralding a later catastrophic bleed.

If infection supervenes, the pseudoaneurysm may expand rapidly and risk of rupture is high. Alternatively, septic emboli into the distal circulation may threaten viability of the limb. Infection may also cause systemic symptoms, such as sweats and fever as well as a raised white cell count. Prompt surgical debridement is essential.

DIAGNOSIS

Recent technological advances in non-invasive imaging have achieved greater diagnostic accuracy in the assessment of pseudoaneurysms. Grey scale and

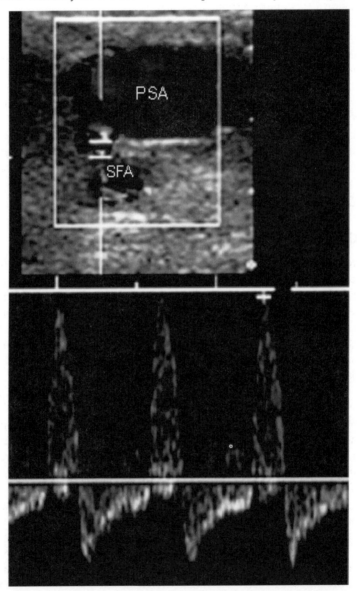

Fig. 1 Colour duplex ultrasound demonstrating a pseudo-aneurysm (PSA) anterior to the proximal superficial femoral artery (SFA) which developed following endovascular intervention. Duplex waveform shows 'to-and-fro' flow through the arterial wall defect, and swirling flow within in pseudo-aneurysm cavity. This was later successfully treated with thrombin injection.

colour duplex ultrasound is now first line imaging modality of choice (Fig. 1) for the majority of pseudoaneurysms but is operator-dependent and performs less well in visceral arteries or where parent vessels are hidden by air or bone. Ultrasound allows real time imaging, assessment of the track and measurement of the overall dimensions of the pseudoaneurysm as well as the width of the neck. Identification of a hypo-echoic cystic structure adjacent to an artery with characteristic swirling ('yin yang' sign) blood flow on colour Doppler imaging and demonstration of 'to-and-fro' duplex waveform pattern in the neck allows confirmation of the diagnosis.

Multidetector CT angiography overcomes some of the operator-dependent and 'blind spot' problems of ultrasound and has high sensitivity (95.1%) and specificity (98.7%) for the detection of pseudoaneurysms.[11] MR angiography does not require the use of nephrotoxic contrast medium or ionising radiation and is, therefore, of greatest value in assessing younger patients and those with renal impairment or contrast allergy. New 'blood-pool' MR contrast agents look promising for the evaluation and detection of pseudoaneurysms as they stay in the vascular compartment and allow a longer imaging window. Conventional digital subtraction angiography allows real-time visualisation of the flow dynamics of feeding and draining vessels and, as such, has greatest advantages in assessing complex pseudoaneurysms and detailed arterial anatomy.

TREATMENT OPTIONS

The treatment of pseudoaneurysms has evolved in the last decade from surgical repair towards less invasive methods. Although surgical repair is curative, it is accompanied by significant morbidity, increased length of hospital stay and increased costs.[12–16] Since the early 1990s, endovascular and radiological techniques have increased the treatment options available for patients with uncomplicated pseudoaneurysms. The choice of method depends upon local interventional expertise and a number of lesions and patient-specific factors (Table 1).

Key point 3

- Treatment choice for pseudoaneurysms is governed by characteristics of the pseudoaneurysm (site, size, symptoms, neck width), patient co-morbidity and anticoagulation status as well as local interventional expertise.

CONSERVATIVE MANAGEMENT

Since the original report by Kotval et al.,[3] several other reports have also indicated that a proportion of pseudoaneurysms may spontaneously occlude; however, this is unpredictable. Small stable asymptomatic pseudoaneurysms with a narrow neck are most likely to be successfully managed in this way with regular observation. In one series, seven pseudoaneurysms ranging in size from 1.3–3.5 cm in diameter following femoral arterial access for percutaneous

Table 1 Factors which affect the choice of technique for pseudoaneurysm treatment

Size and symptoms
Small pseudoaneurysms may occlude spontaneously. We recommend that small uncomplicated asymptomatic pseudoaneurysms (< 6 ml) be managed conservatively with close observation and should only be treated if they become symptomatic, enlarge or fail to resolve following a period of conservative management

Site and accessibility
Limb arteries are more amenable to direct compression or thrombin injection. Visceral artery pseudoaneurysms can often be managed with embolisation or rarely stent grafting as alternatives to surgery

Diameter of the neck
Wide neck pseudo-aneurysms are less likely to thrombose spontaneously or with ultrasound-guided compression. Thrombin injection techniques run the risk of distal embolisation hence these are more likely to require embolisation or suturing of the arterial wall defect

Expendability of parent artery
If the parent artery supplies non-essential tissues such as profunda femoral arterial branch supply to the lateral thigh, embolisation can be performed (assuming a patent SFA). If patency of the parent artery is essential to be maintained, a stent graft may be appropriate if points of flexion and branch vessels can be avoided

Complicated pseudo-aneurysms
For example, infection, pressure effects on nearby structures. These should be treated by surgery

Anticoagulation status
Patients on anticoagulants and/or antiplatelet agents are more likely to develop and maintain flow within a pseudo-aneurysm irrespective of small initial size. In these patients, conservative treatment is unlikely to succeed

Patient co-morbidities
Due to the higher morbidity and mortality associated with surgery, multiple co-morbid patients are more suited to less invasive methods of treatment, if appropriate.

trans-luminal angioplasty, were followed up with weekly duplex scans. All had thrombosed spontaneously within 4 weeks of detection.[8] In another study, 147 patients with small (< 3 cm), stable pseudoaneurysms were managed conservatively with a spontaneous thrombosis rate of 86% and mean duration to closure of 23 days. Strict criteria were, however, used to select which pseudoaneurysms should undergo immediate surgical repair including patients receiving long-term anticoagulation, initial size > 3 cm, evidence of expansion, pain, groin infection, nerve compression, ischaemic symptoms and those patients who could not be followed up with repeat duplex ultrasound scanning.[9]

Patient selection is the key to identify which pseudoaneurysms can be managed in this way. Two studies have indicated a high likelihood of spontaneous resolution for smaller pseudoaneurysms compared to larger ones.[17,18] Flow characteristics on colour duplex do not predict which aneurysms will thrombose spontaneously.[9] Although there is no definite size criteria by which pseudoaneurysms should all be treated, many interventionalists use 6 ml volume as an upper limit for conservative management in uncomplicated asymptomatic cases.[17] Beyond this, the risk of rupture is thought to be too high. Lesions smaller than this can be followed up with duplex ultrasound 2–3 times weekly and treatment instigated if the pseudoaneurysm fails to resolve.

Key point 4

- Small uncomplicated pseudoaneurysms (< 6 ml) can be managed conservatively with regular observation and will usually thrombose spontaneously.

ULTRASOUND-GUIDED COMPRESSION

Ultrasound-guided compression (USGC) of femoral pseudoaneurysms (FPAs) was first described in 1991 by Fellmeth et al.[19] It requires compression of the arterial defect against an underlying bone such as the common femoral artery over the femoral head or the distal brachial artery over the distal humerus. Firm transducer pressure is applied over the pseudoaneurysm track or neck until there is cessation of colour flow within the pseudoaneurysm sac on real-time colour duplex ultrasound imaging. This is usually maintained for 10-min intervals up to 50 min until thrombosis is achieved or as long as the patient can tolerate. The patient is confined to bed rest for 6–12 h with a pressure dressing applied.

Review of several studies revealed an overall success rate of 59–98%.[19–23] In two of these studies, initial success rate was 85–88%. In patients in whom treatment had failed, the procedure was repeated and an overall success rate of 95–98% was achieved.[22,23] Recurrence rate after initial therapy may be as high as 20–30%. The main risk factors for recurrence are anticoagulation and the size of the pseudoaneurysm.[22,24,25]

The advantage with ultrasound-guided compression is that it is non-invasive, clinically effective, safe to perform and cost effective. Disadvantages include poor tolerability by some patients, despite the use of analgesia, with a proportion unable to tolerate the procedure. Rupture of the pseudoaneurysm is a rare complication. It is also less effective in patients on anticoagulants.

ULTRASOUND-GUIDED THROMBIN INJECTION

Thrombin injection was first described in 1986,[26] but it was not until much later that reports emerged of its efficacy.[27] Thrombin is central to the coagulation cascade by converting fibrinogen to fibrin which then covalently cross-links leading to fibrin polymerisation. This strengthens and stabilises the clot. Thrombin may be human or bovine in origin (bovine thrombin has been associated with an increase risk of anaphylactic reactions).[28] Under sterile conditions and using real-time ultrasound imaging, the probe is centred over the pseudoaneurysm and thrombin injected very slowly to reduce the incidence of distal embolisation (Fig. 2). Thrombosis usually occurs within seconds of the start of injection. If the pseudoaneurysm fails to thrombose completely, a second injection into the remaining cavity may be required. The dose of thrombin required varies from around 100–2000 IU.[21,27,29] Dose

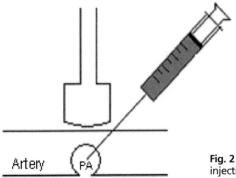

Fig. 2 Diagrammatic illustration of thrombin injection into a pseudoaneurysm under ultrasound control.

Artery PA

depends on whether the pseudoaneurysm is complex or simple rather than on absolute size.[21] More recent studies have used smaller doses of thrombin than earlier ones with similar efficacy.[29] Rather than give a fixed dose, it is recommended that the operator should inject until flow ceases in the pseudoaneurysm sac.

In-patient stay is not required. However, repeat duplex ultrasound examination should be carried out the following day and at 1 week and 4–6 weeks because of the risk of recanalisation of the pseudoaneurysm. The technique is effective in over 90% and safe when used by well-trained or experienced operators. In the majority of cases, a single injection will suffice although a second injection may be required particularly for pseudoaneurysms with a complex anatomy.[29] Recurrence rates range between 0–4% and usually occur in 1–7 days following treatment.[27,30] Several studies, including a small randomised trial,[31] have shown the superiority of ultrasound-guided thrombin injection (USTI) over USGC with respect to higher technical success rates, shorter procedure times and less analgesic requirements.[20,32] Another advantage with USTI is that patients may remain on anticoagulation during treatment.[30] For this reason, USTI has replaced USGC as the first line treatment for pseudoaneurysms in many institutions.

Disadvantages of USTI include the potential risks of introducing infection and of distal embolisation which has been reported to occur in up to 2% of cases.[32] However, in most series, all patients improved spontaneously without recourse to surgery or endovascular intervention. Attention to sterile technique and low-dose thrombin injection reduce these risks. The technique is not recommended for arteries with wide necks due to the risk of embolisation, although balloon protection during thrombin injection may be an alternative (see below).

Key point 5

- Ultrasound-guided thrombin injection is superior to ultrasound compression for the treatment of postcatheterisation pseudoaneurysms with respect to efficacy, recurrence rate, duration of treatment and analgesic requirements.

evidence and issued guidelines in support of thrombin injection of pseudoaneurysms in May 2004. In the guideline, NICE state that the current evidence on the safety and efficacy of thrombin injections for pseudoaneurysms appears to support the use of this procedure, provided that the normal arrangements are in place for consent, audit and clinical governance.

EMBOLISATION

In trans-catheter embolisation, the artery from which the pseudoaneurysm originates is selectively catheterised and embolised with coils (Fig. 3) packed just distal and proximal to the neck of the pseudoaneurysm (the 'sandwich' or 'front and back door' embolisation method). Alternatively, a small pseudoaneurysm can be packed tight with embolisation coils. Rarely other liquid embolisation materials such as Onyx™, cyanoacrylate glues or a combination can be used. Onyx™ (Micro Therapeutics Inc.) is an ethylene–vinyl alcohol copolymer (EVOH) – a black opaque micronised tantalum powder that is dissolved in dimethyl sulphoxide. On contact with blood, it forms a spongy polymeric cast precipitate which solidifies from the outside in. The centre continues to flow allowing filling of a vascular space (AVM or aneurysm). It is biocompatible, non-adhesive, but cohesive, and is prepared at different viscosities allowing controllable and complete filling of the vascular space to be embolised.

This approach allows the parent artery to remain patent but requires special care, and sometimes protection balloons, to ensure there is no compromise to the parent artery. Embolisation is particularly useful for visceral artery aneurysms (*e.g.* splenic, pancreatic, and hepatic). Untreated, these lesions have a high mortality; therefore, repair is generally suggested at a diameter ≥ 2 cm or if symptoms arise. Surgery carries a high mortality, quoted at 16–50% for pancreatic pseudoaneurysms.[33] Various embolisation techniques have been

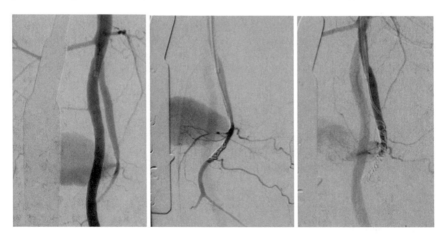

Fig. 3 Large iatrogenic pseudoaneurysm of the profunda femoris artery secondary to orthopaedic drill injury sustained during insertion of a dynamic hip screw for a fractured neck of femur. Percutaneous thrombin injection was initially successful; however, this had recanalised after 4 days. Coil embolisation was then performed using the 'front and back door' technique. Complete thrombosis of the pseudo-aneurysm was confirmed using ultrasound at the end of the procedure.

used depending on the clinical state of the patient, visceral artery anatomy (particularly in relation to the end organ supplied), and the geometry of the aneurysm. Selective angiography and catheterisation is required followed by embolisation with various occluding materials. Potential complications result from embolisation of normal vessels causing end-organ infarction. The degree to which this may occur is related to specific arterial anatomy. For example, the liver can tolerate considerable arterial embolisation without sequelae due to a rich inflow supplied by a patent portal vein.[34] Conversely, the small and large bowel are at considerable jeopardy in the event of non-targeted embolisation.

COVERED STENTS (STENT GRAFTS)

This form of endovascular repair consists of placing a stent graft in the parent artery crossing the pseudoaneurysm neck to exclude it from the circulation. The stent graft consists of a metal frame, usually made of nitinol (nickel-titanium alloy) covered by graft material, *e.g.* PET (polyethylene tetraphthalate) or ePTFE (expanded polytetraflouroethylene). Stent grafts can be divided into two types – balloon expandable or self-expanding. Although balloon expandable stent grafts may allow more accurate placement and have greater radial strength, self-expanding stent grafts such as the Wallgraft™ (Boston Scientific, Natick, MA, USA), Fluency plus™ (Bard Limited, Murray Hill, USA) or Hemobahn (WL Gore and Associates, Flagstaff, AZ, USA) allow more flexibility and are resilient to external compressive forces. There are

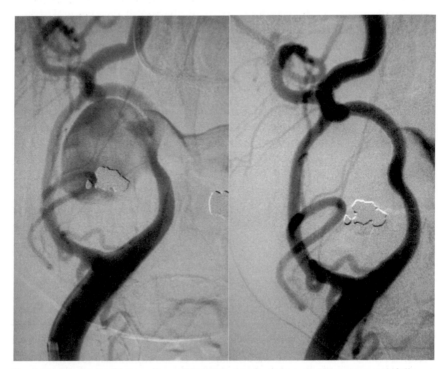

Fig. 4 Moderate-sized internal carotid artery pseudoaneurysm. This was successfully treated using a covered stent graft. At 6-week follow-up, the patient was well and symptom-free.

many differences between these devices but all require relatively large introducer sheaths and hence run the risk of complications relating to their site of insertion. They are usually oversized by 1–2 mm greater diameter than the intended vessel and, ideally, the shortest length of stent graft is chosen to avoid occluding side branches. At least a centimetre of extension proximal and distal to the arterial defect is required to ensure that a good seal is formed with apposition between the graft material and the vessel wall and to reduce the risk of an endoleak developing (see below).

An advantage of stent grafts is that they maintain flow in the parent vessel from which the pseudoaneurysm arises and are preferred in, for example, carotid artery pseudoaneurysms following penetrating trauma or iatrogenic injury (Fig. 4). Not all lesions are suitable for stent grafting with contra-indications including suspected infection, extreme tortuosity of the access arteries and lesions near essential branch points.

Disadvantages are that stent grafts usually require larger access sheaths (10–12 French for large iliac artery stent grafts). Coronary stent grafts such as the monorail™ symbiot™ covered stent (Boston Scientific, Natick, MA, USA) is lower profile but currently only has a coronary artery indication. There is little long-term data on the patency of stent grafts. Potential complications include, nitinol strut fracture causing perforation of the graft material, stent misplacement and migration with side branch occlusion, kinking, in stent stenosis, occlusion, thrombosis and infection.

Despite some limited success, there is little evidence for the use of stents or stent grafts in the common femoral artery due to the risks of stent occlusion, thrombosis, stent kinking, and strut fracture across the hip joint. Surgical alternatives are preferable due to these potential complications and in view of easy arterial access.

BALLOON-PROTECTED THROMBIN INJECTION

In this technique, a compliant, semicompliant or regular (slightly oversized) angioplasty balloon is placed across the arterial wall defect to isolate the pseudoaneurysm from the circulation. Thrombin is then injected under ultrasound guidance percutaneously in the pseudoaneurysm sac.[35] Some interventionalists have modified this approach using the same protection technique but with a second catheter through the neck and into the pseudoaneurysm cavity, with catheter injected thrombin. Both techniques require the balloon to be let down after pseudoaneurysm thrombosis has occurred, and run the risk of distal embolisation at this time.

SURGICAL TREATMENT

Pseudoaneurysms have traditionally been treated by surgery. Surgery may be technically difficult and hazardous and is associated with considerable morbidity and mortality. Complications include local complications such as bleeding, damage to surrounding structures, lymph leak, presence of scar and general complications such as anaesthetic risks, myocardial infection and death.

Surgery is reserved for pseudoaneurysms causing local pressure effects such as a neuropathy, venous compression and damage to overlying skin.

Surgery is indicated for infected pseudoaneurysms since this requires drainage and debridement of the arterial wall and surrounding tissue. Another indication for surgery is cases in which intervention techniques have failed or are not available locally.

The available surgical treatments include repair of the defect with or without a patch (vein or synthetic patch), surgical bypass if the artery is badly damaged, simple ligation or, in the case of some visceral pseudoaneurysms located within the organ, removal of part or all of the organ. The choice of surgery depends upon the expendability of the artery and the presence of infection. Small non-vital arteries can simply be ligated whereas larger vital arteries may require closure of the defect or bypass. For example, pseudoaneurysms arising from the radial or ulnar artery at the wrist following insertion of an arterial line may be ligated provided the palmar arch is intact. The presence of infection or evidence of sepsis is a contra-indication to endovascular or percutaneous techniques and requires surgical debridement of the arterial wall, local tissues and drainage of abscess to eradicate infection. An extra anatomic arterial bypass through a clean field may also be required following excision of an infected artery or graft and, in this circumstance, autologous vein is the preferred conduit over prosthetic material.

Key point 6

- Surgery is now rarely required for iatrogenic pseudoaneurysms and is reserved for pseudoaneurysms that are infected, causing local pressure effects or those in which minimally invasive techniques have failed.

CONCLUSIONS

Pseudoaneurysms are most commonly encountered following endovascular interventions but may also occur following surgery, trauma or infection. The incidence has risen due to the increase in range and complexity of endovascular procedures. They may be completely asymptomatic or may present with massive haemorrhage following rupture. Duplex ultrasound is a reliable, easily accessible and cost-effective way of diagnosing and monitoring femoral pseudoaneurysms and plays a smaller but important role in visceral artery pseudoaneurysm assessment. Multidetector CT allows 3-dimensional visualisation and treatment planning. Treatment of pseudoaneurysms has evolved over the past decade with the vast majority now treated using guidance or andovascular techniques. Provided there are no contra-indications to this approach, the choice of treatment depends on the size and location of the arterial defect and associated pseudoaneurysm, operator experience with each technique together with patient specific factors (including patient tolerance, allergy history and treatment choice). A step-wise progression from least invasive to most invasive treatment is recommended. The majority of uncomplicated, small pseudoaneurysms will spontaneously thrombose. First-line treatments for non-infected pseudoaneurysms include ultrasound-guided compression or thrombin injection. Pseudoaneurysms with wider necks and in which the patency of the native artery must be maintained may be suitable for endovascular stent grafting. Surgery is now rarely required for these pseudoaneurysms but plays an important role in endovascular treatment failure, the presence of infection, local tissue compromise, neurological and ischaemic symptoms.

Key points for clinical practice

- The majority of pseudoaneurysms occur following femoral artery catheterisation. Most uncomplicated pseudoaneurysms can be managed either conservatively or with minimally invasive techniques.

- Arteriotomy closure devices are in wide-spread use but remain controversial in the prevention of access-site related complications. Newer generations of devices appear to be as safe and effective as manual compression.

- Treatment choice for pseudoaneurysms is governed by characteristics of the pseudoaneurysm (site, size, symptoms,neck width), patient co-morbidity and anticoagulation status as well as local interventional expertise.

- Small uncomplicated pseudoaneurysms (< 6 ml) can be managed conservatively with regular observation and will usually thrombose spontaneously.

- Ultrasound-guided thrombin injection is superior to ultrasound compression for the treatment of postcatheterisation pseudoaneurysms with respect to efficacy, recurrence rate, duration of treatment and analgesic requirements.

- Surgery is now rarely required for iatrogenic pseudoaneurysms and is reserved for pseudo-aneurysms that are infected, causing local pressure effects or those in which minimally invasive techniques have failed.

References

1. Demirbas O, Batyraliev T, Eksi Z, Pershukov I. Femoral pseudo-aneurysm due to diagnostic or interventional angiographic procedures. *Angiology* 2005; **56**: 553–556.
2. Katzenschlager R, Ugurluoglu A, Ahmadi A *et al*. Incidence of pseudo-aneurysm after diagnostic and therapeutic angiography. *Radiology* 1995; **195**: 463–466.
3. Kotval PS, Khoury A, Shah PM, Babu SC. Doppler sonographic demonstration of the progressive spontaneous thrombosis of pseudo-aneurysms. *J Ultrasound Med* 1990; **9**: 185–190.
4. Lazarides MK, Tsoupanos SS, Georgopoulos SE *et al*. Incidence and patterns of iatrogenic arterial injuries. A decade's experience. *J Cardiovasc Surg (Torino)* 1998; **39**: 281–285.
5. Morgan R, Belli AM. Current treatment methods for postcatheterization pseudo-aneurysms. *J Vasc Intervent Radiol* 2003; **14**: 697–710.
6. Koreny M, Riedmuller E, Nikfardjam M, Siostrzonek P, Mullner M. Arterial puncture closing devices compared with standard manual compression after cardiac catheterization: systematic review and meta-analysis. *JAMA* 2004; **291**: 350–357.

7. Nikolsky E, Mehran R, Halkin A *et al*. Vascular complications associated with arteriotomy closure devices in patients undergoing percutaneous coronary procedures: a meta-analysis. *J Am Coll Cardiol* 2004; **44**: 1200–1209.

8. Kresowik TF, Khoury MD, Miller BV *et al*. A prospective study of the incidence and natural history of femoral vascular complications after percutaneous transluminal coronary angioplasty. *J Vasc Surg* 1991; **13**: 328–333, discussion 333–325.

9. Toursarkissian B, Allen BT, Petrinec D *et al*. Spontaneous closure of selected iatrogenic pseudo-aneurysms and arteriovenous fistulae. *J Vasc Surg* 1997; **25**: 803–808, discussion 808–809.

10. Onal B, Kosar S, Gumus T, Ilgit ET, Akpek S. Postcatheterization femoral arteriovenous fistulas: endovascular treatment with stent-grafts. *Cardiovasc Intervent Radiol* 2004; **27**: 453–458.

11. Soto JA, Munera F, Morales C *et al*. Focal arterial injuries of the proximal extremities: helical CT arteriography as the initial method of diagnosis. *Radiology* 2001; **218**: 188–194.

12. Graham AN, Wilson CM, Hood JM, Barros D'Sa AA. Risk of rupture of postangiographic femoral false aneurysm. *Br J Surg* 1992; **79**: 1022–1025.

13. Perler BA. Surgical treatment of femoral pseudo-aneurysm following cardiac catheterization. *Cardiovasc Surg* 1993; **1**: 118–121.

14. Roberts SR, Main D, Pinkerton J. Surgical therapy of femoral artery pseudo-aneurysm after angiography. *Am J Surg* 1987; **154**: 676–680.

15. Babu SC, Piccorelli GO, Shah PM, Stein JH, Clauss RH. Incidence and results of arterial complications among 16,350 patients undergoing cardiac catheterization. *J Vasc Surg* 1989; **10**: 113–116.

16. Omoigui NA, Califf RM, Pieper K *et al*. Peripheral vascular complications in the Coronary Angioplasty Versus Excisional Artherectomy Trial (CAVEAT-I). *J Am Coll Cardiol* 1995; **26**: 922—930.

17. Kent KC, McArdle CR, Kennedy B, Baim DS, Anninos E, Skillman JJ. A prospective study of the clinical outcome of femoral pseudo-aneurysms and arteriovenous fistulas induced by arterial puncture. *J Vasc Surg* 1993; **17**: 125–131, discussion 131–123.

18. Paulson EK, Hertzberg BS, Paine SS, Carroll BA. Femoral artery pseudo-aneurysms: value of color Doppler sonography in predicting which ones will thrombose without treatment. *AJR Am J Roentgenol* 1992; **159**: 1077–1081.

19. Fellmeth BD, Roberts AC, Bookstein JJ *et al*. Postangiographic femoral artery injuries: nonsurgical repair with US-guided compression. *Radiology* 1991; **178**: 671–675.

20. Lonn L, Olmarker A, Geterud K *et al*. Treatment of femoral pseudo-aneurysms. Percutaneous US-guided thrombin injection versus US-guided compression. *Acta Radiol* 2002; **43**: 396–400.

21. Taylor BS, Rhee RY, Muluk S *et al*. Thrombin injection versus compression of femoral artery pseudo-aneurysms. *J Vasc Surg* 1999; **30**: 1052–1059.

22. Hajarizadeh H, LaRosa CR, Cardullo P, Rohrer MJ, Cutler BS. Ultrasound-guided compression of iatrogenic femoral pseudo-aneurysm failure, recurrence, and long-term results. *J Vasc Surg* 1995; **22**: 425–430, discussion 430–423.

23. Steinkamp HJ, Werk M, Felix R. Treatment of postinterventional pseudo-aneurysms by ultrasound-guided compression. *Invest Radiol* 2000; **35**: 186–192.

24. Brophy DP, Sheiman RG, Amatulle P, Akbari CM. Iatrogenic femoral pseudo-aneurysms: thrombin injection after failed US-guided compression. *Radiology* 2000; **214**: 278–282.

25. Dean SM, Olin JW, Piedmonte M, Grubb M, Young JR. Ultrasound-guided compression closure of postcatheterization pseudo-aneurysms during concurrent anticoagulation: a review of seventy-seven patients. *J Vasc Surg* 1996; **23**: 28–34, discussion 34–35.

26. Cope C, Zeit R. Coagulation of aneurysms by direct percutaneous thrombin injection. *AJR Am J Roentgenol* 1986; **147**: 383–387.

27. Kang SS, Labropoulos N, Mansour MA *et al*. Expanded indications for ultrasound-guided thrombin injection of pseudo-aneurysms. *J Vasc Surg* 2000; **31**: 289–298.

28. Sultan S, Nicholls S, Madhavan P, Colgan MP, Moore D, Shanik G. Ultrasound guided human thrombin injection. A new modality in the management of femoral artery pseudo-aneurysms. *Eur J Vasc Endovasc Surg* 2001; **22**: 542–545.

29. Kruger K, Zahringer M, Sohngen FD *et al*. Femoral pseudo-aneurysms: management with percutaneous thrombin injections – success rates and effects on systemic coagulation. *Radiology* 2003; **226**: 452–458.

30. Lennox AF, Delis KT, Szendro G, Griffin MB, Nicolaides AN, Cheshire NJ. Duplex-guided thrombin injection for iatrogenic femoral artery pseudo-aneurysm is effective even in anticoagulated patients. *Br J Surg* 2000; **87**: 796–801.
31. Lonn L, Olmarker A, Geterud K, Risberg B. Prospective randomized study comparing ultrasound-guided thrombin injection to compression in the treatment of femoral pseudo-aneurysms. *J Endovasc Ther* 2004; **11**: 570–576.
32. Paulson EK, Nelson RC, Mayes CE, Sheafor DH, Sketch Jr MH, Kliewer MA. Sonographically guided thrombin injection of iatrogenic femoral pseudo-aneurysms: further experience of a single institution. *AJR Am J Roentgenol* 2001; **177**: 309–316.
33. Mandel SR, Jaques PF, Sanofsky S, Mauro MA. Nonoperative management of peripancreatic arterial aneurysms. A 10-year experience. *Ann Surg* 1987; **205**: 126–128.
34. Charnsangavej C, Chuang VP, Wallace S, Soo CS, Bowers T. Angiographic classification of hepatic arterial collaterals. *Radiology* 1982; **144**: 485–494.
35. O'Connor PG, Samet JH, Stein MD. Management of hospitalized intravenous drug users: role of the internist. *Am J Med* 1994; **96**: 551–558.
36. Royal College of Radiologists. Standards in Vascular Radiology. London: Royal College of Radiologists, Ref. No. BFCR (99) 9.

Michael J. Gough

12

Endovenous laser therapy for varicose veins

Superficial venous incompetence resulting in the development of truncal varicosities is common, occurring in up to 32% of women and 40% of men (Edinburgh Vein Study[1]). The majority (60–70%) of primary varicose veins develop as a result of saphenofemoral junction (SFJ) incompetence and great saphenous vein (GSV) reflux whilst some 10% are due to saphenopopliteal (SPJ) and small saphenous (SSV) incompetence. Of the remainder, most arise as a result of perforator incompetence whilst a small number arise from pelvic veins or from a deep vein in the groin or leg without connection to the greater or small saphenous veins.

Although most varicose veins are asymptomatic and only a relative minority present for treatment, it was estimated that the cost of performing around 40,000 National Health Service operations in the UK in 2001 was £20–25 million. This assumed that the majority of patients were treated on a day-case basis (£557/patient) and did not include the indirect, non-hospital, costs relating to community nursing care or absence from work. For patients admitted for overnight stay or longer, the cost of surgery will be increased.

Abolition of venous reflux is crucial to successful treatment and the cost of therapy is largely incurred in undertaking conventional surgery (flush ligation of the SFJ or SPJ, GSV or SSV stripping and stab avulsions of the varicosities). Recently, a number of minimally invasive techniques for the treatment of varicose veins has been developed. Although this chapter will focus on the safety and efficacy of endovenous laser ablation (EVLA) in treating superficial venous incompetence, the technique will be compared to foam sclerotherapy and radiofrequency venous ablation, two alternative minimally invasive techniques for abolishing superficial venous incompetence.

Michael J. Gough ChM FRCS
Consultant Vascular Surgeon, The General Infirmary at Leeds, Great George Street, Leeds LS1 3EX, UK
E-mail: michael.gough@leedsth.nhs.uk

EPIDEMIOLOGY

Many readers will be surprised by the findings of the Edinburgh Vein Study which showed that, in the general population, varicose veins were more prevalent in men. Whilst other studies have found the gender difference reversed, with a prevalence of 20–25% in women and 10–15% in men,[2] these often depended on self-reporting, confirming that women are more likely to present with varicose veins and more likely to undergo treatment.

At a time when those responsible for funding healthcare are considering rationing treatment for varicose veins, it is important to consider the relationship between varicose veins and symptoms. Whilst common symptoms include aching, heaviness, pruritis, and oedema, asymptomatic superficial venous reflux may be present in up to 39% of the population.[3] Further, the Edinburgh Vein Study found that almost half of all women complained of aching legs irrespective of the presence of varicose veins and that the majority of lower limb symptoms had a non-venous cause.[4] Finally, there was a poor correlation between symptoms and the existence of truncal varices. This calls into question the rationale of varicose vein surgery for the treatment of symptoms.

For patients who develop complications (thrombophlebitis, varicose eczema, lipodermatosclerosis, ulceration) from their varicose veins, the case for intervention is much clearer. Although the true incidence of these is uncertain, they probably occur in about 5% of patients.[5]

MANAGEMENT

Regardless of the method of treatment, success depends upon accurate identification of the site or sites of superficial venous incompetence. The chosen intervention should abolish venous reflux, relieve symptoms attributable to this, prevent complications, improve cosmesis, and should be associated with low morbidity and recurrence rates. Additional advantages would include a rapid return to normal activity and work and reduced treatment costs. Most, if not all, of these aims appear to be achieved by the newer methods of minimally invasive therapy for varicose veins which were principally developed to abolish GSV reflux. These include endovenous laser ablation (EVLA), radiofrequency ablation (RFA) and foam sclerotherapy (FS). Further, both EVLA and FS have been used to treat SSV reflux.

The remainder of this chapter will consider the relative merits of conventional surgery and EVLA with reference to the reported outcomes for RFA and FS. For an overview of other treatment options for varicose veins, including variations in surgical technique, the reader is referred to a recent review.[6]

ENDOVENOUS LASER ABLATION

Technique

EVLA can be performed as an out-patient procedure in a clean treatment room. This obviates the need for an operating theatre, although in some institutions, purely for logistic reasons, EVLA is performed in a day-case surgery unit. For

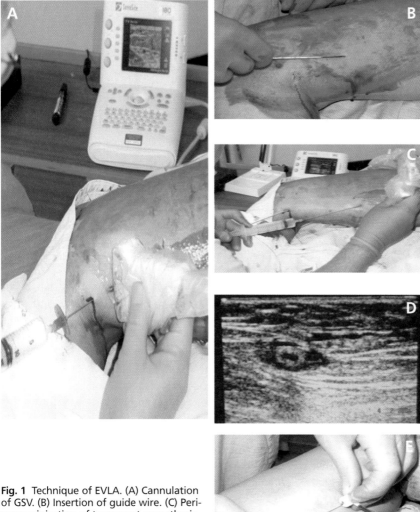

Fig. 1 Technique of EVLA. (A) Cannulation of GSV. (B) Insertion of guide wire. (C) Perivenous injection of tumescent anaesthesia. (D) 'Halo' of tumescent anaesthesia around GSV on ultrasound. (E) Insertion of laser fibre.

GSV ablation, patients lie supine on a tilting table (*e.g.* theatre transport trolley or ultrasound couch) with the leg to be treated flexed and externally rotated at the hip, and the knee slightly flexed. GSV cannulation (Fig. 1) is facilitated by placing the patient in the Trendelenberg position. The skin overlying the vein for ablation is prepared with povidine-iodine solution and a sterile, disposable drape placed beneath it. Using ultrasound guidance, the GSV is cannulated just above or below the knee (mid-calf for SSV) and a guide-wire is passed beyond the SFJ or SPJ. A 5-Fr catheter is then passed over the guide-wire and its tip is positioned (ultrasound control) 0.5–1 cm distal to the junction. If ultrasound imaging of the catheter tip proves difficult, its position can be confirmed by visualisation of a jet of saline flushed through the catheter. The table is now placed in the horizontal position.

185

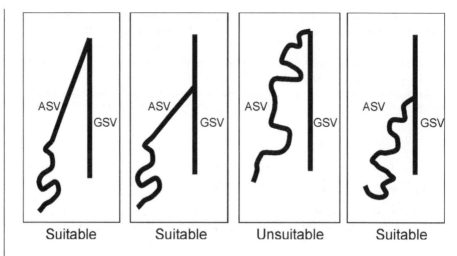

Fig. 2 Suitability of anterior saphenous vein (ASV) for EVLA.

Up to 200 ml of 0.1% lignocaine is infiltrated along the length of the GSV/SSV to be ablated (ultrasound guidance) until the vein is surrounded by tumescent anaesthetic solution (this provides anaesthesia, compression of the vein around the catheter, and absorption of heat). The laser fibre is inserted as far as the tip of the catheter following which the latter is withdrawn by 2 cm so that the laser fibre protrudes beyond the catheter.

The laser fibre is fired during stepwise withdrawal (one second pulses, 12 W energy, 810 nm diode laser; one second intervals allowing withdrawal by 2 mm). During treatment, manual pressure is exerted over the vein.

Following laser removal, the exit wound is closed with a suture-strip and a compression bandage is applied for 1 week followed by a class II compression stocking for a further week. Patients mobilise immediately, are encouraged to resume normal activity as soon as possible and are discharged 20–30 min following the procedure. Usual treatment times are around 35 min/leg. Bilateral GSV/SSV ablation is performed at a single visit.

Patient suitability

Assessment of patient suitability for EVLA requires ultrasound confirmation of the sites of venous incompetence. In our own practice, this is done with a portable ultrasound during the first out-patient visit. For the efficient selection of patients and the subsequent performance of EVLA, it is preferable, though not mandatory, that clinicians offering the service are competent ultrasonographers.

Not all patients with varicose veins due to SFJ/SPJ incompetence are suitable for EVLA. Although uncommon, a very tortuous GSV or SSV may be a relative contra-indication due to difficulties in advancing the guide-wire. Both veins are usually reasonably straight with varicosities confined to the tributaries. However, if varicosities arise from a proximal incompetent tributary, most often the anterior saphenous vein (ASV) in the groin, laser ablation may not be appropriate unless the ASV can be cannulated and its proximal 10 cm ablated or if it arises from the GSV in the thigh ≥ 10 cm below the SFJ (Fig. 2).

Finally, a significant proportion of patients presenting with recurrent varicose veins following previous SFJ or SPJ ligation without stripping may have a persistent GSV or SSV which is suitable for laser ablation. These patients may also benefit from trans-catheter delivery of foam sclerotherapy when neovascularisation leads to refilling of the truncal vein.

In a pilot study, we have assessed the proportion of patients presenting to our venous clinic with truncal varicosities who were suitable for EVLA. Of 591 patients, 365 of 515 (71%) with primary varicose veins and 34 of 76 (45%) with recurrent varicosities were offered EVLA.

Key points 1–3

- Endovenous laser ablation can be provided in a 'one-stop' new patient clinic which includes diagnostic venous ultrasound and treatment to enhance efficiency.

- Knowledge of anatomical variations of the great saphenous vein and the anterior saphenous vein is required.

- About 70% of primary and 45% of recurrent varicose veins are suitable for endovenous laser ablation.

Laser type and mechanism of action

Most studies of EVLA have used either 810 nm or 940 nm diode lasers based upon a haemoglobin absorption peak to red/infrared light of 800–1000 nm. The heat generated by the laser is believed to produce steam bubbles that cause thermal damage to the endothelium and sub-endothelial layer resulting in focal coagulative necrosis and shrinkage leading to thrombotic occlusion of the vein.[7] Histological studies at 3 and 6 months following EVLA indicate failure of endothelial regeneration and progressive damage to the muscle layers of the vein wall resulting in further shrinkage.[8]

The high temperature generated by the laser (average temperature of 729°C at the tip) may cause local perforation of the vein with extravasation of blood. In an animal model, comparison of the histological results for RFA and EVLA found fewer vein wall perforations after RFA which the authors claimed correlated with a lower incidence of haematoma with this technique.[9] However, the protective effect of perivenous tumescent anaesthesia was not examined. Data from our own studies indicate a median temperature of 34.5°C (maximum 43.3°C) immediately adjacent to the vein and this is likely to be of benefit in reducing the frequency of perforations and other temperature-related complications. In contrast, RFA generates a constant temperature of 85°C with the catheter being withdrawn much more slowly down the vein. This is likely to generate higher perivenous temperatures and may account for a higher incidence of nerve injuries and skin burns with this technique.

A single report describes the use of a 1064 nm Nd:YAG laser for EVLA. The laser energy delivered in this study was 10-fold more than that in other EVLA studies and resulted in a high incidence of temporary paraesthesia and thermal injury (36% and 5%, respectively) making it unsuitable for clinical use.[10]

RESULTS OF TREATMENT

GSV occlusion

Endovenous laser therapy for varicose veins was initially described by Navarro and Min in 2001.[11] In publications relating to their experience, the procedure was subsequently termed endovenous laser therapy (EVLT). Whilst this abbreviation is commonly used to describe EVLA it is a registered trademark for a specific laser kit (EVLT®; Diomed Inc, Andover, MA, USA). This equipment utilised an 810 nm diode laser and arguably has been more widely used than other laser devices. In this and other publications, Min and colleagues described the use of laser powers varying from 10–14 W delivered as intermittent pulses (12-W power, 1-s pulses, 1-s intervals, stepwise withdrawal, 4 pulses/cm) or by continuous laser (14-W power) with continuous withdrawal (2 mm/s). These techniques delivered around 50 J/cm of treated vein.

Observational studies report GSV closure rates of 94–100% (assessed by duplex ultrasound) with relief of symptoms and improvement in the appearance of superficial varicosities. For most studies, follow-up was less than a year,[11-14] whilst that for the study reporting 100% success was only 2 weeks.[15] In a later report, Min et al.[16] described the outcome in almost 500 patients followed for up to 3 years. GSV occlusion rates were 98% at 1 month and 93% at 2 years ($n = 121$). Interestingly, 8 of the 9 patients whose GSV was patent were successfully re-treated by laser. No new recurrences were found in a further 40 patients who were followed up at 3 years.

Recently, we have assessed a number of factors that might influence the success of EVLA. Amongst those examined were: GSV diameter, the length of vein ablated, total laser dose, joules of energy delivered per centimetre of vein and body mass index. Thus, the GSV was fully occluded/non-visible (duplex ultrasound) in 432/476 (91%) limbs completing 6-month follow-up. In the remaining 44 limbs, the GSV was partially occluded ($n = 18$) or patent ($n = 26$). Occlusion rates were not influenced by body mass index, which might affect the efficacy of post-treatment compression, GSV diameter or the total laser dose after correction for differences in the length of vein ablated. However, there was a significant difference in the median energy delivery to occluded (61.2 J/cm [range, 50.4–68.4 J/cm]) and partially occluded or patent veins (43.2 J/cm [range, 36.0–55.2 J/cm; $P < 0.01$). Further, successful occlusion was achieved in all veins treated with ≥ 60 J/cm (≥ 5 pulses/cm with protocol described above).

Key points 4 & 5

- To achieve adequate energy delivery, 810 or 940 nm diode laser should be used.

- Delivery of 60–70 J/cm results in optimum great saphenous vein/small saphenous vein occlusion rates.

Small saphenous vein occlusion

Whilst the majority of studies describe the outcome of EVLA for GSV reflux, the technique has also been used in the treatment of SPJ and SSV reflux. A potential risk to the use of EVLA at this site is the effect of heat on the common peroneal nerve and its branches that are in close proximity to the SPJ and proximal SSV. To assess the risk of irreversible nerve damage that may occur at temperatures above 45°0C, we measured the temperature 3 mm, 5 mm, and 10 mm from the GSV following perivenous injection of tumescent anaesthesia during laser fibre withdrawal. The results of this study have been described earlier. Given that tumescent anaesthesia should eliminate the potential for significant nerve injury, 45 SSVs have been ablated to date. All received ≥ 60 J/cm resulting in 100% occlusion rates. Three patients experienced transient paraesthesia or numbness in the distribution of the sural nerve. The risk of sural nerve injury can be further minimised by cannulating the SSV at or above the mid-point of the calf, the point at which the nerve normally joins the vein.

There are two additional reports of SSV ablation in a total of 78 limbs which describe success rates of 95% and 97%.[14,15] Although follow-up was relatively short in these studies (median of 3 months), the results are encouraging given that conventional surgery (SPJ ligation) is associated with high recurrence rates (up to 50%), many of which are the result of inadequate surgery.[17]

A potential criticism of both EVLA and RFA is that, although SFJ ligation is avoided, the GSV tributaries in the groin may remain patent. Ligation of these has been suggested as being pivotal to reducing recurrence rates.[18] In our experience of > 700 ablations of the GSV, the vein is occluded up to the level of the SFJ in almost all patients provided that ablation is commenced within 1 cm of the junction, thus protecting these veins from the effects of SFJ reflux. Further, Chandler *et al.*[19] suggested that avoiding surgical disruption of the SFJ may reduce the risk of neovascularisation and thus recurrence rates may be lower. Preliminary data from our prospective audit appear to confirm that neovascularisation is much less common after EVLA although longer follow-up is required.

The results of EVLA have been reviewed in a recent systematic review.[20] It was concluded that although EVLA seems beneficial, its effectiveness and safety cannot be judged without comparative data from randomised clinical trials. We have recently completed such a trial (GSV EVLA versus conventional surgery) which confirms that laser therapy is as effective as surgery in eliminating reflux, improving symptoms and enhancing cosmesis but with advantages in terms of post-procedure recovery and complication rates. This is discussed further below.

Treatment of residual varicosities

Conventional surgery for GSV (or SSV) varicose veins aims at eliminating the source of superficial venous reflux (SFJ ligation, stripping GSV) and removing the varicosities (multiple phlebectomies). In contrast, EVLA only achieves the primary aim of eliminating reflux. In most centres, patients are subsequently reviewed after 6–12 weeks at which time any residual varicosities that have not disappeared spontaneously following abolition of reflux are treated by injection sclerotherapy. Following GSV or SSV ablation, sclerotherapy is required in 45% and 11% of patients, respectively (Leeds' data). Although previous results for sclerotherapy as a primary treatment for truncal varicosities have been disappointing, long-term efficacy is much more likely in the absence of GSV or SSV reflux.

Table 1 Potential advantages and cost factors relating to EVLA

Potential advantages	Cost factors for EVLA	Cost factors for surgery
Out-patient procedure	Equipment £50,000	Surgical instruments
Avoid general anaesthesia	Disposables/case £275	Disposables
'No scars'	1 'surgeon'	1 anaesthetist/1 ODA,
Reduced risk of complications	2 nurses	2 surgeons
More rapid recovery	Waiting room	2 nurses
Potential reduction in	Treatment room	Day unit/IP bed
direct and indirect costs		Recovery room + staff

Alternative approaches to the management of the residual varicosities have been proposed. These include multiple phlebectomies either at the time of EVLA or after 6–12 weeks or early sclerotherapy. The latter strategy results in up to 95% of patients requiring injections whilst the former does not seem logical and negates much of the benefit of a minimally invasive therapy.

Outcome after EVLA

The potential advantages of EVLA are listed in Table 1. Data from our randomised trial and from our prospective audit confirm that EVLA (compared to surgery) is associated with the same reduction in venous symptoms (Aberdeen Venous Symptom Score), a more rapid return to normal activity and a reduced complication rate. These results are summarised in Table 2. Further, at least 93% of patients would chose EVLA again rather than surgery.

Table 2 Outcomes following EVLA or surgery

	GSV EVLA (n = 66)	SSV EVLA (n = 45)	Surgery (n = 31)
Abolition of reflux	91%*	100%	88%
Time to normal activity (days)	3.5 (0–8)	0 (0–7)	14 (3–28)
Return to work (days)	4 (2–10)	Not recorded	17 (5–32)
Analgesia requirement (days)	2 (1–7)	3 (0–14)	3 (2–8)
Sclerotherapy	45%	11%	–
AVSS	13.83 (10.21–2.3) v 6.05 (2.70–11.64)	14.23 (10.2 – 21.1) v 6.02 (2.5–10.1)	14(9.3–18.2) v 5.3 (1.4–7.4)
Complications			
Phlebitis	12%#	2.6%	
Nerve 'injury'	3.8%	7.8%	15%
DVT/PE	0.29%	0	0
Wound problems	–	–	6.7%
Other	–	–	1 ARDS
Would choose EVLT again	93%	97%	

Values given as median ± IQR.
*Includes patients treated prior to establishing requirement of ≥ 60 J/cm.
#Includes patients treated prior to routine prescription of diclofenac (50 mg tds x 72 h).
Time to normal activity: $P = 0.016$ GSV EVLA v surgery.
Return to work: $P = 0.011$.
AVSS, Aberdeen Venous Symptom Score: $P = 0.001$, pre- v post-treatment for all groups.

Key points 6–8

- Symptom reduction and cosmetic improvement after EVLA are equivalent to surgery.

- Endovenous laser ablation allows a rapid return to normal activity and employment with no requirement for community nursing care.

- Endovenous laser ablation has lower complication rates than surgery, particularly in respect of nerve injury and wound problems.

Potential complications

The commonest complication following EVLA is symptomatic 'phlebitis' of the treated vein. The severity of this can be minimised by the routine prescription of a non-steroidal anti-inflammatory agent such as diclofenac (50 mg tds) for 72 h following the procedure. Rarely, patients may also develop superficial thrombophlebitis in calf varicosities, presumably secondary to stasis, following EVLA. If this occurs, a more prolonged course of anti-inflammatory therapy is usually required.

A further minor complication of EVLA is local bruising along the line of the treated vein. This is uncommon and, when it occurs, it is much less severe than the bruising associated with surgical stripping of the GSV after which haematoma and wound infection are relatively common (up to 10%).

Although skin burns were reported in the study using the 1064 nm Nd:YAG laser,[10] and have also been described after RFA, such injuries have not occurred in EVLA patients, presumably because of the protective effect of the tumescent infiltration. Numbness or paraesthesia in the distribution of either the saphenous or sural nerve may also occur following EVLA although this is much less common than after surgery (Table 2). Further, all neurological symptoms that have occurred after laser therapy in our own series have resolved within 3 months. In contrast, surgery is associated with permanent neurological sequelae after GSV stripping and multiple phlebectomies in 5–7% of patients.[21]

It should also be considered that, although varicose vein surgery is a relatively minor procedure for a non-life-threatening condition, it is the commonest reason for litigation in general/vascular surgery, accounting for 17% of settled claims, including the highest Medical Defence Union settlement for these specialities between 1990–1998. Further, the UK National Health Service Litigation Authority (NHSLA) has paid almost £5.5 million in compensation to varicose vein patients since 1995. Most settled claims result from a failure to warn patients of the risk of sensory nerve injury, thus highlighting the importance of fully informed consent. More disabling nerve injuries may also occur with at least 12 cases of foot drop after saphenopopliteal ligation being recorded on the NHSLA database. Ligation or injury to either the femoral vein or artery may also occur and are impossible to defend. The absence of these complications following EVLA is thus of considerable importance.

It is also important to consider the relative risk of thrombo-embolic complications. Whilst it is a potential risk following varicose vein surgery, there is no evidence to suggest that this risk is greater than with comparable surgery and the suggested incidence of pulmonary embolism is in the order of 0.2–0.5%.[22] In our own series of > 700 GSV EVLA procedures, a single patient has suffered a non-fatal pulmonary embolus. This would suggest that the risk is similar to that for surgery. However, there has been some discussion about propagation of thrombus from the GSV into the common femoral vein after both EVLA and RFA. A recent report by Puggioni et al.[23] found evidence of this in 3 of 54 (5.6%) EVLA patients who underwent early post-procedure ultrasound scans (precise time not stated). Although none had an occlusive thrombus in the common femoral vein, all were anticoagulated and one received a temporary IVC filter. None of the patients suffered a pulmonary embolus and the thrombus had lysed on a subsequent scan. These authors concluded that DVT prophylaxis should be considered for patients ≥ 50 years old.

Although this is an important finding, patients included in this study differed from the majority treated with EVLA in two important ways – all underwent concomitant phlebectomies and all received a general or spinal/epidural anaesthetic. The latter will have precluded immediate ambulation which might explain the discrepancy between this and other observational series of EVLA.

A final complication of EVLA, described in a single patient after SSV ablation, is the development of an arteriovenous fistula in the popliteal fossa between the SSV and the superficial sural artery.[24] This risk should be minimised by careful infiltration of tumescent anaesthesia around the SSV to separate it from adjacent structures. Relatively larger volumes are advised compared to that used during GSV ablation.

COMPARISON OF RESULTS (EVLA/RFA/SURGERY)

RADIOFREQUENCY ABLATION

RFA (VNUS Medical Technologies Inc., Sunnyvale, CA, USA) of the GSV was described by Goldman in 2000.[25] The manufacturer suggests that the technique is suitable for ablation of a non-tortuous GSV of < 12 mm diameter and is thus applicable to 30–58% of varicose vein patients.[26,27]. Although there are anecdotal reports of its use in larger veins, there is no published data to confirm this.

During RFA, the GSV is exposed to a much lower temperature (85°C) than during EVLA but for a longer period of time. This is likely to result in higher perivenous temperatures although there is no data on this. The putative mode of action is endothelial denudation, collagen denaturation and acute vein constriction.[9]

RFA has usually been performed under general or regional anaesthesia and combined with phlebectomy, although it can be performed using local anaesthesia. A multicentre study found that 85% of GSVs were obliterated at 2 years,[28] with other series reporting occlusion rates of 88–100% at up to 2 years' follow-up.[26–29].

There are two randomised, controlled trials comparing radiofrequency ablation with surgery. In the multicentre EVOLVeS study,[30] GSV occlusion was achieved in 81% of patients, with treatment times being slightly shorter than for surgery. Patients recovered more rapidly after RFA and, although there were fewer overall complications, post-treatment paraesthesia was more common in the RFA patients (16% versus 6%).

In a second smaller trial,[26] both RFA and surgery were performed under general anaesthetic and all patients underwent phlebectomies. RFA was successful in all patients and, although postoperative pain scores were significantly lower than for surgery, 3 (20%) thermal injuries were observed in the RFA group. Paraesthesia rates were similar in both groups (RFA 13%, surgery 23%) but symptomatic thrombophlebitis occurred in 20% of RFA patients. Finally, treatment costs for VNUS patients were significantly higher because of the cost of disposables. Individual series reporting experience with VNUS suggest rather lower complication rates (saphenous neuritis, 3–49%; skin burns, 2–-7%; haematoma and phlebitis).[26-29]

Although DVT has been reported in about 1% of RFA patients (0.3% incidence of pulmonary embolus),[31] a recent study involving rigorous duplex examination 10 days after the procedure reported a 16% DVT rate.[32] In 11 of 12 patients this was due to extension of thrombus from the GSV. Although early thrombus resolution was noted following anticoagulation, the authors recommend early duplex scans in all patients following RFA. These authors also reported that the FDA website included four reports of pulmonary embolism and 22 of DVT or ascending thrombosis following RFA. Thus the issue of the thrombo-embolic risk associated with RFA (and perhaps EVLA) remains controversial and good prospective data are required.

One of the difficulties in assessing the reported outcomes for RFA is the variability of the techniques employed. Thus, the procedure has been performed using general, locoregional or local anaesthesia, with or without tumescent anaesthesia, and frequently in combination with multiple phlebectomies. These variations in technique may influence the prevalence of some of the reported complications and make it difficult to assess its safety and efficacy. A comparison of the treatment methods and results for EVLA and RFA are shown in Table 3.

Table 3 Comparison of EVLA and RFA

	EVLA	RFA
Anaesthetic	Local	General, regional, local
Treatment for varicosities	Delayed sclerotherapy	Phlebectomy
GSV diameter	Any size	≤ 12 mm
Patient suitability	> 70%	30–58%
Success	94–100%	85–100%
Mode of action	Heat/steam/endothelial & sub-endothelial damage	Endothelial and collagen damage, venoconstriction
Paraesthesia	Up to 7.8%	13–16%
Thrombophlebitis	Up to 12%	Up to 20%
DVT	Up to 5.6% if under GA	Up to 16%
Skin burns	None	Up to 20% in early studies
Costs	Less expensive OP procedure, LA	RFA catheter ≥ 2x laser fibre ± GA, operating theatre *etc*. More expensive than surgery

GA, general anaesthesia.

Key points 9 & 10

- Endovenous laser ablation is more cost effective than radiofrequency ablation.

- Compared to radiofrequency ablation, endovenous laser ablation may be feasible in a larger proportion of patients, may be more effective and may be associated with fewer complications.

FOAM SCLEROTHERAPY

Sclerotherapy, which initiates a chemical thrombophlebitis, occlusion and subsequent fibrosis of the treated vein was described by Chassaignac in 1855.[1]. Although a variety of sclerosants have been employed (ferric chloride, hypertonic saline, polidocanol, iodine, glycerine), sodium tetradecyl sulphate (STD) is most widely used for saphenous varicosities.[33] When the varicosities themselves are treated, recurrence rates are high in patients who have saphenofemoral or saphenopopliteal incompetence.[34] Reported complications are few, although tissue necrosis following dermal or intra-arterial injection and haemosiderin deposition (skin staining) can occur.[35]

More recently, ultrasound-directed GSV obliteration by sclerotherapy has been attempted in anticipation that the long-term success might be superior to that of injection of the tributaries alone. Thus, in 50 patients using 3% liquid STD, Min and Navarro[36] reported 100% occlusion rates and high patient satisfaction at a mean of 8 months' follow-up.

More recently, it has been suggested that foam sclerotherapy, which allows a smaller quantity of sclerosant to cover a greater surface area and to displace blood from the GSV, might be more effective and have fewer complications.[37] In a randomised trial comparing foam with liquid polidocanol in the treatment of GSV incompetence (GSV < 8 mm diameter), foam was more successful in abolishing reflux as judged by duplex ultrasound at 3 weeks (84% versus 40%).[38] In other studies, GSV occlusion rates of 90% at 28 days and 81% at 3 years have been reported.[39,40]

The complications of sclerotherapy are generally relatively minor and include haematoma formation, skin staining, ulceration and necrosis, matting, and superficial thrombophlebitis. More serious adverse events have also been reported, including DVT, anaphylaxis, visual disturbance, stroke and cardiac events. The last three complications occur more frequently with foam than after liquid sclerosant, presumably because of its increased use in the GSV and the risk of the foam entering the femoral vein. If this occurs then a paradoxical embolus through a patent foramen ovale is possible, thus accounting for cerebral and cardiac complications.

Key point 11

- Published data suggest superior long-term great saphenous vein/small saphenous vein occlusion rates for endovenous laser ablation compared to foam sclerotherapy.

SURGERY

Comparison of the minimally invasive techniques with surgery in randomised trials is limited. In terms of short-term efficacy, data that is available would suggest that the aims of treatment (abolition of reflux, resolution of varicose veins) are achieved equally well by both the conventional and newer methods of treatment. However, there is fairly strong evidence to suggest that the risk of serious complications and of more minor morbidity such as 'nerve injury' is lower with EVLA in particular.

There also seems to be little doubt that the initial recovery and return to normal activity and employment are more rapid after both EVLA and RFA. This has important implications in relation to the cost-effectiveness of the treatment options. In addition, EVLA performed under local anaesthesia in an out-patient setting is almost certainly less expensive than conventional surgery.

The outstanding issue is, therefore, that of the long-term results for EVLA and RFA. Certainly, recurrent GSV/SSV reflux beyond the first year is uncommon and, in the majority of patients, the truncal vein can no longer be identified by ultrasound. Similarly, our own observations would suggest that the other tributaries of the saphenofemoral and popliteal junctions are no longer in continuity with the deep vein and are unlikely to promote the development of further varicose veins. Thus, as far as recurrent varicosities are concerned, the most important factor may be the development of neovascularisation. Long-term follow-up after surgery suggests that this may occur in up to 52% of patients. Data from our own series indicate that there was evidence of this phenomenon in 4% of patients 1 year after EVLA. It is, therefore, tempting to suggest that the risk of recurrent varicosities in patients treated with laser ablation may be less than that for conventional surgery. Data from long-term follow-up are required to confirm this.

Key point 12

- Further evidence regarding long-term efficacy is required for all minimally invasive therapies.

CONCLUSIONS

At present, endovenous laser ablation of both the GSV and SSV shows considerable promise in the treatment of varicose veins. The principal advantages are avoidance of general anaesthesia and the potential complications of surgery, a more rapid return to normal activity and employment, and potentially a lower risk of recurrent varicosities. It is clear, however, that rigorous long-term follow-up is required to confirm this.

A large, multicentre, randomised trial against surgery would provide the best evidence about treatment efficacy. From our experience it is difficult to recruit patients to such a trial since many decline randomisation and opt for EVLA. It is difficult to see how this problem can be overcome.

On the assumption that minimally invasive treatment will, in due course, replace conventional surgery for those patients in whom it is appropriate, there remains the difficulty of selecting the most appropriate method of those currently available. Whilst it might be argued that EVLA has some advantages over RFA in terms of cost and the frequency of complications, there is no clear evidence that one or the other should be the preferred procedure. Again, a randomised trial might answer this question although, without corporate sponsorship, the cost of equipping centres to undertake both procedures make this unlikely. Further, since any differences between the two techniques may be small, a large study is likely to be required. Finally, the information derived from such a trial may not be attractive to the relevant manufacturers.

For foam sclerotherapy there is certainly an advantage in terms of cost, although its durability is unlikely to match that of EVLA or RFA. The technique might also be less appropriate for patients with larger diameter veins, although this is disputed. Further, serious complications have been reported following foam sclerotherapy which, although rare, may mitigate against its routine use for a largely benign and often cosmetic intervention. If a randomised trial of EVLA versus RFA were to take place, then foam sclerotherapy could be included as a third arm in the study.

Key points for clinical practice

- Endovenous laser ablation can be provided in a 'one-stop' new patient clinic which includes diagnostic venous ultrasound and treatment to enhance efficiency.

- Knowledge of anatomical variations of the great saphenous vein and the anterior saphenous vein is required.

- About 70% of primary and 45% of recurrent varicose veins are suitable for endovenous laser ablation.

- To achieve adequate energy delivery, 810 or 940 nm diode laser should be used.

- Delivery of 60–70 J/cm results in optimum great saphenous vein/small saphenous vein occlusion rates.

- Symptom reduction and cosmetic improvement after EVLA are equivalent to surgery.

- Endovenous laser ablation allows a rapid return to normal activity and employment with no requirement for community nursing care.

- Endovenous laser ablation has lower complication rates than surgery, particularly in respect of nerve injury and wound problems.

- Endovenous laser ablation is more cost effective than radiofrequency ablation.

- Compared to radiofrequency ablation, endovenous laser ablation may be feasible in a larger proportion of patients, may be more effective and may be associated with fewer complications.

- Published data suggest superior long-term great saphenous vein/small saphenous vein occlusion rates for endovenous laser ablation compared to foam sclerotherapy.

- Further evidence regarding long-term efficacy is required for all minimally invasive therapies.

References

1. Evans C, Fowkes FG, Ruckley CV, Lee A. Prevalence of varicose veins and chronic venous insufficiency in men and women in the general population: Edinburgh Vein Study. *J Epidemiol Community Health* 1999; **53**: 149–153.
2. Callam MJ. Epidemiology of varicose veins. *Br J Surg* 1994; **81**: 173.
3. Labropoulos N, Delis KT, Nicolaides AN. Venous reflux in symptom-free vascular surgeons. *J Vasc Surg* 1995; **22**: 150–154.
4. Bradbury A, Evans CJ, Allan P, Lee AJ, Ruckley CV, Fowkes FG. The relationship between lower limb symptoms and superficial and deep venous reflux on duplex ultrasonography: The Edinburgh Vein Study. *J Vasc Surg* 2000; **32**: 921–931.
5. Tibbs DJ. *Varicose Veins and Related Disorders*, 1st edn. Oxford: Butterworth-Heinemann, 1992.
6. Beale RJ, Gough MJ. Treatment options for primary varicose veins – a review. *Eur J Vasc Endovasc Surg* 2005; **30**: 83–95.
7. Proebstle TM, Sandhofer M, Kargl A *et al.* Thermal damage of the inner vein wall during endovenous laser treatment; key role of energy absorption by intravascular blood. *Dermatol Surg* 2002; **28**: 596–600.
8. Bush RG, Shamma HN, Hammond KA. 940-nm laser for treatment of saphenous insufficiency: histological analysis and long-term follow-up. *Photomed Laser Surg* 2005; **23**: 15–19.
9. Weiss RA. Comparison of endovenous radiofrequency versus 810 nm diode laser occlusion of large veins in an animal model. *Dermatol Surg* 2002; **28**: 56–61.
10. Chang CJ, Chua JJ. Endovenous laser photocoagulation (EVLP) for varicose veins. *Lasers Surg Med* 2002; **31**: 257–262.
11. Navarro L, Min RJ, Bone C. Endovenous laser: a new minimally invasive method of treatment for varicose veins – preliminary observations using an 810 nm diode laser. *Dermatol Surg* 2001; **27**: 117–122.
12. Bush RG. Regarding 'Endovenous treatment of the greater saphenous vein with a 940-nm diode laser: thrombolytic occlusion after endoluminal thermal damage by laser-generated steam bubbles'. *J Vasc Surg* 2003; **37**: 242.
13. Min RJ, Zimmet SE, Isaacs MN, Forrestal MD. Endovenous laser treatment of the incompetent greater saphenous vein. *J Vasc Intervent Radiol* 2001; **12**: 1167–1171.
14. Proebstle TM, Gul D, Kargl A, Knop J. Endovenous laser treatment of the lesser saphenous vein with a 940-nm diode laser: early results. *Dermatol Surg* 2003; **29**: 357–361.
15. Perkowski P, Ravi R, Gowda RC *et al.* Endovenous laser ablation of the saphenous vein for treatment of venous insufficiency and varicose veins: early results from a large single-center experience. *J Endovasc Ther* 2004; **11**: 32–38.
16. Min RJ, Khilnani N, Zimmet SE. Endovenous laser treatment of saphenous vein reflux: long-term results. *J Vasc Intervent Radiol* 2003; **14**: 991–996.
17. van Rij AM, Jiang P, Solomon C, Christie RA, Hill GB. Recurrence after varicose vein surgery: a prospective long-term clinical study with duplex ultrasound scanning and air plethysmography. *J Vasc Surg* 2003; **38**: 935–943.
18. Browse NL, Burnand KG, Irvine AT, Wilson NM. *Diseases of the Veins*, 2nd edn. London: Arnold, 1999.
19. Chandler JG, Pichot O, Sessa C, Schuller-Petrovic S, Osse FJ, Bergan JJ. Defining the role of extended saphenofemoral junction ligation: a prospective comparative study. *J Vasc Surg* 2000; **32**: 941–953.
20. Mundy L, Merlin TL, Fitridge RA, Hiller JE. Systematic review of endovenous laser treatment for varicose veins. *Br J Surg* 2005; **92**: 1189–1194.
21. Holme JB, Skajaa K, Holme K. Incidence of lesions of the saphenous nerve after partial or complete stripping of the long saphenous vein. *Acta Chir Scand* 1990; **156**: 145–148.
22. Critchley G, Handa A, Maw A, Harvey A, Harvey MR, Corbett CR. Complications of varicose vein surgery. *Ann R Coll Surg Engl* 1997; **79**: 105–110.
23. Puggioni A, Kalra M, Carmo M, Mozes G, Gloviczki P. Endovenous laser therapy and radiofrequency ablation of the great saphenous vein: analysis of early efficacy and complications. *J Vasc Surg* 2005; **42**: 488–493.
24. Tiperman PE. Arteriovenous fistula after endovenous laser treatment of the short saphenous vein. *J Vasc Intervent Radiol* 2004; **15**: 625–627.

197

25. Goldman MP. Closure of the greater saphenous vein with endoluminal radiofrequency thermal heating of the vein wall in combination with ambulatory phlebectomy: preliminary 6-month follow-up. *Dermatol Surg* 2000; **26**: 452–456.

26. Rautio T, Ohinmaa A, Perala J *et al.* Endovenous obliteration versus conventional stripping operation in the treatment of primary varicose veins: a randomized controlled trial with comparison of the costs. *J Vasc Surg* 2002; **35**: 958–965.

27. Sybrandy JE, Wittens CH. Initial experiences in endovenous treatment of saphenous vein reflux. *J Vasc Surg* 2002; **36**: 1207–1212.

28. Merchant RF, DePalma RG, Kabnick LS. Endovascular obliteration of saphenous reflux: a multicenter study. *J Vasc Surg* 2002; **35**: 1190–1196.

29. Manfrini S, Gasbarro V, Danielsson G *et al.* Endovenous management of saphenous vein reflux. Endovenous Reflux Management Study Group. *J Vasc Surg* 2000; **32**: 330–342.

30. Lurie F, Creton D, Eklof B *et al.* Prospective randomized study of endovenous radiofrequency obliteration (Closure procedure) versus ligation and stripping in a selected patient population (EVOLVeS Study). *J Vasc Surg* 2003; **38**: 207–214.

31. Merchant RF, Kistner RL, Kabnick LS. Is there and increased risk for DVT with the VNUS closure procedure? *J Vasc Surg* 2003, **38**: 628.

32. Hingorani A, Ascher E, Markevich N *et al.* Deep venous thrombosis after radiofrequency ablation of greater saphenous vein: a word of caution. *J Vasc Surg* 2004; **40**: 500–504.

33. Partsch H, Baccaglini U, Stemmer R. Questionnaire regarding the practice of sclerotherapy. *Phlebology* 1997; **12**: 43–55.

34. Jakobsen BH. The value of different forms of treatment for varicose veins. *Br J Surg* 1979; **66**: 182–184.

35. Kern P. Sclerotherapy of varicose leg veins. Technique, indications and complications. *Int Angiol* 2002; **21**: 40–45.

36. Min RJ, Navarro L. Transcatheter duplex ultrasound-guided sclerotherapy for treatment of greater saphenous vein reflux: preliminary report. *Dermatol Surg* 2000; **26**: 410–414.

37. Belcaro G, Nicolaides AN, Errichi BM, Cesarone MR. Superficial thrombophlebitis of the legs: a randomised, controlled, follow-up study. *Angiology* 1999; **50**: 523.

38. Ascer E, Lorensen E, Pollina R, Gennaro M. Preliminary results of a non-operative approach to saphenofemoral junction thrombophlebitis. *J Vasc Surg* 1995; **22**: 616–621.

39. Tessari L, Cavezzi A, Frullini A. Preliminary experience with a new sclerosing foam in the treatment of varicose veins. *Dermatol Surg* 2001; **27**: 58–60.

40. Cabrera J, Cabrera J, Garcia-Olmedo MA. Treatment of varicose long saphenous veins with sclerosant in microfoam: long-term outcomes. *Phlebology* 2000; **15**: 19–23.

Adel H. Rateme Reza Mansouri
Mohammed Keshtgar

13

Gynaecomastia evaluation and management

Gynaecomastia (from the Greek words *gyne* [female] and *mastos* [breast]) is an enlargement of the male breast, secondary to proliferation of both epithelial and stromal components. It presents as palpable or visible, unilateral or bilateral, breast enlargement, which can be tender. Patients seek medical advice because of anxiety and social embarrassment and also fear of cancer.

PREVALENCE

Gynaecomastia is a common condition. In two case series, gynaecomastia was detected on physical examination in 36% of healthy younger adult men, 57% of healthy older men,[1] and more than 70% of hospitalised elderly men.[2] At autopsy, its prevalence was as high as 55%.[3]

There are three peak periods for physiological gynaecomastia – in neonates, at puberty and in the elderly.

The neonatal period

An estimated 60–90% of infants have transient gynaecomastia due to transplacental transfer of maternal oestrogens. This stimulus for breast growth ceases as the oestrogens are cleared from the neonatal circulation, and the

Adel H. Rateme MB BCh FRCS(Glasg)
Senior SpR in Breast and General Surgery, Department of Surgery, University College London, 2nd Floor, Charles Bell House, 67–73 Riding House Street, London W1W 7EJ, UK

Reza Mansouri MD
Senior House Officer, Department of Surgery, University College London, 2nd Floor, Charles Bell House, 67–73 Riding House Street, London W1W 7EJ, UK

Mohammed Keshtgar BSc MBBS FRCSI FRCS(Gen) PhD (for correspondence)
Senior Lecturer and Consultant Surgical Oncologist, Department of Surgery, University College London, 2nd Floor, Charles Bell House, 67–73 Riding House Street, London W1W 7EJ, UK
E-mail m.keshtgar@ucl.ac.uk

breast tissue gradually regresses over a 2–3 week period.[5] It usually regresses completely by the end of the first year.[4]

Puberty

Transient gynaecomastia may occur in up to 60% of boys at puberty. It may first appear as early as 10 years of age, with a peak onset between 13–14 years, followed by an involution that is generally complete by 16–17 years.[5–9]

Late in life

The incidence of gynaecomastia increases with advancing age, with the highest prevalence found in the 50–80 year age range.[1,2,5] Ageing is associated with progressive testicular dysfunction, with reduction in serum testosterone levels and, in some cases, elevated luteinising hormone (LH).[10]

Total and free serum oestradiol concentrations remain normal. The exact mechanism of testicular failure remains unknown. Ageing is also associated with accumulation of adipose tissue, which maintains normal serum oestrogen levels, since adipose tissue is an important site of aromatisation of androgens to oestrogens.[4]

Key point 1

- Gynaecomastia is an enlargement of the male breast secondary to proliferation of both epithelial and stromal tissue. It is a prevalent condition with three peak incidences – in neonates, at puberty and later in life.

CAUSES

Most cases of gynaecomastia appear to result from an imbalance between the stimulatory effects of oestrogen and inhibitory effects of androgens on the growth of breast tissue.[12] Table 1 summarises the common causes.

IDIOPATHIC GYNAECOMASTIA

Even with exhaustive evaluation, no underlying cause is identifiable in about 25% of patients.[11] Unwitting exposures to substances with oestrogen-like activity

Table 1 Causes of gynaecomastia[5,11]

Idiopathic gynaecomastia	25%
Pubertal gynaecomastia	25%
Drug-induced gynaecomastia	25%
Cirrhosis or malnutrition	8%
Primary hypogonadism	8%
Testicular tumours	3%
Secondary hypogonadism	2%
Hyperthyroidism	1.5%
Renal disease	1%

and breast tissue oversensitivity to normal levels of oestrogen have been proposed as possible causes of idiopathic gynaecomastia.[13]

PUBERTAL GYNAECOMASTIA

There are periods during puberty when the balance of sex hormone secretion favours oestrogen,[13] despite an increase in androgen production. This ratio attains normal adult values as puberty advances. The condition is usually asymptomatic and self-limited, and regresses spontaneously after about 2 years.

DRUG-INDUCED GYNAECOMASTIA

Up to 25% of gynaecomastia cases may be drug-induced.[11] There are several mechanisms by various drugs reported which include as summarised in Table 2.

CIRRHOSIS OF THE LIVER

Cirrhosis, especially alcoholic cirrhosis, is commonly associated with gynaecomastia. A number of factors may explain this link: (i) alcohol can inhibit the hypothalamic–pituitary–testicular axis, leading to low serum testosterone levels; (ii) peripheral aromatisation of androgens to oestrogens increases in liver disease; (iii) serum human binding globulin (SHBG) levels are often elevated, causing a further decrease in free testosterone levels; and (iv) some alcoholic beverages contain phyto-oestrogens that may contribute to relative oestrogen excess.[4,13]

MALNUTRITION AND RE-FEEDING GYNAECOMASTIA

This phenomenon was first noted in World War II, when men liberated from prison camps developed gynaecomastia within a few weeks of resuming an adequate diet. The mechanism is not known but may be similar to that of pubertal gynaecomastia. Significant weight loss and malnutrition are often accompanied by hypogonadism, as a result of decreased gonadotrophin secretion. With weight gain, gonadotrophin secretion and gonadal function return to normal, resulting in a 'second puberty'.[4]

PRIMARY HYPOGONADISM

Primary hypogonadism from any cause is commonly associated with gynaecomastia.[4] Congenital hypogonadism is seen in anorchia, Klinefelter's syndrome, hermaphroditism, hereditary defects in testosterone synthesis. Acquired hypogonadism is caused by mumps orchitis, trauma, castration, granulomatous disease (including leprosy) and cytotoxic chemotherapy.

OESTROGEN-PRODUCING TUMOURS

Leydig cell tumours are rare testicular tumours that secrete oestradiol; about 90% are benign. Most patients are young to middle aged.[13,15] Oestrogen-producing adrenal tumours are rare, usually malignant and are often quite large when discovered.[16]

Table 2 Mechanisms of drug-induced gynaecomastia

Mechanism	Drug	Details
Direct action of oestrogens or oestrogen-like substances	Oestrogens, digoxin, isoniazid, cannabis (marijuana)	Direct breast stimulation (bind to oestrogen receptors)
Increased oestrogen production	Human chorionic gonadotrophins	Stimulation of testicular Leydig cell oestrogen secretion
	Androgens	Therapeutic doses of testosterone can be peripherally aromatised to oestrogen*
	Anabolic steroids	The exogenous testosterone, used by athletes or body builders, suppresses the endogenous testosterone and leads to increased production of oestrogens.
Decreased oestrogen metabolism	Cimetidine	
Oestrogen displacement from SHBG	Spironolactone, ketoconazole	
Inhibition of testosterone/DHT biosynthesis	Cancer chemotherapy agents (alkylating agents, vincristine, nitrosoureas, methotrexate)	Primary hypogonadism due to Leydig cell damage
	Leuprolide, ketoconazole, metronidazole, finasteride, alcohol	
	Spironolactone	At high doses[14]
Androgen receptor antagonism	Cimetidine, flutamide, cyproterone acetate, zanoterone, spironolactone	
	Cannabis	Phyto-oestrogens
Elevated serum prolactin	Phenothiazines	
Unknown	Calcium channel blockers (verapamil, nifedipine, diltiazem)	
	Angiotensin-converting enzyme inhibitors (captopril, enalapril)	
	Central nervous system agents (amphetamines, diazepam, haloperidol, phenytoin, tricyclic antidepressants)	
	Antihypertensives (amlodipine, clonidine, doxazosin, felodipine, methyldopa, prazosin, reserpine)	
	Intensive anti-retroviral treatment for HIV	
	Amiodarone, domperidone, D-penicillamine, metoclopramide, ethionamide, thiacetazone, sulindac, theophylline, omeprazole, ranitidine, growth hormone, heroin, methadone	

*Other mechanisms may be involved, since non-aromatisable androgens such as methyltestosterone or dihydrotestosterone can also cause gynaecomastia.

SECONDARY HYPOGONADISM

Androgen deficiency due to partial hypopituitarism is another cause of gynaecomastia. In this condition, peripheral aromatisation of adrenal androgens to oestrogens is unaffected and, therefore, serum oestrogen levels remain normal.[4]

HYPERTHYROIDISM

Gynaecomastia has been reported in up to 40% of men with hyperthyroidism. Serum human binding globulin (SHBG) is often increased in hyperthyroidism, resulting in high-normal or elevated total serum testosterone and decreased free testosterone levels. Peripheral conversion of androgens to oestrogens by aromatase may also be enhanced in hyperthyroidism. Breast enlargement usually resolves after the euthyroid state is restored.[4]

RENAL FAILURE AND DIALYSIS

Men with chronic renal failure have a variety of hormonal abnormalities, including low levels of serum testosterone, raised oestradiol and LH levels, and modest increases in serum prolactin. The hormonal abnormalities are often reversed with renal transplantation but are not altered by dialysis.[13] Dialysis-associated gynaecomastia may be pathogenetically similar to re-feeding gynaecomastia. Before dialysis, renal failure patients must follow restricted diets and tend to lose weight. With dialysis, diet is liberalised and patients often regain weight. Dialysis-associated gynaecomastia has been reported to improve spontaneously after 1–2 years.[4]

HYPERPROLACTINAEMIA

Increased serum prolactin level is not believed to play a direct role in gynaecomastia, although prolactin receptors have recently been demonstrated in gynaecomastia tissue. Most patients with gynaecomastia have normal serum prolactin levels.[17] Moreover, not all patients with hyperprolactinaemia have gynaecomastia. Elevated prolactin levels may, however, suppress gonadotrophin release, producing secondary hypogonadism, which then contributes to the development of gynaecomastia.[4]

Key point 2

- There are several causes for gynaecomastia – 25% of cases occur during puberty and another 25% are drug-induced. The cause is unknown in a further 25%. Other causes include cirrhosis of liver, primary and secondary hypogonadism, testicular tumours, hyper-thyroidism and renal disease.

CLINICAL FEATURES AND DIAGNOSTIC EVALUATION

Most patients with gynaecomastia are asymptomatic. It may be an incidental finding during routine physical examination. The main presenting symptom in patients with recent onset of gynaecomastia is usually breast or nipple pain and tenderness; and in those who present late, usually complain of breast enlargement.

Since palpable breast tissue is so prevalent in the normal male population, an otherwise healthy man with asymptomatic, incidentally discovered gynaecomastia should not be subjected to an exhaustive endocrine evaluation. The breasts should be carefully examined in detail, however, and if the findings are suspicious, breast ultrasound/mammogram and fine needle aspiration or core-cut biopsy needs to be performed to rule out breast cancer. Biochemical assessments of liver, kidney, and thyroid functions should be performed as well. In a patient with normal results, no further tests are necessary, but re-evaluation after 6 months is usually advised.[5]

Men with recent-onset breast enlargement or who present with breast pain and tenderness require a more detailed evaluation to search for a possible underlying cause. Additional studies including measurements of serum concentrations of human chorionic gonadotrophins, oestradiol, testosterone, and luteinising hormone should be done.[5]

One-half of patients have bilateral and symmetric gynaecomastia (Fig. 1). Unilateral gynaecomastia seems to be more common on the left side (Fig. 2).[18] Histological studies have shown that virtually all patients have some bilateral involvement.[3] This discrepancy may be explained by asynchronous growth of the two breasts and differences in the amount of breast glandular and stromal proliferation.[5]

HISTORY

About 10–15% of patients recall a history of breast trauma just before, or at the time of discovery of, the breast enlargement.[19] Trauma itself is unlikely to be the cause of gynaecomastia and it seems that the breast pain from the trauma prompts the patient to examine his breast and consequently leads to the detection of a pre-existing gynaecomastia.

Specific points that need to be outlined in the history include the duration of breast enlargement, presence of breast pain or tenderness, drug history (prescription, over-the-counter, occupational, or recreational). In addition, in adult gynaecomastia, sexual functioning and symptoms of hypogonadism (loss of libido, impotence, decreased strength) and changes in virilisation, changes in weight and symptoms of hyperthyroidism need to be assessed.

PHYSICAL EXAMINATION

In addition to general examination, special attention should be given to the masculine features including body hair, voice, and muscles. Signs of hyperthyroidism are

Table 3 Simon's classification of gynaecomastia (1973)

Group 1	Minor but visible breast enlargement without skin redundancy
Group 2A	Moderate breast enlargement without skin redundancy
Group 2B	Moderate breast enlargement with minor skin redundancy
Group 3	Gross breast enlargement with skin redundancy that looks like a pendulous female breast

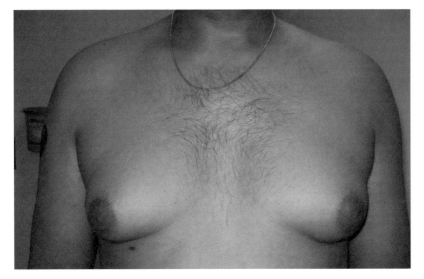

Fig. 1 A 43-year-old man with drug-induced gynaecomastia. For the last 4 years, he has been on cyproterone acetate for treatment of priapism.

looked for. On abdominal examination, hepatomegaly and the presence of an abdominal mass (*i.e.* adrenal) are significant. Examination of genitalia includes testicular examination with particular attention to the size (testicular atrophy) and presence of any testicular mass (tumours). Breast examination needs to include assessment of the size of the breast and presence of lumps and other suspicious findings suggestive of malignancy. The severity is classified as shown in Table 3.

INVESTIGATIONS

Investigations of gynaecomastia include blood tests and imaging studies. The blood tests that need to be considered are serum creatinine, liver function test,

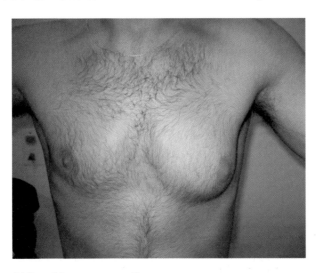

Fig. 2 Unilateral idiopathic gynaecomastia.

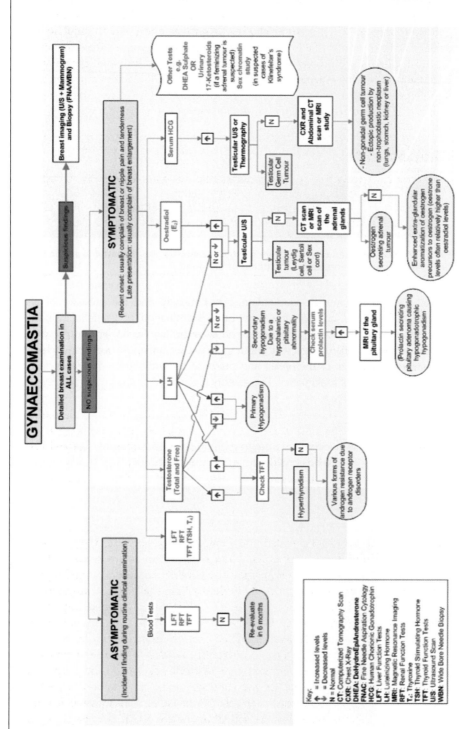

Fig. 3 Assessment, investigations and interpretation of results to determine the cause of gynaecomastia.[5,11]

thyroid function tests, serum total and free testosterone, luteinising hormone, follicle-stimulating hormone, oestradiol and prolactin. Additionally, other investigations may be considered, including serum β-human chorionic gonadotrophin (β-hCG), serum dehydroepiandrosterone (DHEA) sulphate or urinary 17-ketosteroids (if a feminising adrenal tumour is part of the differential diagnosis). Imaging studies should not be ordered unless indicated clinically or by blood results. These include ultrasound scan of the breast and mammography. If indicated, testicular ultrasound scan or thermography, CT scan of the adrenal glands and MRI scan of pituitary gland may be required (Fig. 3).

Key point 3

- The main presenting symptom of recent onset gynaecomastia is breast pain and those who present late usually complain of breast enlargement, social embarrassment and fear of cancer. Clinical examination includes general, breast, abdominal and genital examination. Breast imaging and fine needle cytology may be necessary. Other investigations if indicated include hormonal profiles, LFT, TFT and RFT.

DIFFERENTIAL DIAGNOSIS

Other conditions can mimic gynaecomastia including pseudogynaecomastia, breast carcinoma, dermoid cysts, lipomas, haematomas, neurofibromas and lymphangiomas.[5]

Pseudogynaecomastia

Enlargement of the breasts due to fat deposition rather than to glandular proliferation (pseudogynaecomastia) is common in obese men and needs to be differentiated from true gynaecomastia. Patients with this condition often have generalised obesity and do not complain of breast pain or tenderness. With careful breast examination, it is usually possible to differentiate true from false gynaecomastia.

Breast cancer

Breast cancer accounts for only 0.2% of all malignancies in men, and generally presents as a unilateral hard mass, often eccentric in location rather than subareolar. Patients with carcinoma may also exhibit skin dimpling and nipple retraction, are more likely to have a nipple discharge (60%) than are patients with gynaecomastia (2%), and may present with axillary lymphadenopathy.[19] If the two conditions cannot be differentiated on clinical grounds, then mammography, fine-needle aspiration for cytological examination, or open biopsy should be done. With the exception of Klinefelter's syndrome, no well-established data indicate that gynaecomastia predisposes to the development of carcinoma. Klinefelter's syndrome (phenotypic male, XXY karyotype) is associated with gynaecomastia in about 80% of cases. The unusual feature about this gynaecomastia is that the patient may develop lobular structures. It is the only cause of gynaecomastia that clearly carries an increased risk of breast cancer which is 10–20-fold greater than normal.[4,5,15]

Key point 4

- With the exception of Klinefelter's syndrome, no well-established data indicate that gynaecomastia predisposes to the development of carcinoma.

HISTOLOGICAL FEATURES AND PATHOPHYSIOLOGY

The hormonal milieu, the duration and intensity of stimulation, and the individual's breast tissue sensitivity determine the type and degree of glandular proliferation.[5]

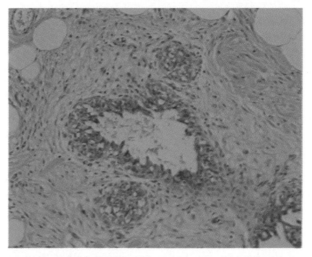

Fig. 4 A photomicrograph of hematoxylin & eosin stained tissues of an early stage gynaecomastia. There is ductal hyperplasia of usual type, periductal myxoid changes and increased cellularity in the stroma. Courtesy of Dr Mary Falzon FRCPath (×40).

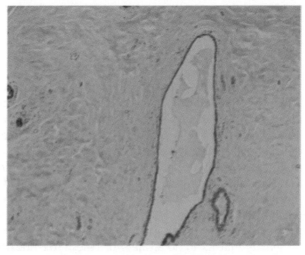

Fig. 5 A photomicrograph of hematoxylin & eosin stained tissues of a late stage gynaecomastia. There is stromal fibrosis and scattered dilated ducts, some of which contain secretions. There is no appreciable epithelial hyperplasia. Courtesy of Dr Mary Falzon FRCPath (×40).

In the early/proliferative/florid stage, ductal proliferation and ductal epithelial hyperplasia are extensive while the stroma is loose and oedematous. Oestrogen leads to elongation and branching of ducts, hyperplasia of ductal epithelium, proliferation of periductal fibroblasts and increased vascularity (Fig. 4). Acinar development is not seen in males, as it requires progesterone in concentrations found during the luteal phase of the menstrual cycle.[5,20] In the proliferative stage, patients may complain of breast pain and tenderness. This stage persists for a variable period but usually lasts less than a year and is followed by spontaneous resolution or enters an inactive stage.

In the late/quiescent stage (over about 12 months) there is a reduction in the epithelial proliferation, the ductules become less prominent, and there is dilatation of the ducts, and hyalinisation and fibrosis of the stroma (Fig. 5).[3,21,22] This inactive stage is usually asymptomatic. This histological picture predominates in men whose gynaecomastia is detected during a routine physical examination.

The microscopic findings are the same regardless of the cause of the gynaecomastia.[3,18]

Key point 5

- Gynaecomastia has two distinct histological stages: an early proliferative and a late quiescent stage. Pain and tenderness are the main symptoms in the proliferative stage. The inactive stage is usually asymptomatic.

TREATMENT

When considering treatment for gynaecomastia, it is important to realise that most gynaecomastia regresses spontaneously. In a group of patients with gynaecomastia from various causes, 85% of untreated patients had spontaneous improvement.[19] It is equally important to appreciate that, after the inactive stage is reached, the gynaecomastia is unlikely to regress spontaneously and is also unlikely to respond to medical therapies.[5]

If the patient is at the pubertal age and has an otherwise normal general physical and testicular examination, he probably has transient or persistent pubertal gynaecomastia. Re-examination at 6-month intervals should determine whether the condition is transient or persistent. At this time, medical or surgical therapy should be considered.[5]

If the patient is on a drug causing gynaecomastia, this should be stopped or changed to another medication if possible, and the patient re-examined after one month. If the drug was the cause, then a reduction in breast pain and tenderness should occur during that time. Similarly, breast enlargement following cytotoxic chemotherapy may also resolve spontaneously.

Treatment of hyperthyroidism and surgical removal of testicular, adrenal, or other causative tumours may lead to regression. In patients with hypogonadism, treatment with testosterone may produce regression by providing androgen and suppressing LH-stimulated oestradiol secretion.[4]

The indications for therapy are severe pain, tenderness, or social embarrassment sufficient to interfere with the patient's normal daily activities.

MEDICAL TREATMENT

As gynaecomastia has a high frequency of spontaneous regression, the decision of when to treat is often difficult. It is also difficult to assess the effectiveness of most medications that have been tried, given the small sample sizes and non-blinded, uncontrolled designs of most studies. Nevertheless, with the exception of early pubertal gynaecomastia that has been present for less than 3 months, a trial of medical therapy for patients with moderate-to-severe symptoms may be effective.

Trials of medical therapy should be limited to only 6 months, due to limited experience and unknown long-term side effects of the drugs. When gynaecomastia has been present for more than 2 years, medical therapy is unlikely to be effective, and surgery may be the only useful treatment.[4]

Options include androgens (testosterone, danazol), anti-oestrogen (clomiphene, tamoxifen), and aromatase inhibitors.

Androgens

Testosterone administration has not been shown to be more effective than placebo in patients with pubertal or idiopathic gynaecomastia and carries the risk of exacerbating the condition by being aromatised to oestradiol.[19] However, micronised testosterone has been shown in a double-blind, placebo-controlled trial to reduce the prevalence of gynaecomastia in men with liver cirrhosis after 6 months of therapy.[27]

Dihydrotestosterone, a non-aromatisable androgen, given either by injection or percutaneously, has been followed by a reduction in breast volume in 75% of patients, with complete resolution in about one quarter.[28] Responders had a decrease in breast tenderness within 1–2 weeks without side effects.

Danazol is a weak androgen that inhibits pituitary secretion of LH and FSH. It is the only drug licensed for the treatment of gynaecomastia in the UK. It has also been evaluated in uncontrolled trials and in a randomised, double-blind, placebo-controlled study, with the latter showing a complete resolution in 23% of patients who received danazol and only a 12% response in those given placebo. The drug was safe and well tolerated.[29] The recommended course of treatment for danazol lasts 6 weeks and the patient is then assessed for response to treatment with clinical examination and ultrasound scan of the breast. Clinical photographic documentation can also be included. If required, the course of treatment can be repeated.

Anti-oestrogen

Clomiphene citrate has been tried mainly in uncontrolled studies, in which it had variable efficacy with response rates of 36–95%. In some of the systemic studies, fewer than 50% of patients had a decrease in breast volume of 20% or more, or were satisfied with the results.[30–33]

Tamoxifen, at a dose of 10 mg twice daily, is associated with statistically significant reduction in pain and breast size.[34,35] Complete regression of gynaecomastia was reported in 70–80% of patients studied in uncontrolled studies.[36] In a head-to-head study, 78% of patients receiving tamoxifen 20 mg daily showed complete regression of gynaecomastia versus 40% in patients receiving danazol 400 mg daily.[37]

In a retrospective study tamoxifen at 10 mg per day given for 3 months seems to be safe and effective in men with painful idiopathic or physiological gynaecomastia.[42]

Aromatase inhibitors

Theoretically, this class of drugs should be useful in patients whose gynaecomastia is primarily the result of enhanced extraglandular aromatisation of oestrogen precursors.

Testolactone was tried in a small uncontrolled study in patients with pubertal gynaecomastia who were treated for 6 months, with good results (decrease in breast size after 2 months of therapy).[33]

Insufficient data currently exist to recommend this drug as a first-line treatment. In addition, there have been no studies of the newer, more potent, aromatase inhibitors anastrozole, letrozole or exemestane in the treatment of gynaecomastia.

Key point 6

- It is difficult to assess the effectiveness of most medications that have been tried, given the small sample sizes and non-blinded, uncontrolled designs of most studies. Trials of medical therapy should be limited to only 6 months, due to limited experience and unknown long-term side effects of the drugs. When gynaecomastia has been present for more than 2 years, medical therapy is unlikely to be effective, and surgery may be the only useful treatment.

SURGERY

Surgical treatment is indicated in patients in whom the gynaecomastia causes distress and psychological trauma, when there is no underlying treatable condition and when hormonal treatment has failed. Operative techniques (individually or in combination) include: (i) open subcutaneous mastectomy; (ii) endoscopic-assisted subcutaneous mastectomy; (iii) liposuction-assisted mastectomy; and (iv) ultrasound-assisted liposuction.

Surgical correction of small-to-moderate size gynaecomastia (Simon's grades I, IIA and IIB) will leave the nipple in its normal position. Grade III cases require skin resection and repositioning of the nipple-areola, otherwise there will be redundant skin folds and a nipple-areola in a lower position than normal.

Open subcutaneous mastectomy

This commonly performed procedure is carried out through a circumareolar incision between 3- and 9-o'clock positions. The length of the incision varies. This approach is used for grade I and IIA gynaecomastia.

The Letterman skin resection and nipple transposition technique is used for moderate grade IIB gynaecomastia. After the skin is resected, the nipple-areola complex is rotated superiorly and medially based on a single dermal pedicle.

The complete circumareolar approach, with a maximum of 2-cm wide ring of de-epithelialised skin, can be used for grade IIB and grade III gynaecomastia.[39]

Cases of massive gynaecomastia (grade III) are treated by similar techniques used for reduction mammoplasty in women including *en-bloc* resection of excessive skin and breast tissue and free nipple grafting.

Haemostasis is secured, and a surgical drain is placed. Subcutaneous tissues are re-approximated, and the skin is closed subcuticularly.[40]

Endoscopic-assisted subcutaneous mastectomy
With this technique it is possible to excise the glandular breast tissue through very small, distant incisions, thus avoiding a breast or areola scar.

Liposuction-assisted mastectomy
This is the most popular method used to correct for pseudogynaecomastia. Advantages compared to the over subcutaneous mastectomy include reduced risk of nipple/areola ischaemia (as blood supply is better preserved), reduced chance of nipple distortion, lower risk of saucer deformity, and reduced risk of haemorrhage, haematoma, seroma and infection.

This technique is not recommended for pure glandular gynaecomastia (unless it is assisted with ultrasound). Incisions are 3–4 mm in length and can be made in the axillary fold, inframammary fold or peri-areolar. Approximately 10–15 mm of tissue, depending on the thickness of the chest wall fat, is left on the flaps and slightly more beneath the nipple-areola to avoid depression in this region, contour irregularities and skin retraction.

Postoperatively, compression garments are applied for at least 2 weeks. The final results are not fully appreciated for up to a year.[40]

Ultrasound-assisted liposuction
This permits emulsification and cavitation of the glandular tissues, which can then be followed by standard liposuction to remove excess fat and the liquefied tissue.

Technical considerations
The following points are important to maximise the chance of a good result:

1. Avoid inframammary incisions in the young, as this will leave visible scar which has the tendency to become keloid.

2. Leave a small amount of breast tissue and subcutaneous fat behind the nipple-areola complex. This is to preserve their blood supply, and to reduce the chance of nipple inversion.

3. Ensure adequate thickness of skin flaps with good volume of subcutaneous fat.

4. Facilitate dissection by dividing up the breast tissue into two or four pieces.

5. It is important to preserve the pectoralis fascia, to prevent skin fixation.

Complications of surgery

In discussing surgery with patients, it must be emphasised that the results can be cosmetically unsatisfactory in up to 50% of patients and there may be a need for further corrective surgery.[4,40] Complications include: bleeding and haematoma (most common); seroma; nipple-areola related complications (inversion, distortion, alteration of sensitivity and necrosis); scar-related complications (painful, conspicuous, hypertrophic or keloid scar); breast asymmetry; contour irregularities (palpable breast tissue edges on the chest wall, and rippling or denting of the skin); skin redundancy; skin necrosis; and infection.

Key point 7

- Surgery is indicated in patients in whom the gynaecomastia causes social embarrassment and psychological trauma, when there is no underlying treatable condition and when trial of hormonal treatment have failed.

PREVENTION

Two situations exist in which gynaecomastia can be prevented. The first is by avoiding drugs that can cause gynaecomastia. If unavoidable, and you have a choice of drugs, then try to use the drug that has the weakest association with gynaecomastia, as not all drugs cause gynaecomastia to the same extent. For example, when considering the use of a calcium channel blocker in an older man, one should remember that nifedipine has been associated with the highest frequency of gynaecomastia, followed by verapamil, with diltiazem having the lowest association.[23,24] Similarly, the incidence of gynaecomastia in patients receiving histamine receptor or proton-pump inhibitors is highest with cimetidine, then ranitidine, and least with omeprazole.[23,25]

The second area of prevention applies to patients with prostate cancer who are about to receive oestrogen therapies or anti-androgen therapy. Several studies have shown that prophylactic breast irradiation (with low-dose of 900 rad) is effective in preventing gynaecomastia and mastodynia in patients with prostate cancer.[4,26,41]

PROGNOSIS

Regardless of the aetiology of gynaecomastia, the prognosis is excellent. Studies have shown that 90% of physiological gynaecomastia involutes spontaneously within 2 years. In drug-induced gynaecomastia, withdrawal of the medication leads to regression in 60% of patients. If the gynaecomastia is of long duration, it is unlikely to regress spontaneously.[40]

Key points for clinical practice

- Gynaecomastia is an enlargement of the male breast secondary to proliferation of both epithelial and stromal tissue. It is a prevalent condition with three peak incidences – in neonates, at puberty and later in life.

- There are several causes for gynaecomastia – 25% of cases occur during puberty and another 25% are drug-induced. The cause is unknown in a further 25%. Other causes include cirrhosis of liver, primary and secondary hypogonadism, testicular tumours, hyperthyroidism and renal disease.

- The main presenting symptom of recent onset gynaecomastia is breast pain and those who present late usually complain of breast enlargement, social embarrassment and fear of cancer. Clinical examination includes general, breast, abdominal and genital examination. Breast imaging and fine needle cytology may be necessary. Other investigations if indicated include hormonal profiles, LFT, TFT and RFT.

- With the exception of Klinefelter's syndrome, no well-established data indicate that gynaecomastia predisposes to the development of carcinoma.

- Gynaecomastia has two distinct histological stages: an early proliferative and a late quiescent stage. Pain and tenderness are the main symptoms in the proliferative stage. The inactive stage is usually asymptomatic.

- It is difficult to assess the effectiveness of most medications that have been tried, given the small sample sizes and non-blinded, uncontrolled designs of most studies. Trials of medical therapy should be limited to only 6 months, due to limited experience and unknown long-term side effects of the drugs. When gynaecomastia has been present for more than 2 years, medical therapy is unlikely to be effective, and surgery may be the only useful treatment.

- Surgery is indicated in patients in whom the gynaecomastia causes social embarrassment and psychological trauma, when there is no underlying treatable condition and when trial of hormonal treatment have failed.

References

1. Nuttall FQ. Gynecomastia as a physical finding in normal men. *J Clin Endocrinol Metab* 1979; **48**: 338–340.
2. Niewoehner CB, Nuttal FQ. Gynecomastia in a hospitalized male population. *Am J Med* 1984; **77**: 633–638.
3. Andersen JA, Gram JB. Male breast at autopsy. *Acta Pathol Microbiol Immunol Scand [A]* 1982; **90**: 191–197.
4. Bembo SA, Carlson HE. Gynecomastia: its features, and when and how to treat it. *Cleveland Clin J Med* 2004; **71**: 511–517.
5. Braunstein GD. Management of gynecomastia. In: Harris JR, Lippman ME, Morrow M, Osborne CK. (eds) *Diseases of the Breast*, 2nd edn. Williams & Wilkins, 2000.

6. Bulard FM, Lucky AW, Huster GA *et al*. Hormonal studies and physical maturation in adolescent gynaecomastia. *J Pediatr* 1990; **116**: 450.

7. Gooren E, Papandreou L, Evangelopoulou C *et al*. Incidence of gynaecomastia in 954 young males and its relationship to somatometric parameters. *Ann Hum Biol* 1994; **21**: 579.

8. Moore DC, Schlaepfer LV, Paunier L, Sizonenko PC. Hormonal changes during puberty: V. Transient pubertal gynecomastia: abnormal androgen-estrogen ratios. *J Clin Endocrinol Metab* 1984; **58**: 492–499.

9. Rose M, Bustos J, Dale Jr JH *et al*. Gynaecomastia in adolescent boys. *JAMA* 1961; **178**: 449.

10. Hall A, Feldman HA, McKinley JB *et al*. Age, disease, and changing sex hormone levels in middle-aged men: results of the Massachusetts male aging study. *J Clin Endocrinol Metab* 1991; **73**: 1016–1025.

11. Braunstein GD. Gynecomastia. *N Engl J Med* 1993; **328**: 490–495.

12. Ando S, De AF, Rago V, Carpino A *et al*. Breast cancer: from estrogen to androgen receptor. *Mol Cell Endocrinol* 2002; **193**: 121–128.

13. Hershkovitz E, Leiberman E. Gynaecomastia: a review. *Endocrinologist* 2002; **12**: 321–332.

14. Mertani DL, Menard R, Taylor A, Pita JC, Santen R. Spironolactone and endocrine dysfunction. *Ann Intern Med* 1976; **85**: 630–636.

15. Korenman SG. The endocrinology of the abnormal male breast. *Ann NY Acad Sci* 1986; **464**: 400–408.

16. Zayed A, Stock JL, Liepman MK *et al*. Feminization as a result of both peripheral conversion of androgens and direct estrogen production from an adrenocortical carcinoma. *J Endocrinol Invest* 1994; **17**: 275–278.

17. Turkington RW. Serum prolactin levels in patients with gynecomastia. *J Clin Endocrinol Metab* 1972; **34**: 62–66.

18. Bannayan GA, Hajdu SI. Gynecomastia: clinicopathologic study of 351 cases. *Am J Clin Pathol* 1972; **57**: 431–437.

19. Treves N. Gynecomastia; the origins of mammary swelling in the male: an analysis of 406 patients with breast hypertrophy, 525 with testicular tumors, and 13 with adrenal neoplasms. *Cancer* 1958; **11**: 1083–1102.

20. Zayed JD, Aiman J, MacDonald PC. The pathogenesis of gynaecomastia. *Adv Intern Med* 1980; **29**: 1.

21. Nicolis GL, Modlinger RS, Gabrilove JL. A study of the histopathology of human gynecomastia. *J Clin Endocrinol Metab* 1971; **32**: 173–178.

22. Williams MJ. Gynecomastia. Its incidence, recognition and host characterization in 447 autopsy cases. *Am J Med* 1963; **34**: 103–112.

23. Thompson DF, Carter JR. Drug-induced gynecomastia. *Pharmacotherapy* 1993; **13**: 37–45.

24. Tanner LA, Bosco LA. Gynecomastia associated with calcium channel blocker therapy. *Arch Intern Med* 1988; **148**: 379–380.

25. Lindquist M, Edwards IR. Endocrine adverse effects of omeprazole. *BMJ* 1992; **305**: 451–452.

26. Waterfall NB, Glaser MG. A study of the effects of radiation on prevention of gynaecomastia due to oestrogen therapy. *Clin Oncol* 1979; **5**: 257–260.

27. The Copenhagen Study Group for Liver Diseases. Testosterone treatment of men with alcoholic cirrhosis: a double-blind study. *Hepatology* 1986; **6**: 807.

28. Kuhn JM, Roca R, Laudat MH, Rieu M, Luton JP, Bricaire H. Studies on the treatment of idiopathic gynaecomastia with percutaneous dihydrotestosterone. *Clin Endocrinol (Oxf)* 1983; **19**: 513–520.

29. Jones DJ, Holt SD, Surtees P, Davison DJ, Coptcoat MJ. A comparison of danazol and placebo in the treatment of adult idiopathic gynaecomastia: results of a prospective study in 55 patients. *Ann R Coll Surg Engl* 1990; **72**: 296–298.

30. Stepanas AV, Burnet RB, Harding PE, Wise PH. Clomiphene in the treatment of pubertal-adolescent gynecomastia: a preliminary report. *J Pediatr* 1977; **90**: 651–653.

31. Plourde PV, Kulin HE, Santner SJ. Clomiphene in the treatment of adolescent gynecomastia. Clinical and endocrine studies. *Am J Dis Child* 1983; **137**: 1080–1082.

32. LeRoith D, Sobel R, Glick SM. The effect of clomiphene citrate on pubertal gynaecomastia. *Acta Endocrinol (Copenh)* 1980; **95**: 177–180.

33. Zachmann M, Eiholzer U, Muritano M, Werder EA, Manella B. Treatment of pubertal gynaecomastia with testolactone. *Acta Endocrinol Suppl (Copenh)* 1986; **279**: 218–226.

34. McDermott MT, Hofeldt FD, Kidd GS. Tamoxifen therapy for painful idiopathic gynecomastia. *South Med J* 1990; **83**: 1283–1285.

35. Parker LN, Gray DR, Lai MK, Levin ER. Treatment of gynecomastia with tamoxifen: a double-blind crossover study. *Metabolism* 1986; **35**: 705–708.

36. Alagaratnam TT. Idiopathic gynecomastia treated with tamoxifen: a preliminary report. *Clin Ther* 1987; **9**: 483–487.

37. Ting AC, Chow LW, Leung YF. Comparison of tamoxifen with danazol in the management of idiopathic gynecomastia. *Am Surg* 2000; **66**: 38–40.

38. Daniels IR, Layer GT. Gynaecomastia. *Eur J Surg* 2001; **167**: 885–892.

39. Persichetti P, Berloco M, Casadei RM, Marangi GF, Di LF, Nobili AM. Gynaecomastia and the complete circumareolar approach in the surgical management of skin redundancy. *Plast Reconstr Surg* 2001; 107: 948–954.

40. Ali A, Bain J. Gynecomastia. *eMedicine* 2005 Available from: <http://www.emedicine.com/plastic/topic125.htm>.

41. Picker AP. The safety and tolerability of low-dose irradiation for the management of antiandrogen monotherapy. *Lancet Oncol* 2003; **4**: 30–36.

42. Hanavadi S, Banerjee D, Monypenny IJ, Mansel RE. The role of tamoxifen in the management of gynaecomastia. *Breast* 2005.

Richard A. Cassell   Bashar Zeidan
Emma-Kate Lacey   Colin D. Johnson

14

Randomised clinical trials in surgery 2005

This chapter reviews the randomised clinical trials published in major surgical and other journals during 2005. The literature search was conducted during December 2005, so some publications may have been overlooked at the end of the year. A small number of meta-analyses has also been included as these provide powerful evidence to help guide practice.

BREAST AND ENDOCRINE SURGERY

The efficacy of fibrin glue over suction drainage in the prevention of seromas following breast surgery was assessed in a randomised, controlled trial.[1] Precise details of the randomisation method were not provided. Of the originally planned 250 patients, only 82 patients participated in the study. The incidence of seroma was 45.5% in the group undergoing drainage compared with 36.8% in the fibrin glue group. The authors concluded that this was not significant and there was no advantage of using fibrin glue over surgical drainage. However, there was failure to blind the surgeons and the patients to the two treatment arms, inability to recruit the planned number of patients and premature termination of the study.

Richard A. Cassell BSc
Medical Student, University Surgical Unit, Southampton University Hospitals, Southampton, UK

Bashar Zeidan MD
Senior House Officer, University Surgical Unit, Southampton University Hospitals, Southampton, UK

Emma-Kate Lacey BM
Senior House Officer, University Surgical Unit, Southampton University Hospitals, Southampton, UK

Colin D. Johnson MChir FRCS (for correspondence)
Reader and Consultant Surgeon, University Surgical Unit, Southampton University Hospitals, Southampton, UK
E-mail: c.d.johnson@soton.ac.uk

217

ADJUVANT THERAPY OF BREAST CANCER

The long-term effectiveness of adjuvant chemotherapy in patients who had undergone surgery but were at risk of relapse was assessed in a recent cohort study[2] using three randomised, controlled trials and an observational study. Women were considered for inclusion into the first three studies if they had undergone surgery for unilateral breast cancer and had histological evidence of axillary node involvement. The other study considered patients who had no axillary node involvement and oestrogen receptor-negative neoplasms. The results suggested that there were statistically significant, long-term benefits of adjuvant chemotherapy in terms of reduced risk of relapse (29%) and relative risk of death (21%). The study also found differences in the response to treatment from premenopausal and postmenopausal women and two patients were lost to follow-up.

Survival outcomes of premenopausal patients with lymph node positive breast cancer treated by radiation therapy and adjuvant chemotherapy following radical breast surgery were assessed in a randomised trial.[3] The authors randomly assigned 318 premenopausal women who had undergone radical mastectomy to either radiation and chemotherapy or to chemotherapy alone treatment arms using a computer. After 20 years of follow-up, the results demonstrated a statistically significant 32% reduction in breast cancer mortality in patients treated by both radiation and chemotherapy as well as a 27% reduction in overall mortality. However, 8 patients in the chemotherapy only group had radiation therapy and, in the radiation and chemotherapy group, 12 patients did not receive radiation therapy and there were a greater number of cases of toxicity associated with radiation and chemotherapy.

Discussion of whether adjuvant chemotherapy programmes in breast cancer treatment should be identical in patients of all age groups[4] arose from the Early Breast Cancer Trialists' Collaborative Group study of women with early stage disease which demonstrated an 8% reduction in mortality in women aged 60–69 years with several months of combination chemotherapy compared with a 27% risk reduction in women aged under 50 years. Other evidence discussed argued that younger and older women gained similar benefit from chemotherapy with respect to both survival and disease recurrence but the older patients have increased treatment-related mortality. The authors suggest that gene expression profiling may offer an answer as to who responds best to therapy.

Elderly breast cancer patients with node-positive disease have been shown to have improved disease-free survival from epirubicin-based chemotherapy in addition to tamoxifen as adjuvant treatment following surgery compared with tamoxifen alone.[5] In a randomised trial of 338 patients over the age of 65 years with node-positive breast cancer, the 6-year, disease-free survival rates were 69.3% and 72.6% in the tamoxifen only and the epirubicin-based treatment, respectively ($P = 0.14$). No details of the randomisation process were provided. Overall survival advantage was not demonstrated in the epirubicin-based treatment arm: longer follow-up would be required to evaluate this.

High-dose chemotherapy with cyclophosphamide, cisplatin and carmustine and stem cell support has not been shown to be superior to intermediate-dose treatment in overall survival of women with high-risk breast cancer.[6] The prospective, randomised study involved 785 women with disease affecting at least 10 axillary nodes who had undergone surgery and adjuvant chemotherapy. Details of randomisation were not provided. Following treatment, patients were followed up and results at 5 years showed no significant differences between the two treatment arms in terms of event-free survival. Moreover, there were 33 treatment-related deaths in the high-dose group compared with none in the other group. The lack of a control group prevents comparison of outcomes being made with conventional adjuvant chemotherapy programmes.

Efficacy of pre-operative systemic therapy was compared with the same regimen given postoperatively in patients with breast cancer as part of a meta-analysis.[7] Data from nine randomised trials including 3861 patients were used to compare pre-operative with postoperative adjuvant therapy, evaluated using two-sided statistical tests. The authors were unable to find any statistically significant difference between the therapies with respect to death, disease progression or distant recurrence. However, pre-operative therapy was associated with a statistically significant increased risk of regional recurrence. The authors, however, were unable to exclude the possibility of publication bias and failed to include recent data from large randomised studies. Furthermore, there was considerable diversity in the treatment programmes used in each of the studies.

The effectiveness of different pre-operative chemotherapies in breast cancer patients was also evaluated in a randomised, parallel study in which 200 previously untreated patients aged 18–65 years were randomly assigned to either combined doxorubicin plus paclitaxel (AP) or doxorubicin plus cyclophosphamide (AC) treatments.[8] Details of the randomisation process were not provided. Eradication of invasive carcinoma in tumour and axillary nodes was achieved in 16% of patients in the AP arm compared with 10% in the AC arm although these figures fell to 8% and 6%, respectively, following independent expert review. Furthermore, not all patients received all the courses of planned chemotherapy.

The effects of using menopausal hormone therapy following a diagnosis of breast cancer were assessed in the Stockholm trial in which 378 postmenopausal women were randomly assigned to receive either therapy or no therapy.[9] Randomisation was performed using balanced lists prepared with permuted blocks of six. Patients were followed up every 6 months; at a median follow-up of 4.1 years, there were 11 patients with breast cancer recurrence in the menopausal hormone therapy group and 13 in the control group. The trial was prematurely closed for patient entry on issues relating to patient safety and, owing to the limited number of patients, no definitive conclusions were made.

THYROID SURGERY

Evaluation of bilateral subtotal thyroidectomy with unilateral total and contralateral subtotal throidectomy in preventing recurrence of hyperthyroidism in patients with Graves' disease has been performed;[10] 340 patients were randomised into two groups and underwent either one of the two procedures above, with all surgery performed by one surgeon. The groups had similar characteristics with respect to age, sex and follow-up. At long-term follow up, recurrent hyperthyroidism was significantly lower in the group undergoing unilateral total and contralateral subtotal thyroidectomy; however, the incidence of hypothyroidism was higher in this group but the difference was deemed to not be significant. Temporary postoperative hypocalcaemia was also more severe in this group.

Comparison of the harmonic scalpel with electrocoagulation in thyroidectomy found that the former requires less operative time.[11] A randomised study was performed of 60 patients who were assigned into two surgical groups using either of above techniques to achieve haemostasis. A permuted block method was used for randomisation and sequential numbers were assigned to opaque envelopes which contained assigned treatment groups and were opened in the surgical suite. There were no statistical differences between the groups in terms of intra-operative bleeding, pain control or length of in-patient stay. However, an average reduction of operative time of 25 min was found in the harmonic scalpel group.

SURGICAL ONCOLOGY

A novel approach to the treatment of cancer cachexia using the TNF-α synthesis inhibitor thalidomide was evaluated as part of a randomised, placebo controlled trial involving 50 patients with advanced pancreatic cancer.[12] Randomisation was performed through sealed envelopes which contained a computer generated code. A third party opened the envelopes and dispensed the drug to achieve double blinding. Results at 4 weeks demonstrated that patients in the treatment group gained a mean mass of 0.37 kg compared with a mean loss of 2.21 kg in the placebo group and data at 8 weeks also showed that thalidomide was effective in attenuating weight loss. However, only 43% of patients were available for analysis at 8 weeks and the authors failed to demonstrate that treatment led to an improved quality of life.

The effectiveness of erythropoietin in treating anaemia in cancer patients was assessed in a systematic review.[13] The review included data from 27 trials which involved a total of 3287 patients. The findings were that the use of erythropoietin was associated with a lower relative risk of having a blood transfusion than in those who were untreated. However, there was no significant evidence that overall survival was improved with erythropoietin treatment. Furthermore, there was an increased risk of hypertension and thrombo-embolic complications with erythropoietin treatment but these were not statistically significant.

The addition of surgery to chemoradiation treatment in patients with locally advanced squamous cell carcinoma (SCC) of the oesophagus had been found to improve local tumour control but not survival.[14] A total of 172 patients under the age of 70 years with histologically proven SCC of the upper and mid-third oesophagus were randomly assigned, unblinded, into either the chemoradiotherapy and surgery or chemoradiotherapy without surgery. At 2 and 3 years, overall survival was equivalent in both groups, although 34% of patients did not proceed to surgery. However, treatment-related mortality was significantly higher in the group who underwent surgery but local tumour control was significantly increased and there was a lower chance of death from cancer.

GASTROINTESTINAL SURGERY

ANORECTAL

A prospective, randomised, controlled, single-blind, clinical trial[15] compared stapled technique with the conventional Milligan-Morgan haemorrhoidectomy in Indian patients. Patients were randomly allocated to the stapled (n = 42) or open (n = 42) groups. All patients were operated on using spinal anaesthesia. Follow-up was for a range of 2–19 months. The mean operative time was shorter in the stapled group. The blood loss, pain scores, requirement of analgesics and mean hospital stay were significantly less in the stapled group. The patients in the stapled group returned to work or routine activities earlier and a higher percentage were satisfied with the stapled compared to open technique. Stapled haemorrhoidectomy is a safe and effective day-care procedure for the treatment of Grade III and IV haemorrhoids. It is a minimally invasive, faster technique and ensures less postoperative pain, early discharge, less time off work, complications similar to open technique, and a more satisfied patient with no peri-anal wound. This study does not advocate stapled haemorrhoidectomy in patients with large external components.

A randomised trial comparing the use of local and regional anaesthesia in circular stapled haemorrhoidectomy found no differences in analgesia requirements or pain scores.[17] A total of 60 consecutive patients with third or fourth degree haemorrhoids were randomised in a non-blinded fashion into two equal groups and underwent circular stapled haemorrhoidectomy performed under either local or spinal anaesthesia. Postoperative pain levels were assessed using a visual analogue scale and analgesia requirements were measured. The study also demonstrated that procedures performed under local anaesthesia were associated with considerable financial savings compared with those using regional anaesthesia and admission.

A prospective randomised trial[16] aimed to compare the effectiveness and morbidity of surgical versus chemical sphincterotomy in the treatment of chronic anal fissure with a 3-year follow-up. Patients with chronic anal fissure were treated by either open lateral internal sphincterotomy (n = 40) or chemical sphincterotomy (n = 40) with 25 U Botulinum toxin injected into the internal sphincter. Clinical and manometric results were analysed at 1 week, 2, and 6 months, and 1-, 2-, and 3-year follow-up visits. Overall healing was 92.5% in the open group and 45% in the Botulinum group ($P \leq 0.001$). Recurrence or persistence of the fissure was recorded in 12 patients in the chemical group and two in the surgical group after 6 months ($P \leq 0.05$). There were no new recurrences at 2- and 3-year follow-up. The final percentage of incontinence was 5% in the open compared to none in the Botulinum groups ($P > 0.05$). There is a group of patients with clinical and manometric features associated with a higher rate of anal fissure. This trial recommends surgical sphincterotomy as the first therapeutic approach in patients with clinical and manometric features which predict recurrence. Botulinum use is preferred in patients older than 50 years or with risk factors for incontinence, despite the higher rate of recurrence, since it avoids the greater risk of incontinence found in the surgical group. This is the first prospective randomised study with a long-term (36 months) clinical and manometric follow-up.

COLORECTAL

A multicentre, randomised trial[18] compared the participation and detection rates achievable through different strategies of colorectal cancer screening. Subjects aged 55–64 years were randomly assigned to 5 different screening groups: (i) biennial faecal occult blood test (FOBT) by mail; (ii) biennial FOBT by GP or a screening facility; (iii) patient-choice of FOBT or once-only sigmoidoscopy; (iv) once-only sigmoidoscopy; or (v) sigmoidoscopy followed by biennial FOBT; 26,682 patients were randomised. Of the FOBT group, 4.3% had a positive test result, 3.5 per 1000 had cancer and 1.4% had advanced adenoma. Of the sigmoidoscopy group, 7.4% were referred to colonoscopy and of these 4 per 1000 had cancer and 5.1% advanced adenoma. In both FOBT and sigmoidoscopy groups, participation rate was between 22–40%. The detection rate for advanced neoplasia was 3 times higher following screening by sigmoidoscopy than by FOBT. The positive predictive value of a FOBT for advanced neoplasia was 45.3% and it was statistically significantly higher among those aged 60–64 years compared to those aged 55–59 years. The higher yield of lesions achieved with sigmoidoscopy than with FOBT screening supports the hypothesis that sigmoidoscopy screening might have a larger impact on colorectal cancer incidence than FOBT screening. Possible deficiencies of the study include that the absolute number of colorectal cancers detected in the study was too low to allow precise estimates of the relative performances of the tests. Also, the detection rate of FOBT was reported after only one round of screening – several screening rounds should be considered.

A prospective randomised study[19] assigned 329 patients to two groups who had colorectal surgery with ($n = 164$) and without ($n = 165$) mechanical bowel preparation (MBP) using Sofodex (a phosphate-based purgative). All patients were treated with antibiotics prior to surgery; 81.5% underwent surgery for colorectal cancer and 18.5% for benign disease. Complications were registered daily after surgery, and patients were re-examined at the out-patient clinic 1, 3, and 6 weeks following surgery. The hospitalisation period was longer in the MBP group but this was not statistically significant. The time until the first bowel movement was similar between the 2 groups. Postoperative complications were not different between the 2 groups. No advantage was gained by pre-operative MBP in elective colorectal surgery and MBP failed to show any benefit in reducing the rate of complications. This study, however, does not examine the benefit of antibiotic prophylaxis in colorectal surgery in addition to MBP. Sub-group analysis did suggest the need for MBP in patients who need low anterior resections and for those with polypoid lesions where localisation by palpation and intra-operative colonoscopy is necessary.

FAST-TRACK GASTROINTESTINAL SURGERY

In this randomised, observer-and-patient, blinded trial[20] patients underwent either laparoscopic ($n = 30$) or open ($n = 30$) colonic resection with fast-track rehabilitation and planned discharge after 24 h. Functional recovery was assessed in detail during the first postoperative month. Median postoperative hospital stay was 2 days in both groups, with early and similar recovery to normal activities as assessed by many organ functions. Duration of surgery was significantly longer in the laparoscopic group. Intra-operative blood transfusion was given more frequently in the open group. Three patients had their operations converted from laparoscopic to open. There were no significant differences in postoperative stay, morbidity, mortality, or re-admissions, although 3 patients in the open group died compared to none in the laparoscopic group. This may be related to the higher ASA scores in the open group. In conclusion, functional recovery after colonic resection is rapid with a multimodal rehabilitation regimen and without differences between open and laparoscopic operations. This is the first randomised, blinded study to combine appropriate blinding with 'fast-track' care in laparoscopic surgery, and it shows that functional recovery of a large variety of organ functions is fast, but similar, between laparoscopic and open procedures. These findings emphasise that postoperative outcome may merely depend on principles of postoperative care rather than single-modality intervention with minimal invasive surgery. Further large-scale studies are required on cost issues, satisfaction, and potential advantages of laparoscopic resection in high-risk patients to decrease serious morbidity and mortality.

Patients undergoing major intestinal resection, and on a fast-track (standardised) postoperative care plan, were randomised to pre-emptive thoracic epidural (TE, $n = 31$) or to patient-controlled analgesia (PCA, $n = 28$).[21] Patients were evaluated at standard time points for pain score, quality of life and complications. Oral analgesia was substituted for TE and PCA on the second postoperative day. The primary goal of the study was to compare the time to discharge from the hospital. Discharge criteria were identical for both groups. Six patients had a failed epidural and there was no significant difference in length of stay, pain scores, quality of life, complications, or hospital costs. TE patients had less pain before oral medication was commenced on day 2. There was no significant reduction in the time taken to achieve gastrointestinal motility or in intestinal transit time. TE offers no advantage over PCA for patients undergoing major intestinal resections who are on a fast-track postoperative care plan using PCA. Possible deficiencies of this relatively small study include randomisation using sealed envelopes.

UPPER GASTROINTESTINAL SURGERY

A prospective, randomised, double-blind trial[22] compared clopidogrel with aspirin plus esomeprazole for the prevention of recurrent bleeding from ulcers in high-risk patients. Patients studied were those who took aspirin to prevent vascular diseases and who presented with bleeding ulcers. After the ulcers healed and patients were *Helicobacter pylori* negative, patients were randomly assigned to receive either 75 mg clopidogrel daily plus esomeprazole placebo twice daily or 80 mg aspirin daily plus 20 mg esomeprazole twice daily for 12 months. The end points were recurrent ulcer and lower gastrointestinal bleeding. A total of 320 patients were studied (161 clopidogrel, and 159 aspirin plus esomeprazole) at months 1 and 3, then 3-monthly thereafter. Thirteen patients in the clopidogrel group had recurrent bleeding and one in the aspirin plus esomeprazole group. There was a significant difference in the cumulative incidence of recurrent ulcer bleeding in the 12-month period among those who received clopidogrel (8.6%) and those who received aspirin plus esomeprazole

(0.7%). However, there was no difference in the cumulative incidence of lower gastrointestinal bleeding between the two groups (both 4.6%). Therefore, in patients with a history of aspirin-induced ulcer bleeding whose ulcers healed, aspirin plus esomeprazole was superior to clopidogrel in the prevention of recurrent ulcer healing. In this study it is not possible to estimate the risk reduction achieved by either clopidogrel or the addition of esomeprazole compared with aspirin alone.

Leontiadis et al.[23] performed a systematic review and meta-analysis of 21 randomised controlled trials of treatment with a proton pump inhibitor (PPI) in patients with ulcer bleeding and determined the impact on mortality, re-bleeding and surgical intervention. PPI was compared with placebo or H2-receptor antagonist for treatment of an endoscopically proven bleeding ulcer. The analysis included trials that reported at least one of: mortality within 30 days of randomisation, re-bleeding, or surgical intervention within 30 days of randomisation. In all, 2915 patients were involved. PPI treatment had no significant effect on mortality but reduced re-bleeding (number needed to treat, NNT = 12) and the need for surgery (NNT = 20). These results were similar when the top 10 trials with the highest methodological quality were compared. After ulcer bleeding, treatment with a PPI reduces the risk of re-bleeding and the requirement for surgery but has no overall benefit on mortality.

A prospective randomised trial[24] compared patients who underwent laparoscopic Nissen fundoplication with simple sutured crural closure ($n = 50$), and patients who underwent laparascopic Nissen fundoplication with simple sutured cruroplasty and onlay of a propylene mesh ($n = 50$). Main outcome measures included recurrence, complications, and results of oesophageal manometry, 24-h pH monitoring, oesohagogastroduodenoscopy, barium swallow and symptomatic outcome. Patients in both groups had similar levels for all tested parameters at 1 week, 6 weeks, and at 3 months. By 1-year follow-up, all functional outcome variables significantly improved. There were no significant differences between the groups in terms of functional variable outcomes except for dysphagia, in which a higher postoperative dysphagia rate was found in the mesh group at 3 months after surgery but by a year there was no difference. An intrathoracic wrap migration occurred in 13 patients in the suture group compared with 4 in the mesh group ($P \le 0.001$). In conclusion, laparoscopic Nissen fundoplication with prosthetic cruroplasty is an effective procedure to reduce the incidence of postoperative hiatal hernia recurrence and intrathoracic wrap herniation. However, longer follow-up of this randomised prospective study is needed to study any late complications.

A prospective randomised study[25] evaluated the results of laparoscopic gastric banding using two different bands; the Lapband Bioenterics, and the Swedish Adjustable Gastric Band (SAGB). The primary end point was weight loss, and secondary end points were correction of co-morbidities, early and long-term complications, importance of food restriction, and improvement of quality of life in morbidly obese patients. In all, 180 patients were randomly assigned to receive the Lapband or the SAGB. All procedures were performed by the same surgeon. Initial weight loss was faster in the Lapband group but eventually was identical in the two groups. There was a trend toward more early band-related complications and more band infections with the SAGB. All other measures were identical between the two groups. Only 55–60% of the patients achieved an excess weight loss of at least 50% in both groups. There was no difference in the incidence of long-term complications. In conclusion, gastric banding can be performed safely with the Lapband or the SAGB with similar short- and mid-term results with respect to weight loss and morbidity. Only 50–60% of patients achieve sufficient weight loss, and close to 10% will develop severe long-term complications. Possible deficiencies of the study include randomisation using sealed envelopes. The study had limited power and the analysis of complications must therefore be regarded with caution. Length of follow-up was limited with a mean of 39 months compared to the minimum standard of 60 months.

Oesphagogastric cancer

One trial of chemoradiation for locally advanced disease has been described above.[14] A meta-analysis[26] aimed to look at the effectiveness in improving survival of neo-adjuvant chemoradiotherapy (NCRT) in patients undergoing surgery for oesophageal carcinoma. Medline, the Cochrane Database of Systemic Reviews, Biosis Previews, and other resources were searched from January 1966 to January 2003. Randomised trials were selected on the basis of study design that included NCRT followed by surgery versus surgery alone. Across 6 studies, 374 patients underwent NCRT(all cisplatin based) followed by surgery and 364 underwent surgery alone. In 5 of the 6 studies, there was a small, insignificant trend towards improved survival with NCRT. Only 1 study demonstrated a statistically significant benefit from NCRT. Overall data from all 6 studies showed a non-significant trend toward improved long-term survival in the NCRT followed by surgery group (P = 0.07). Future, larger, randomised trials should examine whether this benefit is sufficient to warrant the considerable expense and risks associated with NCRT, and should report effects on quality of life.

There are many possible deficiencies of this study. The randomised trials have been small, which limits their power to detect small differences. No individual patient data was obtained and it was, therefore, difficult to obtain time-to-event analyses and gain information about follow-up periods for each patient. Adenocarcinoma and squamous carcinoma groups were combined in this study as there were not enough individual numbers. In the surgery-alone group, there were many more patients with advanced disease. Uncertainty about the true baseline characteristics of patients limited the ability to interpret the effect of the pre-operative disease stage on outcome. Although all chemoradiotherapies were cisplatin based, there were some differences in the agents used and doses given. Surgical techniques were also not uniform across the studies.

The aim of a prospective, randomised, clinical trial[27] was to compare technical feasibility and both early and 5-year clinical outcomes of laparoscopic-assisted and radical subtotal gastrectomy for distal gastric cancer. Patients were randomised to undergo subtotal gastrectomy either open (OG; n = 29) or laparoscopic (LG; n = 30). No significant difference was found in any of the outcome variables studied (number of lymph nodes, complications, survival). Additional benefits for the LG were reduced blood loss, shorter time to resumption of oral intake, and earlier discharge from hospital. In conclusion laparoscopic radical subtotal gastrectomy for distal gastric cancer is a feasible and safe oncological procedure with short- and long-term results similar to those obtained with an open approach. Possible deficiencies of this study include the undocumented method of randomisation.

PANCREAS AND LIVER

The long-term follow-up is reported[28] of a randomised clinical trial comparing pancreatic head resection according to Beger and limited pancreatic head excision combined with longitudinal pancreatico-jejunostomy according to Frey for surgical treatment of chronic pancreatitis. Patients were randomly allocated to Beger ($n = 38$) or Frey ($n = 36$) operations. Median follow-up was 8.5 years. Seven patients were not available for follow-up. There were no significant differences in any of the parameters studied which included quality of life, pain, exocrine and endocrine function. This study also suggests that development of pancreatic insufficiency probably develops independent of the surgical procedure and seems to be related to progression of the disease. The authors conclude that the decision regarding the procedure should be based upon the surgeon's experience.

In a randomised trial,[29] 82 patients scheduled for hepatectomy under selective hepatic vascular exclusion (SHVE) were allocated randomly to either the sharp transection group ($n = 41$) or the clamp crushing group ($n = 41$). Outcome measures included warm ischaemic time, blood loss and transfusions, postoperative morbidity and mortality, and tumour-free margins. The two groups were similar in all variables except that sharp transection yielded better tumour-free margins. In conclusion, after application of SHVE, sharp liver parenchymal transection with a scalpel is equally safe in terms of blood loss and mortality compared with the clamp crushing method. Although it is a technically demanding method, requiring selective hepatic vascular occlusion, it may be recommended when the tumour-free margins are expected to be narrow. Possible deficiencies of the study include no documentation of method of randomisation.

A prospective randomised controlled trial[30] evaluated first the ischaemic damage, and second, the feasibility, safety and efficacy, amount of blood loss, and postoperative complications of selective clamping in patients undergoing minor liver resections. Eighty patients were randomly assigned to intermittent pedicular complete clamping (CC; $n = 39$) or selective clamping (SC; $n = 41$) in minor liver resections (less than 3 liver segments). Overall, the aim of this study was to evaluate whether the use of SC should be generalised to all patients undergoing minor hepatectomies. Haemodynamic parameters, including portal pressure and the hepatic venous pressure gradient (HVPG), were evaluated. No differences were observed in the amount of blood loss or the number of patients requiring transfusion. There were no significant differences in ischaemic period, or postoperative morbidity between groups. Cirrhotic patients with CC had significantly higher ALT and AST values on the first postoperative day compared to the SC group. The multivariate analysis demonstrated that high central venous pressure (HVPG > 10 mmHg) and intra-operative blood loss were independent factors related to morbidity. In conclusion, both techniques of clamping are equally effective and feasible for patients with normal liver and undergoing minor hepatectomies. However, in cirrhotic patients, SC induces less ischaemic injury and should be recommended. SC was feasible in all patients whenever indicated without haemodynamic consequences in 80% of cases. There were no complications related to this technique; thus, SC is a safe and effective vascular occlusion procedure. Even in minor hepatic resections, CVP, HVPG, and intra-operative blood loss are factors related to morbidity and should be considered, particularly in patients with cirrhosis. Randomisation in this study was by sealed envelope, but the authors used stratification to include similar number of cirrhotic patients in each study group.

A randomised clinical trial[31] compared transhepatic intrapartal portosystemic shunt (TIPS) to H-graft portocaval shunts (HGPCS) for bleeding varices. This report of long-term outcome compared actual with predicted survival data when treating patients with cirrhosis, portal hypertension, and variceal haemorrhage. Predicted survival was determined using Model for End-stage Liver Disease (MELD). Patients undergoing TIPS (n = 66) or HGPCS (n = 66) were similar by Child's class, MELD and predicted survival. Actual survival was significantly superior to predicted survival. Up to 24 months, actual survival after HGPCS was superior to actual survival after TIPS. Survival was superior after HGPCS compared with TIPS for patients of Child's class A and B (P = 0.07) and with MELD scores of less than 13 (P = 0.04) with follow-up at 5–10 years. Shunt failure was less following HGPCS (P < 0.01). In conclusion, predicted survival data for patients undergoing TIPS or HGPCS confirms an unbiased randomisation. Actual survival following either of the 2 procedures was superior to predicted survival. Shunt failure was less frequent after HGPCS, and survival was better, particularly for the first few years after shunting and for patients of Child's class A or B or with MELD scores < 13. This trial establishes a role for surgical shunting, particularly HGPCS. TIPS, however, seems well applied to patients in need of portal decompression who are unacceptable operative candidates.

GENERAL SURGERY

Data from a prospective, randomised, double-blind study[32] to compare the effectiveness of different prophylactic antibiotics in abdominal surgery has demonstrated advantages of using ceftriaxone as opposed to cefotaxime. Using a blocked, randomised method, 1013 patients admitted into general surgical units for both acute and elective surgery, requiring antibiotic prophylaxis, were randomised to receive either ceftrixone or cefotaxime intravenously at induction of anaesthesia. In-patient, out-patient and community costs of infection were collected and results demonstrated that frequency of wound infection was similar in both groups but the associated financial costs were less with ceftriaxone. However, 9% of patients were excluded from analysis and cefotaxime was used more in non-elective surgery.

A randomised, double-blind, placebo-controlled prospective trial[33] compared wound infection rates in 360 patients undergoing primary inguinal hernia repair using polypropylene mesh. (180 received prophylactic antibiotics-cefazolin- and 180 received placebo). Infections were evaluated at 1 week, 2 weeks, and 1 month after operation. All complications were recorded.

Groups were well matched for all pre-operative variables. Superficial surgical site infection developed in 3 patients from the antibiotic group and 6 from the placebo group ($P = 0.50$). One from each group developed deep surgical site infection which needed re-operation and resulted in mesh removal. Pre-operative administration or single-dose antibiotic prophylaxis for tension-free inguinal mesh herniorrhaphy did not markedly decrease risk of wound infection. Possible deficiencies of the study include the need for a larger sample to confirm equivalence of the two treatments. The timing of the antibiotic injection given prior to procedure was not made clear: this could have affected the results.

A single-centre, prospective, randomised, double-blind, placebo-controlled study[34] evaluated whether selective digestive decontamination (SDD) reduces mortality from any cause, and the incidence of endogenous pneumonia in patients with severe burns. Patients with burns > 20% of total body surface and/or suspected inhalation injury were assigned to receive SDD or placebo for the total duration of treatment in the burn intensive care unit (ICU; 53 SDD and 54 placebo). The ICU mortality was 2.8% in the placebo group and 9% in the SDD group. Treatment with SDD was associated with a significant reduction in mortality both in the burn ICU and in the hospital, following adjustment for predicted mortality. The incidence of pneumonia was significantly higher in the placebo group. In conclusion, treatment with SDD reduces mortality and pneumonia incidence in patients with severe burns. Possible deficiencies of study include randomisation using sealed envelopes.

VASCULAR SURGERY

The last year has seen important trial reports dealing with technical approaches to major vascular surgery. Chief among these are the reports of endovascular repair of aortic aneurysm, with important data also available for carotid surgery and several other aspects of vascular surgery.

ENDOVASCULAR REPAIR OF AORTIC ANEURYSM

Two papers report linked studies designed to determine the place of endovascular aneurysm repair (EVAR). The EVAR-1 trial[35] compared the mortality, durability, health-related quality of life (HRQL) and costs of EVAR compared to open repair in patients with abdominal aortic aneurysm (AAA). The sample included 1082 patients aged 60 years or older, with aneurysms of at least 5.5 cm in diameter. The primary end point was all-cause mortality. Follow-up at 4 years showed a persistent reduction of aneurysm-related deaths in the EVAR group, yet similar all-cause mortality and negligible difference in HRQL between the groups. EVAR was shown to be more expensive and led to more complications and re-interventions.

Similarly disappointing results were found in patients unfit for open repair of AAA in whom EVAR was compared to no intervention (EVAR-2).[36] The primary end-point was all-cause mortality. After random assignment of 338 patients from 31 UK centres, aged 60 years and more, with an AAA diameter of at least 5.5 cm, no difference was found between the two groups in all-cause and cause-specific mortality rates. On the contrary, the more costly EVAR group needed further surveillance with higher rates of complications and re-intervention. HRQL showed no difference between the 2 groups in the EVAR-2 trial.

Not surprisingly, the EVAR-2 study group showed significantly higher 30-day mortality than the EVAR-1 group, and the EVAR-2 group had a substantially lower HRQL than the EVAR-1 group.

The 2-year outcome of conventional versus endovascular repair of AAA in the DREAM trial[37] showed that the peri-operative survival advantage in patients with endovascular repair compared to open repair is not sustained after the first postoperative year, in addition to similar cumulative survival rates and moderate/severe complications rate. No significant difference was shown in aneurysm-related deaths beyond the 30-day peri-operative period. The sample included 351 patients with an AAA diameter of 5 cm and more, who were suitable for both techniques. The primary end point was operative mortality or moderate/severe complications. Six patients did not undergo repair after randomisation and 6 cross-overs were recorded; 19 patients were lost to follow-up during the first 24 months. An unexplained, non-aneurysm related cluster of deaths occurred about 1 year after randomisation in the endovascular repair group. After endovascular repair, re-intervention was 3 times the rate seen after open repair in the first 9 months, with significant difference beyond the 9-month period.

SCREENING FOR ANEURYSM

The role of screening for AAA in reducing mortality in Danish men aged 65 years or more was assessed in a single-centre, randomised, controlled trial.[38] The sample included 6333 patients with 76.6% attendance rate, and patients with AAA > 5 cm were referred for surgical evaluation. The surgeons assessing trial data were blinded to randomisation and each other's evaluation. Primary outcome measures were specific mortality due to AAA, total mortality, number of operations and their indications, and the number of ruptured aneurysms. The authors concluded that mass screening for AAA reduced specific mortality by 67%, and assumed that the benefits of screening were underestimated given that the incidence ruptured AAA increases with age. The results are limited by short observation period. The data suggest that, in this population, 352 scans resulted in one life saved.

CAROTID ENDARTERECTOMY

A prospective, randomised study[39] compared primary closure to polyurethane patch angioplasty after carotid end arterectomy (CEA) in 404 patients, 305 of whom had undergone CEA under local anaesthesia, followed up for 2.5–5 years. The primary end point was postoperative incidence of residual disease at 3 months and restenosis after 3 months. The clamping time was significantly shorter in primary closure, with significantly less shunt usage as well. Residual stenosis (> 50%) within the first 3 months, and long-term restenosis (> 70%) were significantly lower in the patch group. Women in the patch group had higher rates of restenosis. Stenosis was assessed by blinded duplex ultrasound. Peri-operative mortality and neurological events were similar in the two groups.

The authors point out that a larger sample size would possibly allow further evaluation of the link between patch and gender, in addition to the detection of relatively rare postoperative events. Future studies should consider intra-operative imaging to exclude technical problems.

Embolus after CEA remains a cause for concern. A small trial[40] addressed prevention of embolic events using a single pre-operative dose of 120 mg acetylsalicylic acid (ASA) for patients undergoing CEA. No significant difference in embolic rate was found between treatment and placebo groups. No extra bleeding complications were detected by surgeons in the ASA group. However, a significant difference was noted in embolic rate between men and women in the placebo group, which was not observed in the ASA group.

ENDOVASCULAR STENTS

Early embolic events are also a cause for concern after placement of carotid artery stents. A small trial[41] compared standard treatments with combined aspirin and clopidogrel treatment. They found some possible benefit on reducing adverse neurological events without increase in bleeding complications compared to aspirin and heparin given for 24 h. Outcome measures included 30-day bleeding and neurological complications and 30-day stenosis rates. The restenosis needs to be assessed for longer than the 30-day rate assessment which showed no significant difference in this trial. Weaknesses in the trial include the small sample size (50 patients), non-blinded assessment, and early termination due to high complications with the heparin group.

The attributes of different stent material were investigated in a randomised, double-blind study[42] involving 57 patients with chronic limb ischaemia and superficial femoral artery occlusion or stenosis, with a primary end point of mean stent lumen diameter at 6 months, and a 24-month monitoring plan determined by angiography. No statistically significant differences were found between Sirolimus-eluting and bare Nitinol stents in terms of mean stent lumen diameter after 6 months, restenosis rate or adverse events, most of which were neither device- nor procedure-related. The data from this trial may not be reliable, however, because of its small size, early completion (6 months), and the need to see the final 24-month results. Further, several patients had missing data, leading to exclusion, and half the patients had a Rutherford category between 0 and 2, in whom supervised exercise should be the first line of treatment.

BYPASS SURGERY

Technical aspects of the distal anastomosis were investigated in a comparison[43] between end-to-end versus end-to-side distal femoropopliteal bypasses. In this study, 274 patients were followed up for 36 months, in a non-blinded, prospective, randomised, multicentre trial with the primary outcome being the primary patency rate at 36 months' postoperatively. End –to-end anastomosis did not improve patency compared to end-to-side anastomosis, and major amputations after bypass failure were more frequent after end-to-end anastomosis, even after excluding technical failures. The number of patent run-off vessels significantly correlated with the major amputation rate.

The possible benefits of postoperative anticoagulation after lower limb bypass surgery were assessed in a trial[44] of the effects of 3 months' postoperative treatment with low molecular weight heparin (LMWH, dalteparin), The primary patency was assessed in a prospective, randomised, placebo-controlled, double-blind, multicentre trial including 284 patients from 12 Swedish hospitals. Patency was assessed for a 1-year period during which all the 281 remaining patients received 75 mg ASA daily. The primary outcome was graft patency, 3 and 12 months after surgery. LMWH was started at different intervals, 2–4 days' postoperatively. The authors concluded that long-term dalteparin did not improve patency, graft failure rates, amputations or cardiovascular complications during 12-months' follow-up.

A multicentre, prospective, blind, randomised trial[45] assessed the value of a suction wound drain on postoperative haematomas after carotid and femoral artery surgery. Using duplex scanning, there was no significant difference between the two groups (CEA or groin dissection). A selective drain policy was recommended. However, the sample size was small (70 CEA and 73 groins); a larger trial might be needed to detect differences in clinically significant wound complications

NON-SURGICAL TREATMENTS FOR PERIPHERAL ARTERIAL DISEASE

Surgery is a costly and dangerous treatment for patients with peripheral arterial disease. Secondary prevention, as an alternative strategy in patients who have been diagnosed with stable arterial disease, would be preferable, if effective. Patients who have reached a (combined) cardiovascular end point, especially those with peripheral vascular disease, have a high *Chlamydia pneumoniae* IgA titre. An ambitious randomised, double-blind, placebo-controlled, secondary prevention, clinical trial[46] included 509 patients with stable peripheral arterial disease. This trial tested the hypothesis that *C. pneumoniae* might be related to the progression of the vascular disease, and that a short course of azethromycin would reduce the incidence of subsequent atherosclerotic events of the coronary, cerebral and peripheral arterial circulations. Clinical end points were death, coronary or cerebral events, complications of peripheral arterial disease with decreased ankle-brachial pressure index and/or the need for a re-vascularisation procedure. Azethromycin treatment did not reduce the risk of any event. The patients were followed up for 24 months, and showed 95% compliance rate. The authors concluded that a short-term course of azithromycin offers no benefits for survival or ankle pressure in peripheral arterial disease patients. However, this was a small trial, and the effect of a longer course of antibiotic treatment on cardiovascular risk reduction is not known.

Another prospective, randomised, controlled study[47] aimed at reducing the progression to surgery included 41 stable claudicants, and compared patients treated with 75 mg aspirin plus intermittent pneumatic compression (IPC) of foot and calf compared to patients receiving aspirin alone. IPC was used for 5 months, with continuous follow-up 12 months after IPC cessation. The trial showed a significant improvement in initial and absolute claudication distances, resting and post-exercise ankle-brachial pressure index in the treatment group. In addition, health-related quality of life in the IPC group was better after 5 months and this was sustained 1 year later. Compliance rates were above 80% in the IPC group throughout the first 5 months, which was also complication-free. Deficiencies of this trial include the small sample size, and the fact that unsupervised exercise was encouraged, whereas life style and exercise were not assessed.

VENOUS DISEASE

An open-label, prospective, randomised trial[48] studied the effectiveness and safety of a low molecular weight heparin (tinzaparin) in the long-term treatment of proximal deep vein thrombosis (DVT). Primary outcomes were recanalisation and development of reflux. After 1-year follow-up of 108 patients, the trial showed that tinzaparin was at least as effective and safe as combined unfractionated heparin and acenocumarol treatment, with a significant benefit of recanalisation from 3 months onward in the tinzaparin group. In addition, the tinzaparin group needed no hospitalisation and had fewer major events. Reflux in both groups worsened with time. No significant bleeding complications were seen. Total costs were slightly in favour of the tinzaparin group. Deficiencies of this trial include: (i) the INR was in the target therapeutic range in only two-thirds of measurements; (ii) a double-blinded study was not feasible; and (iii) that patients with a history of asthma were excluded.

Technical advances have allowed new treatments, such as radiofrequency ablation, for the management of varicose veins. In the EVOLVeS study,[49] the outcome of radiofrequency obliteration of the long saphenous vein was compared to stripping and ligation in 85 patients followed up over 24 months. Neovascularisation rates were similar in both groups. Patients reported superior quality of life, return to activity, and return to work in the radiofrequency group from the first 4 months onward. Pain was improved at all stages in the radiofrequency arm of the study. The authors concluded that radiofrequency obliteration of the long saphenous vein was at least equal clinically to stripping and ligation. Despite the better trend in the radiofrequency group, the small sample size prevented any comment on outcomes such as recurrence or neovascularisation. It should be noted that the trial sponsors had reviewed patients' records.

In another small trial,[50] the effect of surgical technology on recurrence of varicose veins in the groin was studied. In this randomised, non-blinded trial including 36 patients followed up for a period of 3 months postoperatively, no significant difference between ultrasonic dissection, electrocoagulation technique or sharp dissection of the groin for recurrent saphenofemoral incompetence other than more frequent, clinically insignificant, lymphatic fistulas on the day of operation with the ultrasound group.

References

1. Johnson L, Cusick TE, Helmer SD, Osland JS. Influence of fibrin glue on seroma formation after breast surgery. *Am J Surg* 2005; **189**: 319–323.
2. Bonadonna G, Moliterni A, Zambetti M *et al*. 30 years' follow up of randomised studies of adjuvant CMF in operable breast cancer: cohort study. *BMJ* 2005; **330**: 217–222.
3. Ragaz J, Olivotto IA, Spinelli JJ *et al*. Locoregional radiation therapy in patients with high-risk breast cancer receiving adjuvant chemotherapy: 20-year results of the British

Columbia randomized trial. *J Natl Cancer Inst* 2005; **97**: 116–126.

4. Gradishar WJ, Xaklaman VG. Adjuvant therapy of breast cancer in the elderly. Does one size fit all? *JAMA* 2005; **293**: 1118–1120.

5. Fargeot P, Bonneterre J, Roche H *et al*. Disease-free survival advantage of weekly epirubicin plus tamoxifen versus tamoxifen alone as adjuvant treatment of operable, node-positive, elderly breast cancer patients: 6-year follow-up results of the French Adjuvant Study Group 08 Trial. *J Clin Oncol* 2004; **22**: 4622–4630.

6. Peters WP, Rosner GL, Vredenburgh JJ *et al*. Prospective, randomized comparison of high-dose chemotherapy with stem-cell support versus intermediate-dose chemotherapy after surgery and adjuvant chemotherapy in women with high-risk primary breast cancer: a report of CALGB 9082, SWOG 9114, and NCIC MA-13. *J Clin Oncol* 2005; **21**: 2191–2200.

7. Mauri D, Pavlidis N, Ioannidis JPA. Neoadjuvant versus adjuvant systemic treatment in breast cancer: a meta-analysis. *J Natl Cancer Inst* 2005; **97**: 188–194.

8. Dieras V, Fumoleau P. Romieu G *et al*. Randomised parallel study of doxorubicin plus paclitaxel and doxorubicin plus cyclophosphamide as neoadjuvant treatment of patients with breast cancer. *J Clin Oncol* 2004; **22**: 4958–4965.

9. von Schoultz E, Rutqvist LE. Menopausal hormone therapy after breast cancer: the Stockholm randomized trial. *J Natl Cancer Inst* 2005; **97**: 533–535.

10. Chi S, Hsei K, Sheen-Chen S, Chou F. A prospective randomized comparison of bilateral subtotal thyroidectomy versus unilateral total and contralateral subtotal thyroidectomy for Graves' disease. *World J Surg* 2005; **29**: 160–163.

11. Cordon C, Fajardo R, Ramirez J, Herrera MF. A randomized, prospective, parallel group study comparing the harmonic scalpel to electrocautery in thyroidectomy. *Surgery* 2005; **137**: 337–341.

12. Gordon JN, Trebble TM, Ellis RD, Duncan HD, Johns T, Goggin PM. Thalidomide in the treatment of cancer cachexia: a randomised placebo controlled trial. *Gut* 2005; **54**: 540–545.

13. Bohlius J, Langensiepen S, Schwarzer G *et al*. Recombinant human erythropoietin and overall survival in cancer patients: results of a comprehensive meta-analysis. *J Natl Cancer Inst* 2005; **97**: 489–498.

14. Stahl M, Stuschke M, Lehmann N *et al*. Chemoradiation with and without surgery in patients with locally advanced squamous cell carcinoma of the esophagus. *J Clin Oncol* 2005; **23**: 2310–2317.

15. Bikhchandani J, Agarwal PN, Kaut R, Malik VK. Randomised controlled trial to compare the early and mid-term results of stapled versus open haemorrhoidectomy. *Am J Surg* 2005; **189**: 56–60.

16. Arroyo A, Perez F, Serrano P, Candela F, Lacuova J, Calpena R. Surgical versus chemical (botulinum toxin) sphincterotomy for chronic anal fissure: long-term results of a prospective randomised clinical and manometric study. *Am J Surg* 2005; **189**: 429–434.

17. Ong CH, Foo ECB, Keng V. Ambulatory circular stapled haemorrhoidectomy under local anaesthesia versus circular stapled haemorrhoidectomy under regional anaesthesia. *Aust NZ J Surg* 2005; **75**: 184–186.

18. Segnan N, Senore C, Andreoni B *et al*. Randomised trial of different screening strategies for colorectal cancer: patient response and detection rates. *J Natl Cancer Inst* 2005; **97**: 347–357.

19. Ram E, Shermany Y, Weil R, Vishne T, Kravarusic D, Dreznik Z. Is mechanical bowel preparation mandatory for elective colon surgery? A prospective randomised study. *Arch Surg* 2005; **140**: 285–288.

20. Basse L, Jacobsen DH, Bardram L *et al*. Functional recovery after open versus laparoscopic colonic resection: a randomised, blinded study. *Ann Surg* 2005; **241**: 416–423.

21. Zutshi M, Delaney CP, Senagore AJ *et al*. Randomised controlled trial comparing controlled rehabilitation with early ambulation and diet pathway versus controlled rehabilitation with early ambulation and diet with pre-emptive epidural anaesthesia/analgesia after laparotomy and intestinal resection. *Am J Surg* 2005; **189**: 268–272.

22. Chan FK, Ching JY, Hung LC *et al*. Clopidogrel versus aspirin and esomeprazole to

prevent recurrent ulcer bleeding. *N Engl J Med* 2005; **352**: 238–244.

23. Leontiadis GI, Sharma VK, Howden CW. Systematic review and meta-analysis of proton pump inhibitor therapy in peptic ulcer bleeding. *BMJ* 2005; **330**: 568–570.

24. Granderath FA, Schweiger UM, Kamolz T, Asche KU, Pointer R. Laparoscopic Nissen fundoplication with prosthetic hiatal closure reduces postoperative intrathoracic wrap herniation. *Arch Surg* 2005; **140**: 40–48.

25. Suter M, McLennan G, Reinhardt JM, Riker D, Hoffman EA. Laparoscopic gastric banding: a prospective randomised study comparing the Lapband and the SAGB: early results. *Ann Surg* 2005; **241**: 55–62.

26. Greer SE, Goodney PP, Sutton JE, Birkmeyer JD. Neoadjuvant chemoradiotherapy for oesophageal carcinoma: a meta-analysis. *Surgery* 2005; **137**: 172–177.

27. Huscher CG, Mingoli A, Sgarzini G *et al.* Laparoscopic versus open subtotal gastrectomy for distal gastric cancer; results of a randomised prospective trial. *Ann Surg* 2005; **2**: 232–237.

28. Strate T, Taherpour Z, Bloechle C *et al.* Long-term follow-up of a randomised trial comparing the Beger and Frey procedures for patients suffering from chronic pancreatitis. *Ann Surg* 2005; **241**: 591–598.

29. Smyrniotis V, Arkapoulos N, Kostopanagiotou G *et al.* Sharp liver transection versus clamp crushing technique in liver resections: a prospective study. *Surgery* 2005; **137**: 306–311.

30. Figueras J, Llado L, Ruiz D *et al.* Complete versus selective portal triad clamping for minor liver resections; a prospective randomised trial. *Ann Surg* 2005; **241**: 582–590.

31. Alexander S. H-graft portacaval shunts versus TIPS. Ten-year follow-up of a randomised controlled trial with comparison to predicted survivals. *Ann Surg* 2005; **241**: 238–246.

32. Woodfield JC, Van Rij AM, Pettigrew RA, van der Linden A, Bolt D. Using cost of infection as a tool to demonstrate a difference in prophylactic antibiotic efficacy: a prospective randomized comparison of the pharmacoeconomic effectiveness of ceftriaxone and cefotaxime prophylaxis in abdominal surgery. *World J Surg* 2005; **29**: 18–24.

33. Perez AR, Roxas MF, Hilvano SS. A randomised, double-blind, placebo-controlled trial to determine effectiveness of antibiotic prophylaxis for tension-free mesh herniorrhaphy. *J Am Coll Surg* 2005; **200**: 393–397.

34. de La Cal MA, Cerda E, Garcia-Hierro P *et al.* Survival benefit in critically ill burned patients receiving selective decontamination of the digestive tract: a randomised, placebo-controlled, double-blind study. *Ann Surg* 2005; **241**: 424–430.

35. EVAR Trial Participants. Endovascular aneurysm repair versus open repair in patients with abdominal aortic aneurysm (EVAR trial 1): randomised controlled trial. *Lancet* 2005; **365**: 2179–2186.

36. EVAR Trial Participants. Endovascular aneurysm repair and outcome in patients unfit for open repair of abdominal aortic aneurysm (EVAR trial 2): randomised controlled trial. *Lancet* 2005; **365**: 2187–2192.

37. Blankensteijn JD, de Jong SECA, Prinssen M *et al.* for the Dutch Randomized Endovascular Aneurysm Management (DREAM) Trial Group. Two-year outcomes after conventional or endovascular repair of abdominal aortic aneurysm. *N Engl J Med* 2005; **352**: 2398–2405.

38. Lindholt JS, Juul S, Fasting H *et al.* Screening for abdominal aortic aneurysm: single centre randomised controlled trial. *BMJ* 2005; **330**: 750–754.

39. Mannheim D, Weller B, Vahadim E, Karmeli R. Carotid endarterectomy with a polyurethane patch versus primary closure: a prospective randomized study. *J Vasc Surg* 2005; **41**: 403–407.

40. Tytgat SHAJ, Laman DM, Rijken AM *et al.* Emboli rate during and early after carotid endarterectomy after a single preoperative dose of 120 mg acetylsalicylic acid – a prospective double-blind placebo controlled randomised trial. *Eur J Vasc Endovasc Surg* 2005; **29**: 156–161.

41. Gaines PA, Tan KT, Venables GS *et al.* The benefits of combined anti-platelet treatment in carotid artery stenting. *Eur J Vasc Endovasc Surg* 2005; **29**: 522–527.

42. Duda SH, Bosiers M, Lammer J *et al.* Sirolimus-eluting versus bare nitinol stent for obstructive superficial femoral artery disease: The SIROCCO II Trial. *J Vasc Intervent Radiol* 2005; **16**: 331–338.

43. Schouten O, Hoedt MTC, Wittens CHA, Hop WCJ, van Sambeek MRHM, van Urk H and on behalf of the VASCAN Study Group. End-to-end versus end-to-side distal anastomosis in femoropopliteal bypasses; results of randomized multicenter trial. *Eur J Vasc Endovasc Surg* 2005; **29**: 457–462.

44. Jivegård L, Drott C, Gelin J *et al.* Effects of three months of low molecular weight heparin (dalteparin) treatment after bypass surgery for lower limb ischemia – a randomised placebo-controlled double blind multicentre trial. *Eur J Vasc Endovasc Surg* 2005; **29**: 190–198.

45. Youssef F, Jenkins MP, Dawson KJ *et al.* The value of suction wound drain after carotid and femoral artery surgery: a randomised trial using duplex assessment of the volume of post-operative haematoma. *Eur J Vasc Endovasc Surg* 2005; **29**: 162–166.

46. Vainas T, Stassen FRM, Schurink GWH *et al.* Secondary Prevention of Atherosclerosis through *Chlamydia* pneumonia Eradication (SPACE trial): a randomised clinical trial in patients with peripheral arterial disease. *Eur J Vasc Endovasc Surg* 2005; **29**: 403–411.

47. Delis KT, Nicolaides AN. Effect of intermittent pneumatic compression of foot and calf on walking distance, hemodynamics, and quality of life in patients with arterial claudication: a prospective randomized controlled study with 1-year follow-up. *Ann Surg* 2005; **241**: 431–441.

48. Daskalopoulos ME, Daskalopoulou SS, Tzortzis E *et al.* Long-term treatment of deep venous thrombosis with low molecular weight heparin (tinzaparin): a prospective randomized trial. *Eur J Vasc Endovasc Surg* 2005; **29**: 638–650.

49. Lurie F, Creton D, Eklof B *et al.* Prospective randomised study of endovenous radiofrequency obliteration (closure) versus ligation and vein stripping (EVOLVeS): two-year follow-up. *Eur J Vasc Endovasc Surg* 2005; **29**: 67–73.

50. Mouton WG, Bessell JR, Zehnder T *et al.* A randomised trial of ultrasonic dissection versus electrocoagulation to reduce lymphatic complications after surgery for recurrent sapheno-femoral incompetence. *Eur J Vasc Endovasc Surg* 2005; **29**: 313–315.

Index

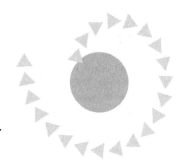